ALCOHOL AND DRUG ABUSE

'THE KNOTTED CORD'

AN UPDATE ON TRANSGENERATIONAL ALCOHOL (2020)

Alcohol and Drug Abuse

Additional books and e-books in this series can be found on Nova's website under the Series tab.

ALCOHOL AND DRUG ABUSE

'THE KNOTTED CORD'

AN UPDATE ON TRANSGENERATIONAL ALCOHOL (2020)

KIERAN D. O'MALLEY

nova
Medicine & Health
New York

Library of Congress Cataloging-in-Publication Data

Names: O'Malley, Kieran D., author.
Title: The knotted cord: an update on transgenerational alcohol/Kieran D. O'Malley.
Identifiers: LCCN 2020016470 (print) | LCCN 2020016471 (ebook) | ISBN 9781536178593 (hardcover) | ISBN 9781536178609 (adobe pdf)
Subjects: LCSH: Alcoholism in pregnancy--Complications. | Children of prenatal alcohol abuse. | Fetal alcohol spectrum disorders.
Classification: LCC RG580.A46 O63 2020 (print) | LCC RG580.A46 (ebook) | DDC 618.3/686--dc23
LC record available at https://lccn.loc.gov/2020016470
LC ebook record available at https://lccn.loc.gov/2020016471

Published by Nova Science Publishers, Inc. † New York

CONTENTS

PREFACE

SYNOPSIS: THE KNOTTED CORD. (2014 BOOK)

Alcohol Related Neurodevelopmental Disorder (ARND) whether dysmorphic, called Fetal Alcohol Syndrome (FAS) or non-dysmorphic, ARND itself, are both trans-generational developmental psychiatric disorders.

The prevalence of ARND continues to be truly unrecognized because this disorder mainly presents as a hidden disability, rather than a dysmorphic disorder. Dysmorphic ARND and non-dysmorphic ARND are not commonly neurodegenerative in nature, but they do reflect each generation's alcohol addiction/misuse, and continued use in pregnancy. The subtle denial and minimization of trans-generational alcohol abuse is aided by only acknowledging the far less frequent dysmorphic ARND, namely FAS, creating a false security across social classes concerning alcohol's true trans-generational epigenetic effect. Thus the financial costs and health care burden of trans-generational ARND with a prevalence of 1 in 100 live births are avoided.

There are no systematic medical management approaches to ARND, and it continues to be managed in a piecemeal fashion with disconnections between the obstetric, pediatric, psychiatric, social service and alcohol addiction services. This book will include an academic review of the current state of the ARND behavioral phenotype recognition, and management. Interwoven in the narrative will be a personal reflection on 25 years psychiatric experience diagnosing and managing these patients in Canada, USA, UK and Ireland, incorporating trans-generational and trans-cultural clinical examples garnered from this unique international 'systems of care ' perspective.

A System of Care Approach to Management Is the Only Way to Go

The principles of systems of care, and with it a wrap–around approach, have been long known in child psychiatry and are well ingrained in training for the modern child and adolescent psychiatrist finishing their training in USA. (Goldman 1999). Systems of care have been one of the core competencies in child and adolescent psychiatry for at least 10 years. It is the foundation stone of medical/psychiatric management in community psychiatry and thus offers a structured, systematized way to manage transgenerational ARND.

At this stage it behooves us to reflect on JD Salinger's seminal book, The Catcher in the Rye' (1945) in which the author, through his book's narrator, Holden Caulfield, presents us the graphic picture of thousands of children playing in a vast field of rye close to a cliff and at risk for falling off. Holden Caulfield has the impossible task of trying to catch these children if they start to fall off the cliff. Sometimes it is the poets and writers who best capture the essence of society's challenges. Almost four decades later Jane Knitzer in her book Unclaimed Children (1982) gave birth to what became the community based systems of care which indicated the urgency and the fundamental duty of care duty in preventing succeeding generations of disenfranchised children with serious emotional disturbances and their equally troubled families falling off life's cliff. Such is the current journey of children with ARND and their families, who continue to be 'orphan' children as they are not deemed the responsibility of any particular medical specialty. It is the final curse of transgenerational alcohol. The systems of care approach attempts to bring these children back to their families, communities, ethnic and socio-cultural roots, strengthening the knot of connection that alcohol has loosened if not broken.

At a personal level the conceptual frame of this book and its approach to management has been nurtured in the feisty but telling debates for nigh on 8-9 years in the American Academy of Child and Adolescent Psychiatry, Work Group on Community Systems of Care.

Finally, this book is written in a Joycean recursive style as a method of mirroring its circular subject. It is best read, slowly, over one sitting and savored as a 30-year-old Port so that you can feel the essence of the aftertaste.

Synopsis. An Update on Transgenerational Alcohol, 2020

This update aspires to bring the link between the epigenetic effect of prenatal alcohol exposure and a long lasting non-IQ, non-face driven global neurodevelopmental disorder to the medical table. I have kept the structure of the 2014 book, and each chapter has an update added, which is fully understood and incorporated into new thinking only after reading the proceeding chapter/section from the original book.

The intervening 5 years have in some ways 'muddied the waters' related to understanding the true legacy of prenatal alcohol. Over 20 years ago the Institute of Medicine in the USA recognized a non-facial dysmorphic clinical condition related to prenatal alcohol exposure, and named it Alcohol Related Neurodevelopmental Disorder (ARND) which was the 2014 book. Now the International Classification Medical/Psychiatric Systems ICD 11 has introduced the Diagnostic term: Neurodevelopmental Disorder associated with Prenatal Alcohol Exposure (NDPAE), code 315.8, DSM 5 and the new ICD 11 has also introduced Neurodevelopmental Disorder associated with Prenatal Alcohol Exposure code: 6AOY; So both systems are now in alignment.

However, in parallel, the older concept of FASD stubbornly remains.

In truth this was never a diagnostic term but a descriptive term of a spectrum of conditions which range from the well-defined facial dysmorphic Fetal Alcohol Syndrome (FAS) to the vastly more prevalent non-facial dysmorphic condition, now defined as NDPAE.

1) The primary aim of the Update is to find a medical home for this "orphan condition" of Neurodevelopmental Disorder Prenatal Alcohol Exposure (NDPAE) which creates a prenatal alcohol brain-injury based deficit in reflective function, planning and decision-making (Hobson 1993, Mattson et al. 2011).
2) I also hope that the societal and biological Roots of transgenerational alcohol dependence will begin to break the glass ceiling of understanding.
3) I still support a Systems of Care approach to management, but would clarify that this approach is not only community-based, but also hospital-based involving adult and child health professionals working in tandem. An example of the "thinking differently" initially articulated by social worker Dianne Malbin in Portland over 20 years ago (Malbin, 1997), and expanded by Densmore, 2011& Rich, 2016.
4) This Update is not an analysis of the transference and counter- transference feelings when treating patients with NDPAE and their families. However, it offers a clinical structural template to begin those therapeutic conversations.

It is also the author's continuing hope that in the coming generation the age related behavioral phenotypes of NDPAE will begin to finally be acknowledged, and we/society will be better saved by their eventual acknowledgement.

This MRI slide done in a standard General Hospital in Canada shows a String Corpus Callosum. Abnormalites in the Corpus Callosum one of the classical pathognomic brain features which can be seen in NDPAE.(O'Malley 2006).

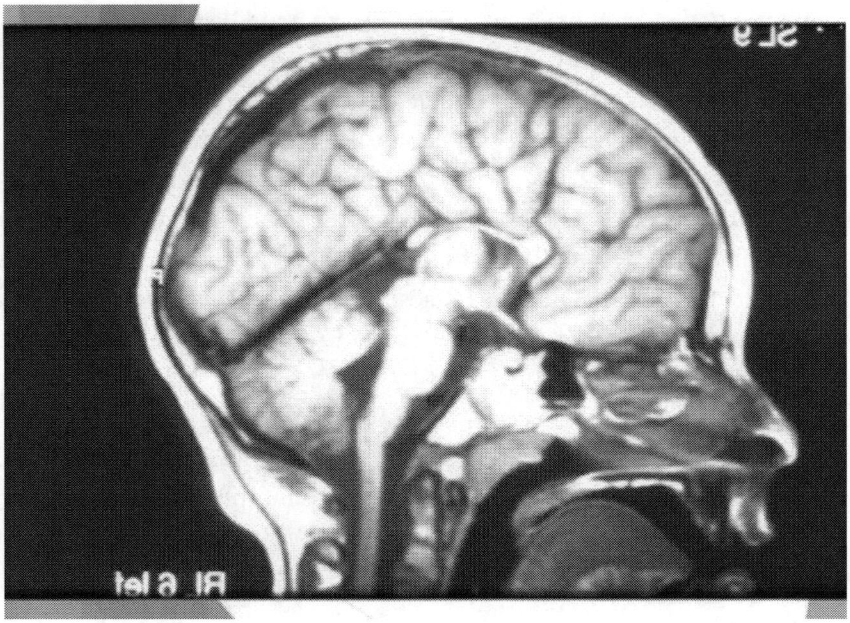

ACKNOWLEDGMENTS

THE KNOTTED CORD. (2014 BOOK)

This book has had a tortuous journey to fruition but has been well supported along the way. Firstly, I wish to thank the team at Nova Science Publishers for keeping me on the straight and steady path. From idea to print, with the help of Nadya, Donna, Trish, Stella Rosa, Rich to name but a few.

As well I wish to thank Professor Ann Streissguth for permission to use her secondary disability slide, Professor Marcus Raichle for permission to use his PET scan slides, and the BMA for permission to use their face and lip/philtrum slides, and Professor Susan Astley Ph.D., University of Washington for permission to use her face and lip/philtrum slides.

Bob Klaehn MD, USA was very helpful in proof reading my chapter on systems of care and helping me place it in a wraparound context.

Judge Desmond Marrinan, N. Ireland also helped in proof reading the early chapters and offered solid advice, and especially Barry Stanley M.D., Canada for saving the day!

A special thank you is due to Charlene and her foster parents for allowing me to use their photograph and especially Charlene's story.

A special thank you is also due to Randy Mc Donald and his adoptive mother Nanci for letting me use their photograph and including their separate narratives.

Last but never least Mollyo's faithful handler and my wife Siobhan who helped test the 'common man/woman' parts of the book! The rest is before you.

THE KNOTTED CORD. AN UPDATE 2020

Bangor Carnegie Library, especially Pamela, Paula and Makk for its peace, tranquility and computer expertise which created the atmosphere for this creative academic work.

Judge Desmond Marrinan for advice on the Ethics and Stigma chapter updates.

Bob Khaelk MD and Fernando Valles MD from AACAP for the updated Systems of Care information especially on ECSII.

Dr. Bill Lockhart, Forensic Psychologist for his sound advice on forensic issues, detailed proof reading, and general encouragement.

American Psychiatric Association (APA) for allowing use of key DSM 5 criteria for SCD and DMDD.

American Academy of Child and Adolescent Psychiatry (AACAP), especially Community Systems of Care Committee for permission to use CASII and ECSII criteria.

Microsoft Editorial Support.

Professor Ann Streissguth, University of Washington for guiding me to look beyond the face towards the whole person.

My wife Siobhan for patiently tolerating my 'epigenetic obsession'!

Finally, the Nova Science Team for tightening my over-inclusive prose, and bringing my book to fruition.

Kieran D. O'Malley, MB BAO BCh DABPN

Chapter 1

PROLOGUE

(2014 BOOK)

The thrust of this book has come from my continuing clinical work in Ireland which is a country still caught up in 'a toxic romance with alcohol'. This romance spans many generations and brings with it the untold legacy of prenatal alcohol exposure. In many ways this book is 'an ode to Ireland' in the hope that this Nation's experience helps wake the rest of the world up to alcohol's pernicious transgenerational effect.

The title of the book harks back to Michael Dorris's seminal book The Broken Cord (1987) which eloquently brought this 'hidden' population to light. However the truth is that the metaphorical umbilical cord is not broken and the unique neurodevelopmental disorder resulting from prenatal alcohol exposure will continue to be one ghost in our delivery rooms and nurseries which will continue to haunt us. (Ghosts, Ibsen, 1888, Ghosts in the Nursery, Fraiberg et al., 1975). Alcohol Related Neurodevelopmental Disorder (ARND), whether dysmorphic and called Fetal Alcohol Syndrome, or the substantially more common, non-dysmorphic condition, ARND itself, both offer an entry in to a complex, tortuous and truly knotted cord of these complex families.

We cannot all escape from our collective histories of colonization and abusive violence, and the trans-generational history of alcohol addiction, abuse and trauma lies embedded in these stories. It is a story repeated in many different countries, cultures and religions. Although I am now working In Ireland, my medical experience has taught me the hidden legacies of transgenerational alcohol abuse and addiction, in Native American, First Nations, disenfranchised minorities and the seemingly invulnerable gentry.

The teratogenic effect of alcohol was first observed by pediatrician Paul Lemoine in Nantes, France in 1968, when he linked facial dysmorphic and growth features with maternal use of alcohol (wine) in pregnancy. His initial series was of 127 infants. Subsequently the syndrome Fetal Alcohol Syndrome was defined in 2 classic papers in

1973 by Ken Jones and David Smith in Seattle (Jones & Smith 1973a, b). Their initial case series were 8 patients. The recognition that prenatal alcohol exposure did not only cause dysmorphic facial features and growth delay was made by Sterling Clarren in Seattle in 1978 (Clarren & Smith 1978a,b) with the introduction of the term Fetal Alcohol Effect (FAE) to describe children with alcohol exposure but no facial features. This descriptive clinical term was changed to Alcohol Related Neurodevelopmental Disorder (ARND) by the American Institute of Medicine in 1996 (Stratton et al., 1996).

I have chosen to write on Alcohol Related Neurodevelopmental Disorder as this is the true essence of the long term legacy of prenatal alcohol exposure. Currently scientific studies continue to map out the minutiae of dysmorphic, anatomical, biochemical, neurophysiological, neuropsychological deficits acquired through prenatal alcohol exposure. However, sadly, 40 years since the dysmorphic Fetal Alcohol Syndrome was named, there continues to be no collective will to actually treat these patients or approach the roots of transgenerational alcohol abuse which form the substrate of the condition.

It is the Alcohol Related Neurodevelopmental Disorder (ARND) whether dysmorphic, Fetal Alcohol Syndrome (FAS), or non-dysmorphic ARND that is the true kernel of understanding the long term consequences of prenatal alcohol exposure. These two conditions have commonly been described under the collective umbrella term Fetal Alcohol Spectrum Disorders (FASDs) plural NOT singular (Streissguth & O'Malley 2000).

Why a 'knot'. Because management becomes knotted with the origins of the infants prenatal life, whether they be inter-country/race adopted, birth, fostered or adopted within the same culture. The 'knot' also speaks to societies continued ambivalence to acknowledging another inconvenient truth. The ghosts of past generations live within our children and our children's children. They are acted out in the primal mother/infant interaction which can become disrupted even before it has a chance to begin (Fraiberg et al., 1975). It is in the collective unconsciousness of the growing children and remains with them through placement changes, adoptions, fostering, through countries and across ethnic groups. The complex dance of identity becomes more unpredictable when the patient is not just physically displaced from their birth parents, but also cognitively displaced as a result of the central nervous system dysfunction inherent to the prenatal alcohol. (Jung, 1959). As children grow defiance can turn to conduct problems to aggressive/violent behaviors. These as well have roots in their own 'ghosts. As Karr-Moore and Wiley have extrapolated from their treatise Ghosts from the Nursery, tracing the roots of violence (Karr-Moore et al., 1999).

There are no safe limits of alcohol in pregnancy, and experimenting with varied alcohol drinking patterns in pregnancy is akin to playing Russian Roulette with the developing fetus. Alcohol is a true teratogen. But for many medical professionals it is still a 'NOT IT', therefore not a teratogen to follow or understand.

Meanwhile the knotted weave continues to deceive and confound our normal paradigms of scientific evidence- based medical management.

This book will include a mixture of an academic review of international psychiatric experience in diagnosis and intervention in Alcohol Related Neurodevelopmental Disorder, (dysmorphic or non-dysmorphic), as well a rich offering of clinical case examples garnered from psychiatric diagnostic and consultation work with patients who have a history of prenatal alcohol exposure. The clinical experience has been gathered the last 25 years working in 4 different country environments namely Canada, the USA, the UK and Ireland. Each country offers its own unique approach to transgenerational alcohol, alcohol use in pregnancy and the recognition of alcohol related neurodevelopmental disorder in exposed infants and children.

The concept of a transgenerational approach to management is embedded in the general 'systems of care' approach, which is a central tenet to the wrap-around approach to management in child and adolescent mental health. Even though this is type of approach is still not widely used in medicine the book will show how in ARND it is really the only viable method of treatment.

Alcohol use and abuse is so socially accepted in many communities and countries, especially binge drinking, that the thought of its transgenerational harm cannot be considered. Countries such as Ireland still 'officially ' have no cases of ARND, whereas the UK and Ireland are internationally recognized as having the highest rates of binge drinking and under age alcohol consumption in the world. Is this plethora of alcohol drinking completely disconnected from pregnancy? I doubt it.

However it is fair to say that both educational and legal systems in Canada, USA, Australia and UK are identifying the particular neuropsychological/learning problems that persons with ARND present. ARND is not confined to indigenous/aboriginal populations as has been a popular myth. In fact it is probably fair to say that only when societies begin to honestly acknowledge the destructive trans-generational effect of alcohol can these complex developmental psychiatric patients be understood for what they are and how they will evolve through life.

Conditions such as ADHD, ASD, and Asperger's Disorder, Mood Instability, so called Conduct Disorder, Intermittent Explosive Disorder, increased suicidality and early alcohol craving are just some of the hidden disabilities presented trans-generationally but still not understood as having their potential roots in prenatal alcohol exposure.

Only recently has there been an international appreciation of environmentally induced developmental disorders. Within this conceptualization is included an understanding of the epigenetic effects of the fetal neurotoxic exposure to alcohol. *Never Forg*et Alcohol *Teratology*. The trans-generational effects of alcohol lie in the legacy of alcohol on fetal programming which can effect genetic transcription and so 'turn on' the very genes that bring alcohol craving to the next generation of potential mothers and fathers, O'Malley 2010, 2011a, c.

In expanding this concept there was the well-recognized Barker's Hypothesis: i.e., 'Biological factors acting during prenatal life are associated not only with the development of common adult cardiovascular and metabolic disorders, but also with neurobehavioral abnormalities and behavioral disorders' (Bell et al., 2002). This fundamental concept had been mooted as far back as 1978 by Battaglia when he wrote about the commonality and diversity of fetal development, describing that the underlying mechanism for this developmental origins phenomenon had been labelled 'programming' and recently tested by Wilhelm –Benartzi et al., 2012. Embedded in this concept is the uncomfortable programmed connection between fetal learning about alcohol and later alcohol responsiveness (Abate et al., 2008). The in utero programming for later alcohol responsiveness and craving had long been well established in animal research. (Bond & Di Gusto 1976, Reyes et al., 1985, Dominguez et al., 1993). Early nutrition has a role as shown by the Dutch Winter Study (Lurney et al., 2007), and more recent work by Lucas 1991, and Waterland et al., 2003.

The book is structured using a developmental frame with an initial overview of the concept of transgenerational approach to management, but acknowledging the unique features of alcohol related disorders which include its romance, stigma and ethical issues in management. Succeeding chapters include examples from the range of age groups, infants, 3-5 years, 5-10 years, 11 to 14 years, 14 to 18 years, single young adulthood, adulthood and parenthood. This patient population is often called 'orphan' patients as no medical specialty wants ownership but they are clearly in the developmental psychiatric and addiction medicine arena.

An Update on Transgenerational Alcohol, 2020

Strangely the five years have not substantially changed the essence of thoughts and aspirations as expressed in the initial Prologue of 2014.

This update is much less 'Irish-centric' but has become more of an appraisal of International attitudes, approaches and attempts to forge a societal management. A recent scientific review of research studies has shown that there is no safe amount of alcohol in pregnancy (Manlak et al., 2020).

It is still the capacity for prenatal alcohol to change the embryological development of the fetal central nervous system that is the heart of this neuropsychiatric, neurodevelopmental disorder. This is especially relevant for the brain areas related to alcohol craving or addiction which animal researchers had shown 45 years ago (Bond, 1976). So, the epigenetic effect of prenatal alcohol consumption can kindle an alcohol craving vulnerability in the developing fetus and later child/adolescent, which underpins the transgenerational impact of the condition NDPAE (or FASD).

Thus, this remains the unspoken life script of transgenerational alcohol. As international researchers have pointed out: Why should there not be an organic basis to addiction? (Tomkins et al., 2001, Volkow et al., 2015, Lingford-Hughes, 2020).

This Update is written as an internal conversation between myself in 2014 and now in 2019. The resultant product will be a book which needs to be seen as a 'whole' rather than the sum of its, separated through time, parts. The wish to see the Joycean recursive style to this story and science, mirroring the subject, is still no less valid. Although its new length may take more than one day's reading!

The book is dedicated to the individuals with FAS, FAE, ARND, Static Encephalopathy, FASD, FASDs and now Neurodevelopmental Disorder Prenatal Alcohol Exposure (NDPAE), DSM 5, whom I have seen, and tried to help over the last 30 years. I hope to ultimately offer a structure of management approach to this pervasive societal transgenerational condition and set that structure within a holistic family – centered frame.

It is also dedicated to the birth, foster and adoptive families, whom I have also have had the pleasure and privilege of joining with them through part of their journey.

The Prologue and this book update is prefaced by highlighting the brain – injured, unknown vulnerable population of children in State Care Systems. The statistics are from Northern Ireland and the UK but the story continues in countries across the world, not least in Australia, Canada and the USA.These are not only the disenfranchised populations of Aboriginals, First Nations, Native American & Irish Travelers, but the product of families devastated by transgenerational alcohol.

Children in Care

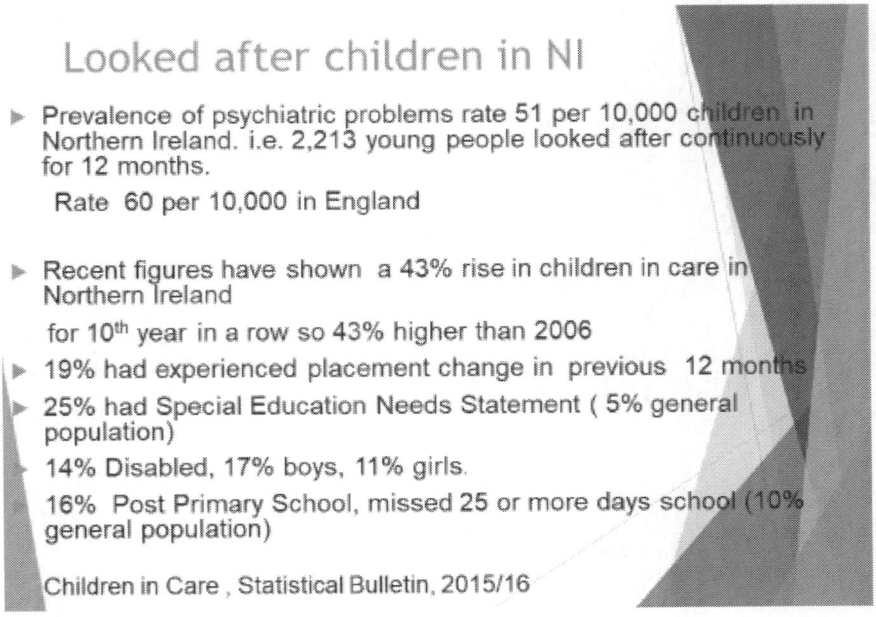

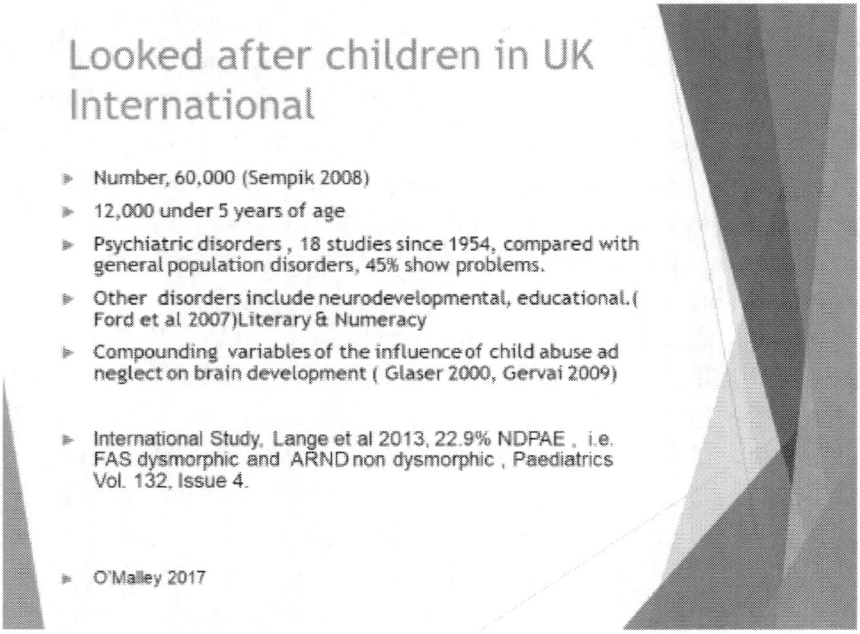
Looked after children in UK
International
Number, 60,000 (Sempik 2008)
12,000 under 5 years of age
Psychiatric disorders , 18 studies since 1954, compared with general population disorders, 45% show problems.
Other disorders include neurodevelopmental, educational.(Ford et al 2007)Literary & Numeracy
Compounding variables of the influence of child abuse ad neglect on brain development (Glaser 2000, Gervai 2009)
International Study, Lange et al 2013, 22.9% NDPAE , i.e. FAS dysmorphic and ARND non dysmorphic , Paediatrics Vol. 132, Issue 4.
O'Malley 2017

Chapter 2

IRELAND'S TOXIC ROMANCE WITH ALCOHOL

THE KNOTTED CORD. (2014 BOOK)

An epidemiological entry into the world of transgenerational alcohol offers an insight into Ireland's unique place in the pantheon of alcohol abuse, addiction, Romanization, denial and minimization.

Alcohol Related Neurodevelopmental Disorders, either non-dysmorphic or dysmorphic (also called FAS) are more prevalent than have been generally recognized or appreciated in many countries. The confusion over prevalence is tied to the pervasive denial and minimization of alcohol use and effects in pregnancy, seen strikingly in countries such as Ireland with no official cases of ARND, the UK with only 128 cases. The generalized accepted prevalence is 1 in 100 live births (1%). Italy has prevalence figures of 2.3 - 4.1%, Croatia 4.7% with 15.5% drinking in pregnancy; Luxembourg has 16% drinking in pregnancy. Some populations namely Aboriginal, Native American, Cape Colored in South Africa, Travelers (Ireland) have been deemed more susceptible to the effects of prenatal alcohol exposure. However the truth is that alcohol does not discriminate between races or social classes so ARND, non-dysmorphic or dysmorphic, appears in all populations whether recognized or not. (May et al., 2009, O'Malley 2011a).

Alcohol Related Neurodevelopmental Disorders, (ARNDs) either non-dysmorphic or dysmorphic are more prevalent than have been generally recognized or appreciated in many countries. The confusion over prevalence is tied to the pervasive denial and minimization of alcohol use and effects in pregnancy, seen strikingly in countries such as Ireland with no official cases of ARND, and as well the UK reporting only 128 cases. (O'Malley 2011a).

However, I decided that I could not begin a book on transgenerational alcohol without placing it in an ethnic context.

I grew up in Ireland, Belfast, and left at the beginning of the so called 'Troubles' to seek my fame and fortune in North America. I returned in 2006 and after 7 years working back here I feel both sadder but a little wiser.

When you grow up you are immersed in your culture its attitudes, social events but in Ireland it was really all about alcohol. Ireland was a true Alcohol Nation. (Sigman 2011). The pub was the epicenter of cultural exchange and the sheanachie (storyteller) and the balladeers the pied pipers of the time.

A popular Irish ballad 'Jug of Punch' tells its own story.

> "When I get drunk, Well my moneys me own,
> And if people don't like it, they can leave me alone
> I'll tune my fiddle and I'll rattle my bone
> And I'll be welcome wherever I roam!"

There's a seductive romance to alcohol in Ireland which is carried in the local music, poetry, song and theatre.

> "When I am dead and in my grave
> No costly tombstone will I crave
> Just lay me down in my native peat,
> With a jug of punch at my head and feet."

Death and drink glorified for the generations.

The weaving of romance and alcohol has a peculiar ring in Ireland. It is as if a celebration of one is a celebration of the other.

> "I wish I was in sweet Dungloe
> And seated on the ground
> And in my arm a bottle of wine
> And on my knee a bride,
> I'd call for liquor of the best
> And I'd pay before I'd go
> And I'd hold my Mary in my arms
> In the town of sweet Dungloe."

Through generations alcohol has colored family gatherings and rituals from births, christenings, first communions, confirmations, weddings, funerals. It is as if there is a drink for every occasion and a story and a song in your heart to boot!

Even hospital care was not immune and a wee drop of the black stuff helped you recover or a wee dram of Irish whiskey or brandy helped you sleep soundly. That was part of my medical training indoctrination in the cultural benefit of alcohol in healing the sick.

Nowadays, people would disremember these cultural niceties. To-day it is binge drinking, fighting, alcohol poisoning, unprotected sexual intercourse and unplanned pregnancies that rule the roost. At a recent case management meeting about an 8 year old girl with ARND a story developed where her mother, the 14th of 14 children born to alcoholic parents had run away from home because of domestic violence. For her 1st communion, at a similar age, she sat on her father's knee in the local pub sharing a whiskey with him in celebration. A number of professionals agreed that the mother wanted to parent her child, but was too overwhelmed, emotionally and cognitively, by the task. Transgenerational ARND comes to life.

The societal denial and minimization of the transgenerational alcohol problem interwoven in the society is borne out in many ways For example in Ireland there are no official notified cases of ARND, dysmorphic, (FAS) or non-dysmorphic ARND but certain statistics belie a different story.

1. In a retrospective chart review study of alcohol use in pregnancy (1999 to 2005) in one of Ireland's major maternity centers

(The Coombe Maternity Hospital in Dublin) a rather revealing prevalence of alcohol use was shown in both Irish and UK mothers.

The study showed the prevalence of alcohol use in pregnancy to range from

Irish 79%;
UK 77%;
EU 68.4%;
Non-EU 25.9%
(Barry, S, et al., 2006)

2. A more recent study reported in the Obstetrics and Gynecology Journal 2013, spotlighted, yet again, the pervasive nature of the alcohol abuse and its link to succeeding generations.

In this study Professor Louise Kenny and her colleagues in Cork found that 80% of women in Ireland drank at some point in their pregnancy.

This compared with 66% for UK women, 53% New Zealand women and 38% for Australian women.

Professor Kenny's group, which included 1, 774 women in the Irish component of the study, showed further striking facts (5,000 in total sample)

Light drinking 1 to 7 unit's week,
Moderate drinking 7 to 14 units a week,
Heavy drinking more than 14 units a week,
Binge drinking 6 or more units on one occasion.

At 15 weeks gestation in pregnancy:

20% admitted to moderate to heavy alcohol drinking

30% admitted to 2 or more binge episodes of drinking (compared with just 4% in the New Zealand sample),

Both of these studies from 2 separate urban centers spanning over 20 years of maternity practice in Ireland bare stark testament to the reality of the problem.

In the meantime Ireland continues to have the highest birth rate in Europe, and had a total of 71, 986 registered births in 2012. (Economic and Social Research Institute (ESRI) Perinatal Statistics Report 2012). As well the average age of Irish women giving birth was 31.9 years with a possibility of a longer history of alcohol consumption prior to pregnancy.

It is as if the country is fiddling and dancing a jig as the house burns.

Further statistics on alcohol consumption place Ireland (and the UK) in an unfortunate light.

It is interesting to see how alcohol consumption has decreased markedly over the last 25 years in France and Italy but the Ireland, of the 'Celtic tiger' has increased progressively.

Table 1. WHO statistics on alcohol consumption per capita liter consumption, population 15 + years old

	1970	2003	2004
Australia	11.5	9.8	
Canada	8.8	7.9	
*France	20.4	14.0	13.0
Germany	13.4	10.2	10.1
IRELAND	7.0	13.5	13.4
*Italy	18.2	8.0	
UK	7.1	11.2	11.5
USA	9.5	8.4	

Table 2. FEMALE drinking patterns – European comparison

France	5
Italy	12
Germany	7
Finland	16
Sweden	16
UK	21
IRELAND	30

Binge drinking per 100 drinking occasions.

BINGE is 6 or more units of alcohol per drinking occasion.

WHO unit = ½ pint beer, 1 small glass wine. I glass of spirits.

Strategic Task Force on Alcohol, Sept 2004.

Table 3. MALE binge drinking patterns – European comparison

France	9
Italy	13
Germany	13
Finland	29
Sweden	31
UK	40
IRELAND	59

Binge drinking episodes per 100 drinking occasions.
Strategic Task Force on Alcohol, Sept. 2004.

Professor Frank Murray, Chair of the Royal College Physicians of Ireland Alcohol Policy Group. Recently said:

> "There is a crisis in problem drinking consumption in Ireland. Increasing death rates from liver cirrhosis and increasing rates of hospital admission in young women tell a story of a bitterly unhappy relationship between the Irish and cheap alcohol" Medical Independent, 2013.

Table 4. High risk drinking by gender

At least one binge weekly	
Females	44%
Males	61%
Binge per 100 drinking occasions	
Females	60%
Males	76%

The Health of Irish Students, Health Promotions Unit, Dept. of Health and Children, 2005.

Table 5. Binge drinking (WHO definition 6 or more units on drinking occasion)

12- 13-year-old:	weekly 3%;	monthly 10%
14-15-year-old:	weekly 9%;	monthly 17%
16-17-year-old:	weekly 14%;	monthly 31%
18-19-year-old:	weekly 36%;	monthly 28%

My World Survey/Headstrong/UCD Dept. of Psychology, 2011, (reported Irish Times, May 16th 2012).

The 21st century romance of alcohol continues in Ireland, as girl buddy TV adverts exhort 25 to 35 year old professional white women to 'shine on', as they knock back the latest sexy Californian wine cooler.

In the recent Hollywood film 'Saving Mr. Banks', the archetypal Irish alcoholic father was played by the archetypal Irish actor Colin Farrell, who had a visceral understanding of the role. The father told his princess daughter that 'this life is an illusion,' and regaled her with Celtic mystical stories which possibly formed the unrecognized substrate of the whimsical Mary Poppins.

Further medical statistics on alcohol related morbidity and mortality, however, tell Ireland's continuing self-destructive story at many levels.

1) There was a 190% increase in liver disease in the period 1995 to 2007.
2) There has been a 247% increase in patients with liver disease treated in hospital from 1995 to 2007.
3) The majority were male, but there was a higher proportion of females in the youngest age group.
4) There has been a 170% increase in deaths in hospital from liver disease from 1995 to 2007, i.e., 2.6 per 100, 000 adult population to 71 per 100,000 population (Mongon et al., 2011).
5) There were 14, 239 people admitted to Saint Vincent's University Hospital Liver Unit, in Dublin, for alcohol dependence in 2011(Medical Independent, December 2013)

"Oh what a tangled tale we weave."

Suicide, used to be the lowest in the world in Ireland 30-35 years ago. It was a mortal sin (in the language and belief of the predominant Catholic Church), and so a person could not be buried in consecrated grave. Societies have a way of 're-framing' problems, so death by misadventure or accidental homicide entered the books.

Now suicide is recognized as a major problem in the island of Ireland North and South. So much so that the particular epidemic of youth suicide has begun to overwhelm medical and psychiatric providers. Only recently, on 21st May 2013, the Irish Times, Ireland's respected paper reported a major study on suicide. It was led by Professor Kevin Malone and was based on interviews of families involving 104 suicides between 2003 and 2008. The majority were male, and 14 took their own lives at 20 years of age. Now Ireland had entered the higher stakes of suicide in the EU. In fact as Professor Malone pointed out in this study discussion, Ireland was now rated 4th highest in suicide rates for people 15 years to 24 years of age.

As in many research studies the details tell different stories.

34 people who completed suicide had attempted it before, with 32 never mentioning intent.

51, or 49% of the sample, had abused alcohol in the 12 months before their death.

24, almost 25% of the sample, had been bereaved by the death of a friend in the last 12 months.

Relatives told of being sent away from A and E (Casualty) departments in hospitals only to have their loved one commit suicide later.

Was this just a product of over worked, harassed hospital triage services? Or could another story be waiting in the wings?

Table 6. Age of onset drinking by gender

Age at onset of drinking	Females	Males	Total
Under 14 years	17.3%	121.4%	18.9%*
15-16 years	48.6%	46.9%	48%
17 years or older	34.0%	31.7%	33.1%

Significant difference between gender p<0.5.
The Health of Irish Students, Health Promotions Unit, Dept. of Health and Children, 2005.

The statistics sometimes don't lie.

They tell a story of the prevalent underage drinking in the island of Ireland and the girls/women quickly catch up to the men by 15 to 16 years. Both of these populations are not too expectantly the mothers and fathers of their next generation of ARND, primed for alcohol craving and disruptive mood disturbance with impulsivity.

Transgenerational alcohol exists. It is very much congruent with the sentiments voiced in the proverbial 'Ghosts in the Nursery' eloquently articulated by Selma Fraiberg and colleagues in 1975. The eloquent rendering of the worlds that infants arrive could not be better articulated than in the author's original words;

> "In every nursery there are ghosts. They are visitors from the unremembered pasts of the parents, the uninvited guests at the christening... these intruders from the past have taken up residence in the nursery, claiming tradition and rights of ownership. They have been present at the christening for two or more generations. While no one has issued an invitation, the ghosts take up residence and conduct the rehearsal of the family tragedy from a tattered script... the baby in these families is burdened by the oppressive past of his parents from the moment he (she) enters the world. The parent, it seems, is condemned to repeat the tragedy of his (her) own childhood with his own baby in terrible and exacting detail."

Ibsen or Yeats could not have said it any better. The poetic lilt of the unremembered past conjures up Carl Jung's concept of collective unconscious and in the historical colonial tragedy of Ireland it continues to resonate. However, in Ireland, the 'ghosts' are washed in alcohol through countless generations. Alcohol has had a double action, as described by Franz Alexander 1965; it helps with the desire to escape from stress and also it serves to release the desire for the regressive gratification of repressed or inhibited impulse. In a country of centuries of violent colonial subjugation, war, dispossessed land, famine and religious oppression and sexual repression alcohol releases many visceral impulses. Mothers mourn their sons who have gone to fight, women mourn their lost loves. Cycles of war, displacement, and poverty famine bring generations of pain and suffering that has no words, but is translated through the centuries, In Ireland it was the oral culture that became the link to the continuity of history. Songs, ballads and poetry told and re-told the archetypal stories of pain, loss, betrayal, war and death. The more heartfelt they were expressed the more alive became the story and the story within the story. Alcohol became the natural conduit for this emotional release. It relaxed the spirit to sing the songs, and soothed the psychic pain that had no cure. In modern Ireland that story includes mourning for 'the Disappeared', a particular type of Irish cruelty whereby the paramilitaries executed so called informers and buried them in hidden graves so their families could never have closure to their deaths.

This 18th century Irish ballad captures some of the historical trans-generational trauma still present in the 21st century. As happens with archetypal ballads they continue to have lives in other times and other continents. (Byrne 2013).

Johnny I Hardly Knew Ye

"While going down the road to sweet Athy,
Harroo! Harroo!
While going down the road to sweet Athy,
Harroo! Harroo!
A stick in my hand and a drop in my eye,
A doleful damsel I heard cry,
"Och Johnny I hardly knew ye!
With your drums and guns and gun and drums
The enemy nearly slew ye.
My darling dear, you look so queer
Och, Johnny I hardly knew ye.!"

"Where are your eyes that looked so mild?
Harroo! Harroo!
Where are your eyes that looked so mild?
Harroo! Harroo!
Where are your eyes that looked so mild?
When my poor heart you first beguiled?
Why did you run from me and the child?
Och, Johnny I hardly knew ye!"
"Where are the legs with which you run?
Harroo! Harroo!
Where are the legs with which you run?
Harroo! Harroo!
Where are the legs with which you run
When you went to carry a gun?
Indeed, your dancing days are done!
Och, Johnny I hardly knew ye!"

Ireland holds many of the keys to unravelling transgenerational trauma interwoven with the pervasive use of alcohol which serves to dull the pain and also give some sense of a false joviality amidst the personal, family and community ruins. Generations of parents have been 'present but absent' for their children. The dual effects of alcohol addiction and unresolved trauma serve to immobilize these mothers and fathers and make them emotionally unavailable. The society has celebrated and in many ways glorified pain and sacrifice. Ireland's colonial history of occupation has been littered with romantic stories of 'heroes' dying for 'the cause of freedom'. They fought valiantly, but lost is the recurring theme. It is no better said than in the modern classic ballad Four Green Fields; "*What have I now said the fine old woman: I have 4 strong sons they fought to save my jewel. They fought and they died. That was my dream said she.*" Through generations this is a narrative that has permeated not just the conscious world but the more complex, subtle, unconscious world. "*Roddy Mc Corley goes to die on bridge of Toome to-day,*" the grass was red with the blood of the Fenian dead in the 1798 Rebellion at Vinegar Hill, Lord Mayor Terence Mc Sweeney dies after along hunger strike, Cromwell slaughters the women and children in the town of Drogheda.

Modern times have their own hunger strikers in Long Kesh prison and the more haunting 'Disappeared', executed so called informers with no marked graves. All these deaths and sacrifices celebrated in ballads and poems. Each one keeping the memory of the sacrifice and death alive for each coming generation. Ireland's particular form of un-remitting grief. Only 90 years have now separated Ireland from colonization, so it is still an emerging Republic finding its own voice and resonance. Unfortunately the programming of generations for alcohol mixed in with trauma has rendered many parts of the country 'frozen in time'. Ireland has married itself to the 'wounded hero' archetype (Jung 1959) whether it be patriot, dying for 'the cause' or the poet, musician or playwright suffering for his/her art such as Patrick Kavanagh, Brendan Behan, Mary Coughlan or Shane Mc Gowan.

However one of the most telling statistics revealing the addiction to addiction in Ireland was brought out in the last year. A previous government which oversaw Ireland's march into complete fiscal crisis, were guided by a leader, not unlike the commander who lead the infamous Charge of the Light Brigade, consumed more than 30% more kegs of Guinness in the Dail/government bar than the subsequent government who were passed the alcohol poisoned chalice. One only wonders how the fiscal decision making process was completed in the midst of Ireland's romance with the bottle or the jug. This points to the societal and not only financial cost of transgenerational alcohol which is almost impossible to fully comprehend and put a value or cost on.

At the most basic of societal levels the very family structure is compromised from the onset. The primary mother/infant bond in Ireland is disrupted for many dispirit reasons even before conception. The alcohol addiction has a two- fold effect, affecting the developing fetus in utero, but also impairing the pregnant mother to prepare mentally and physically for the new baby. The tell-tale signs of prenatal bonding disruption come from missed antenatal appointments, prenatal stress due to the trials and tribulations of a toxic co-dependent relationship, not uncommonly this is with a partner who is also alcohol dependent and sometimes intermittently violent. Well-meaning family members, i.e., the pregnant mother's own mother or father step in to take care of the new born baby, but this only serves to enable the alcohol dependent mother to continue drinking in the postnatal period, and so be unavailable emotionally and physically for her new-born infant. This is a cycle repeated through generations in Ireland, but is fair to say not unique to Ireland. Aboriginal communities in Canada, USA and Australia have similar patterns. The subtle guilt of transgenerational alcohol seeps through generations as the potential grandmother remembers her own alcohol dependence a generation before and so wants to help her, now alcohol addicted, daughter in her own pregnancy. It seems to be a recursive negative loop that has no exit. Irish society continues to be immersed in its catholic value system, so an infant or child removed from an alcohol dependent mother and/or father who is unable to cope will go to an emergency foster care, and later long term foster placement, but in parallel the social service will make sure to keep the infant and child connected with the substance abusing or even violent parent as 'family preservation' trumps child rights or welfare.

Thus in Irish society the negative loop of disadvantage inherent to transgenerational alcohol abuse is maintained by the agents of the government. Whether this is part of the pervasive denial and/or minimization in the society is hard to know. However for each succeeding generation of brain damaged ARND infants and children it perpetuates their life scripts of hardship. It is as if the biological fetal programming dealt by prenatal alcohol is not enough of a disadvantage in life, but society needs to keep the biologically vulnerable child in a postnatal environment of unpredictability and chaos. Seems reminiscent of Sean O' Casey's classic lines to end 'Juno and the Paycock', said as the two alcoholic buddies, Captain Boyle and Joxer, collapse, drunk and bereft on the floor of the empty flat, ' the whole world is in a state of chassis' Indeed. Not the whole world but parts of it where they continue to manufacture their own unique chaos.

We are living in a society in which the environment we inhabit and create changes us. It changes our personalities, our resilience to stressors, our problem solving skills when confronted with life's problems, our emotional reasoning. When fundamental judgement such as cause and effect reasoning are impaired then the likelihood of impulsive self-destructive decision making invariably increases. Then we have the change in our DNA methylation. Now we crave, as a society, alcohol, our delta b fos cells, nucleus accumbens come into the world waiting to be primed. No wonder Ireland has the highest underage drinking in the world. Maybe it is just the availability of alcohol in the local groceries store at ever decreasing costs, or maybe there is another reason?

When I returned in 2006 to Belfast to work as an adolescent psychiatrist the prevalence of impulsive suicide attempts and completions was quite astounding. Here was a small part of the country ravaged by a 30 year war, euphemistically called 'the troubles', which in truth were not over. The historical trauma permeated generations of Catholics and Protestants, washed in no mean way by alcohol to dampen the pain. Young children, teenagers abounded with levels of undiagnosed brain dysfunction due to prenatal exposure to alcohol. They lived in separate ghettoes united by a common lack of direction, support, basic jobs and education. They aspired to live no further than the boundaries of their ghettoes. Alcohol and drug use was rampant. Paramilitaries still controlled the areas, offering their special type of moral justice. Some small stories tell a larger tale.

A. One Yorkshire teenager, threatened by paramilitaries, climbed a crane and threatened to jump off in desperation at his plight. He saw no solution, no way out. He was being seen in the adolescent crisis services, had ARND, ADHD, intermittent explosive episodes and was alcohol dependent from 11 years old. The fire services used their high extending ladders to reach up to communicate and pizza and beer brought the teenager to talk, and eventually to come down to safety. As happened in those times, the non-medical crisis assessment team deemed the teenager not a risk, not suicidal, and safe to return to his traumatized, alcohol washed home environment. The hidden risk of impulsive self-destructive act in a brain damaged patient was not part of the triage decision making.

B. Another teenager, (who had a protestant father and a catholic mother) was harassed by paramilitaries because of his perceived antisocial behavior, drinking and selling drugs and beaten on the leg with a baseball bat. The paramilitaries had become the police of many ghettoes in the city as well as the guardians of moral behavior. The teenager was taken by his residential staff in great distress to A. and E. Dept. in a local Belfast hospital. He impulsively ran into the disabled toilet and tried to hang himself with the longer toilet cord. Fortunately, an alert hospital staff was able to break into the toilet. He was sent back to his residential home, deemed to not be a risk by the crisis intervention team. The next day when interviewed by the consulting psychiatrist he was acutely suicidal and pervasively hopeless and helpless, saying 'what can I do to'? He was admitted to an acute triage psychiatric bed that afternoon. Again he had an ARND/ADHD profile. Again, the organic brain damage/impulsive suicidal risk was not part of his crisis team assessment. Both of these examples are emblematic of the prevalence of impulsive self-destructive behaviors still current in Belfast. The chronic enduring trauma of the war has not remitted. The small 'country' within the larger Island of Ireland is still very much divided and in multiple ways denying its unresolved trauma. The role of transgenerational alcohol in this trauma has not received any consideration. Brain damaged, alcohol, drug abusing teenagers fill out patient and in patient departments. They do not respond to Cognitive Behavioral Therapy (CBT), or insight oriented therapy as they have rooted cognitive disconnections, not the least are decreased processing of information and grossly impaired working memory. (As recently as September/October 2013, Dr. Alaistir Rennie, emergency physician in Manchester, UK spoke of an 88% increase in the last 5 years of women, aged 18 to 34 years old, being admitted through the A and E department with severe alcohol related medical problems). A trend that has been reported in Ireland as well (Cronin et al., 2012).

These clinical examples are just 2 of many that exist in that traumatized part of Ireland. The interaction between transgenerational trauma and transgenerational alcohol brain dysfunction are generally ignored. ARND, whether dysmorphic or non-dysmorphic, have been described as 'orphan' conditions. They are orphaned from society at large and orphaned from medical/psychiatric care as their problems are seen as too vague, too complex, or maybe too many (O'Malley 2008). The crisis team assessors more commonly are becoming non-medical (physician), frequently due to fiscal constraints, and so the medical/neuropsychiatric consciousness of the 'at risk assessment' is minimized or just plainly dismissed. Another hidden disability lies within the medical or mental health staff in traumatized societies such as the North of Ireland. This disability is a form of desensitization, compassion fatigue, burn out, call it what you may. The children and teenagers are unable to communicate the distress, or are not heard when they attempt to communicate it.

C. About 5 or 6 years ago, I saw a teenage Irish/Polish girl who had ARND and severe PTSD. She had been sexually abused (maybe by a relative) but had been in court 4 times as the police would not validate her story. Each time they asked her leading questions and had her contradict herself. She had a significant learning disability with working memory and processing problems. Eventually she took the law into her own hands and compulsively would put ligatures around her neck to kill herself. She confronted the treating psychiatrist saying there was nothing they could do. Which was unfortunately true as she was not able to have an advocate in the room when interviewed by police, and the psychiatrist's report as to her severe PTSD, acute suicidal risk, on top of her ARND was not admissible. In the end, she had to be transferred to a secure unit psychiatric hospital in the UK which dealt with psychiatric disorders and intellectual disability. In some ways her problems were complicated but not complicated. She had been violated and in her simplistic way wanted validation of her life story.

One wonders how many of those patients in Professor Malone's study in the south of Ireland met similar scotomas/blind spots of thinking in their initial suicide risk assessments.

Almost 10 years ago work in University of Washington had been beginning to unravel suicidal risk factors in patients with ARND (Huggins et al., 2008). The underlying brain dysfunction was an essential part of the clinical decision tree of assessment and management.

Within societies such as the North of Ireland the transgenerational legacy of abuse and victimization seethes and is curdled with alcohol. Victims become perpetrators and sometimes it is hard to differentiate those healing from those needing healing. The blurring of boundaries is compounded by the basic denial and minimization of the pervasive dysfunction, sadness, disconnection and psychic numbing. Where transgenerational alcohol fits into this continuum is hard to place, but it seems to have a dual role of dampening down the pain and disconnecting from unsettling events. The cognitive disconnection inherent to ARND serves a perfect foil to 'disremember'. These are stories not unheard of in other countries, both in cities and rural communities. Domestic violence, sexual abuse, neglect, emotional unavailability, abandonment, are all ingredients well known in the transgenerational alcohol world. Unbeknown to many they are not the only purvey of socially disadvantaged but exist across all social classes, religions and ethnic groups.

Ireland has a special place in this self-destructive incubus of a universe and Belfast is its dark moon.

Belfast. A shadow city

The shadows never really left,
They just changed shapes,
As the generations progressed.

Forever slogan chants,
"1690"
"Remember the Fighting 13"
"6 into 26 don't go"
"No surrender"
Cast giant images of hatred
On the red brick tenement houses.

Now,
Enraged callow teenagers
In hoodies and balaclavas
Wrap themselves
In The (Their) Union Flag,
For what?

It is said that a nation that keeps an eye on the past,
Is wise,
Whereas a nation that keeps both eyes on the past,
Is blind.

Similar such words are painted
On a well known pub's outside wall,

A stone's throw from
The embattled Belfast City Hall.

Some people and cities live in the shadows,
Belfast remains in that place and in that time.

(And Thinking Of, 2014, Kieran D. O'Malley)

The recognition of historical trauma and its impact on the collective unconscious in the individual, but also the community, is being seen worldwide. From Native American, First Nation's experiences to Holocaust survivors, Kosovo, Croatia, Iraq and now Syria. Areas such as the North of Ireland serve as templates for the melding of this transgenerational experienced and collectively remembered trauma that can overcome a society/ethnic group and keep it in many ways 'frozen in time'. It is surely no accident that in the socio cultural environment of Ireland alcohol would have a pivotal role in dealing, or not dealing, with this transgenerational trauma. Trauma is known to effect the structure and chemistry of the brain with effects documented in the hippocampus, memory center, as well as effects on the amygdaloid as well as the HPA axis which alter the individual's response to stress and fear/flight response can be triggered by overreaction to facial cues.(Bremner et al., 1996, Meewise et al., 2009). How much of this transgenerational trauma is imprinted in the conscious and unconscious memory is still being explored, but researchers such as Yehuda et al., have demonstrated such a phenomenon is real.

However, in the schizophrenic perversity of thinking and logic that is Ireland there once was a famous Father Matthew who espoused total abstinence from alcohol because of its evils to society. He founded the Total Abstinence Society in Cork on April 10th 1838 and at one stage there were 3 million members, almost half the population of Ireland, before The Great Famine. He was invited to the USA, and visited the city hall with the mayor of New York. He further dined at the White House in Washington DC, as a guest of the then President Zachary Taylor, and was even given a seat at the House of Representatives. His political undoing was a refusal to be part of a debate on 'chattel slavery', saying that it was not mentioned in the Bible. His statue still remains on O'Connell Street, the main street in Dublin, and also in Salem Massachusetts. In modern secular Ireland, disconnecting from its religious history, the influence of the Total Abstinence or Pioneer Society is now quite minimal.

So naturally, it was W.B. Yeats, the developmental psychiatrist, who succinctly summarized the transgenerational angst in Ireland, which is washed down with alcohol and acted out in the primal mother/infant symbiosis.

Out of Ireland,
Have we come,
Great hatred, little room,
Maimed us at the start,

I carry from my mother's womb,
A fanatic heart.

(Remorse for Intemperate Speech).

THE KNOTTED CORD. AN UPDATE, 2020

A further five years living and working in Ireland has re-acquainted me with a cultural collective unconscious of the nation, which is so ingrained in the society's living consciousness as to be unnoticed and so unacknowledged.

"I eat when I'm hungry
I drink when I'm dry,
And if the moonshine don't kill me,
I'll live till I die."

The mythical "uisce beatha" (water of life) from Celtic mythology has now been replaced in modern society by Irish whiskey (the water of life interrupted).

What more to say.

The intervening 5 years has, however, changed some of my thinking.

Now, I would not fully agree that the "Great Hatred. Little room," was the origin of the nation's self-destructive dance with alcohol. It is my old psychoanalytic training that has awakened new understandings.

Ireland nurturing

Maybe it is not
Great hatred
That immobilizes the
mother and father,
As they struggle to decipher
The dreams and nightmares
of their collective memories.
The island's little womb
still constricts these emotions
but it is the profound
unspoken sadness
which each generation
needs to recognize
and slowly release.

KD O'Malley, Travelin' Still, 2018

The younger age range of my clinical work with transgenerational alcohol in Ireland, the clearer the challenges of seminal mother/infant symbiosis.

1) A grandmother becomes the primary parent of her grandson C, as the birth mother, her daughter, is unable to parent C because of alcohol dependence and co-occurring psychiatric disorders. The grandmother is torn between her need to nurture her daughter, and the immediate parenting/nurturing needs of her inherited grandson C. She has to make a decision in the infant's interest, or the daughter's interest, as she is incapable of protecting both of them. In the meantime, the daughter has rejected psychiatric and addiction counselling help, and remains angry because of the loss of her child.
2) A grandmother M. is coerced to work in a residential laundromat, because she was removed from her birth home for protection because of physical abuse, but had also become a binge drinking, single teenage parent.
3) Her daughter, N was taken into state care at 4 weeks of age passing through 3 foster home placements as they were unable to cope with her emotional dysregulation and sensory reactivity problems.
4) The daughter, N had a boy T, when she was 17 years old, and that child was also taken into state care at 6 weeks of age as the single mother, N, was now chronically depressed, alcohol dependent and so judged to be an 'unfit parent'.
5) The boy T, displayed complex developmental problems from an early age and was placed in residential care at 11 years of age with a diagnosis of Oppositional Defiant Disorder, but was intermittently hopeless and suicidal.
6) T craves his birth mother's affection, but N is not able to tolerate his visits as she feels both guilty and angry with him and herself at the same time.
7) An aunt or uncle take over the custody of their 32-year-old sister's son as she is unable to cope with him because of her own alcohol dependence and medical illnesses, such as liver cirrhosis.
8) The birth mother resents the intervention of her sister or brother as kinship carers, but at the same time appreciates that they allow her to maintain a caring, though still alcohol dependent and medically ill, relationship with her son.

(All examples in this Updated Book are amalgams of clinical cases to protect the patient identity).

Ireland's recognition of the transgenerational alcohol problem in its midst.
There remains an almost 'schizophrenic', self-destructive divide in the country.

Separately the National TV stations RTE showcases "Can't Stop Won't Stop," about the lives and loves of 30 something Irish women (Ireland's answer to the wildly popular USA show 'Sex in the City', where sex has become alcohol).

Alcohol statistics change but remain the same.

National Survey of Alcohol Use Cases

- 55,675 Problem Alcohol Cases (2011-2017).
- 6,300 Alcohol Use Cases in 2016 increased to 7,350 Cases in 2017.
- 37% Binge drinking, 22% Binge drinking more than 1 day a week (Binge drinking defined as 6 or more drinks at one occasion).

(Medical Independent, 4/4/2019).

The Costs to Society of Problem Alcohol Use in Ireland was 3.7 Billion Euro
(Byrne Report 2010).

Middle Class parents are more likely to let their children drink alcohol

- 13% of children 11 to 15 years of age admitted alcohol use in the last week from wealthy families.
- 7% of children 11 to 15 years of age admitted to alcohol use in the last week from less wealthy families.
- Overall: 37% of children 11 to 15 years of age reported alcohol use from wealthy families.
- 27% of children 11 to 15 years of age reported alcohol use from less wealthy families.

(Smoking, Drinking and Drug Use Survey of Young People 2018; Reported in the Irish Times 1/8/2019)

*When I asked "Dr. Google" on September 10th 2019 (the day after World FASD Day 2019) the question:

What are the statistics in Ireland on FASD?

The reply I immediately received was "There is no register of children with FASD in Ireland."

The following statistics then appeared, quoted from a recent *National Survey of Pediatricians in Ireland,* (Gill et al., *2018).*

- 81% of Irish women reported drinking alcohol in pregnancy.
- 31.3% of the total sample of women surveyed did not know of the existence of FASD.
- 34% of the total sample of women surveyed felt FASD only existed if there were dysmorphic facial features.

Now, the Black Brew (Ireland's stout of choice) shows us that with their product you are 'made of more'. Old TV newsreels of famous sporting achievements confirm this magical power.

As if Harry Potter has waved his iconic wand.

Ireland, 5 years later, remains just as intoxicated and in love with alcohol.

New statistics still appear:

RTE NEWS, 9/12/2019. Fiachra O Clonnaith, using access under the Freedom of Information Act for new facts.

This revealed that in 2018 Ireland had 113 babies born addicted to drugs or exposed to drugs or alcohol but only five babies in Ireland in 2018 were reported as exposed to alcohol in Ireland. Amazingly, the same reporter revealed that only 5-7 babies each year from 2014 to 2018 had been born exposed to alcohol in Ireland

There is an old Irish saying 'de-Nile' (Denial) is not just a river in Egypt!

THE IMPACT OF COLONIZATION AND STARVATION

Ireland was colonized for 800 years, but as well suffered the loss of 12.5% of its population during the 1845 to 1851 period of the Great Famine or starvation (it has been called a starvation because food was plentiful on the island at the time, but was shipped out of the country to England). This acute loss of population was the largest of any country in the world. (The Killing Fields of Cambodia resulted in 9% total population loss). At the time of the Great Famine Ireland's population had boomed to 8.75 million and was a mainly rural population. The famine resulted in the deaths of 1 to 1.2 million people and a further 1.5 million emigrated to North America. It was the systematic eviction of poor rural tenants by the Anglo-Irish landlords that prompted the disaster. 70,000 homes were evicted with 500,000 adults and numerous children displaced. The English colonial landlords increased their tithes to precipitate evictions and make land available for livestock. So small tenant farmers had to sell their one goat, or one cow which had sustained their families and thus lost their homes. They also had to sell their currachs/boats which had brought the fish to sustain their families with similar effects.

In parallel, the term 'souper' appeared to describe people who sold their identity and Roman Catholic religion for soup and food. When emigrating to America or Australia these 'soupers', because of that shame and stigma, changed their names and dropped the Mac or O' in their surnames.

On the other side of the coin those families who survived the Famine with their name unchanged and Catholic faith intact were seen as true survivors.

The country did not just suffer death and destruction, but survivor guilt and/or loss of identity. This was aptly captured in a series of articles in the Lancet 2019, on the double burden of malnutrition. "Exposure to malnutrition during early critical periods, results in the body reducing its valuation of the future, diverting energy from growth and health to survival and potential reproduction." (Wells et al., 2019).

Also, rarely acknowledged sequelae of the Famine were other destructive, violent actions to themselves or others. These traumatic events became implanted into the nation's psyche. The epigenetic impact on humans of famine has been explored. It is also relevant in the world of transgenerational trauma and alcohol (Heljmans et al., 2008).

In the aftermath of this great human tragedy it was acknowledged that the "laissez faire" attitude of the British Government at the timer that was to shoulder the blame. Subsequently, their approach was described as' catastrophic neglect and ideological blindness'' (Crawley et al., 2012).

Ireland is therefore a country where colonization has had, and continues to have, profound effects. Aboriginals in Australia, Maoris in New Zealand, First Nations in Canada and Native Americans in USA, indigenous Travelers in Ireland all share a self-destructive history of subservience and transgenerational trauma.

Alcohol has played its part, both in healing/soothing but also the continued self-destruction in all these communities and cultures.

This imposed legacy of individual and collective self-destruction shows the mother/infant dyad lying at its very heart (Menninger, 1938). The continuing cycles of pregnancy and birth bring unwritten scripts for generations to come.

They offer the society a chance to see it is still not too late to act, and maybe change for the good.

The Escape from the Pervasive Effect of Colonization and Starvation

The romantic story of the fight for freedom from 800 years of colonization is crystalized in the famous Easter Rebellion in Dublin 1916.

Now, less than 100 years after shedding the straitjacket of colonization and becoming a Republic the country has fled into a secular world. Mammon has now become its primary God and spiritual colonizer.

Into this spiritual void, Time is being redefined in a quaint Irish way as 'Black Brew Time'. All the more to caress and savor its ambrosia, live in the eternal moment, with no thought given to the future. It is living in this Instagram moment that matters.

Nevertheless, it was Samuel Beckett who truly captured the dark 'shadow' of the Irish persona, which presents a 'Jokers' face to the world, but behind this face there lies a troubled, and sometimes destructive heart.

It is within this spirit of lost openness to new, or even old, knowledge, that I offer this recent poem. It is an attempted entry into Ireland's eyeless, guileless, self-destruction, which has not disappeared since it became a Republic.

Easter Sunday 2016

I
The centennial ritual celebrations
of the revolution begin,
England's infamous pyrrhic victory
which crowned the Irish martyrs,
Pearse and Connolly
Clarke and Mac Donough
Ceannt and Mac Diarmad
Joseph Mary Plunkett.

II
One hundred years later,
The Free State/Republic,
enjoys the festivities with no national government,
in place,
for 50 days and counting,
The mantle has passed,
to Kenny and Martin,
Burton and wee Gerry,
who do not stride the world as a Colossus,
but more pygmies in the modern ruins.

III
The two right wing conservative parties,
Fine Gael and Fianna Fail,
Speak hackneyed empty rhetoric,
Diluted in muddy water.

IV
What happened to?
"equal rights and equal opportunities to all citizens,"

While foreign venture capitalists evict
families from their hard earned homes,
and homelessness increases exponentially.

V
What happened to?
"cherishing all the children of the nation equally"
When Ireland has no Charter of Rights for Children.

VI
Now,
International drug gangs
shoot people in broad daylight
and strut around Dublin,
in limited edition silver BMWs,
becoming latter-day "Paycocks."
Now,
Health and Social Care,
are bought and sold in the market place;
And "as you only have one body,"
plastic surgeons are ready,
to sculpt it to perfection,
because, of course, you are worth it.
And your money is most welcome.

VII
Meanwhile;
Children in Care are not cared
Hospitals have stopped functioning,
and flounder unnoticed;
Cherishment is an aspiration,
from an old century.

VIII
Now;
The Adolescent Nation,
twitters and selfies itself,
into malignant fleeting narcissism.
bathed in four-leaf clovered Diageo black brew.

IX
What has been borne in revolution,
Is terrible,
but with no lasting beauty.

X
Nevertheless;
for those with ears that still can hear,
eyes that still can see,
and hearts that still beat
You can till breathe in the strains
of a lone blind uileann piper's
long forgotten Celtic lament
playing in the disappearing twilight.

K D O'Malley, Travelin' Still, 2018.

This commentary exposes the secular world that Ireland has become, where many unnamed vulnerable populations do not even reach the bottom of the proverbial totem pole of care.

Can Irish Society Now Learn from the Lessons of the Past?

1) Maybe, just as suicide, the ultimate self-destructive act, was discovered as real only 30-35 years ago. At that time the suicidal act was deemed a mortal sin by the Dominant Church, so the family could not bury their loved ones in consecrated graves. Deaths were thus registered as 'accidental' or 'by misadventure'. However, it has been discovered and now Ireland is recognized as having one of the highest suicide rates in Europe, but it is not hidden or denied.
2) Child sexual abuse did not exist, as its presence was denied by the Dominant Church. Similarly, it came out of the closet and was discovered 20 to 25 years ago. Now, victims of institutional abuse in the North of Ireland are receiving compensation through the UK government (the South of Ireland is still somewhat ambivalent).
3) Transgenerational Alcohol is the 3rd and last seminal Taboo in Ireland. (The specter of transgenerational alcohol is denied by both secular and non- secular institutions.) Its discovery is more problematic as Ireland rapidly races into a capitalist secular society.

Summary Statement

History has, however, shown Irish society the potential future. The first two taboos, suicide and sexual abuse, have both been 'outed' in the last 20 to 35 years.

Thus, there remains hope that Ireland will begin to open its eyes and ears, and realize the truth of transgenerational alcohol which stands as the ubiquitous 'Green Elephant' in that society.

As I am finishing this chapter just before Christmas 2019 it seemed culturally appropriate to end with a line from 'Fairytale in New York'. This iconic song was co-authored by the stereotypical Irish/English alcohol-troubled, self-destructive singer and poet Shane Mac Gowan. The song begins with a rambling Joycean melancholic monologue by an old man in the drunk tank on Christmas Eve.

However, it ends with the archetypal Irish wish fulfillment dream,

> "I can see a better time when all our dreams come true."

Why not?

Chapter 3

The Stigma of Transgenerational Alcohol

The Knotted Cord. (2014 Book)

> "Sure I wouldn't want to upset his mother by telling her that her son has ARND as she is an alcoholic and just in recovery the last few weeks"

It is rather a strange phenomenon to work in a society which celebrates with gusto its national addiction with Arthur's Day, called after the previously indigenous Black Porter. On the International stage this is quite a unique celebration. No other country makes a party out of its widespread addiction, thereby contributing to the national addiction and in many ways normalizing it.

On the other hand it is frowned on to admit drinking in pregnancy. Medical practitioners collude with this collective shame by removing a diagnosis of FAS or ARND from the medical records. The alcohol abusing parent is protected from this shame and stigma of potentially harming their unborn baby. However the brain damaged infant and child is not protected, and 'bad behaviors' quickly result in censure by the medical and social welfare authorities. In the further perversity of transgenerational alcohol related neurodevelopmental disorder in Ireland, the brain damaged child, with FAS or ARND mostly undiagnosed, grows up programmed for alcohol, becomes pregnant, but is protected in the pregnancy because of the societal shame about alcohol harm to the fetus and the minimization of the alcohol risk.

It seems no problem to disclose smoking in pregnancy, but both alcohol use and exposure to violence/trauma in pregnancy period are taboo subjects. The effects of chronic post-traumatic stress disorder which couple apathy and despair coming to roost. (Lenore Terr 2003, Bessell van der Polk et al., 1995).

Ireland seems to subscribe to the old notion of "stigma" as a mark of social disgrace. This notion then contributes to a process that begins with negative stereotyping, and proceeds to the person being treated with prejudice, discrimination and creates a true power imbalance in inter-relationships for the stigmatized individual.

The old notion of stigma dates back in modern times to Goffman's classic book in 1963. More recently the steady work of Sartorius has reviewed and revealed the situation from an International perspective. (Goffman 1963, Sartorius 2007). The words of Goffman echo and resonate some 50 years later in society's such as Ireland. "Blemishes of individual characters are perceived as a weak will, domineering, unnatural passions" ... "records of addictive illnesses are also seen." (Goffman 1963). The stigma of mental illness and alcohol addictive disorder and it's blemish on the family is so prevalent in modern day Ireland that mothers still can refuse to let the diagnostic report of a child with ARND be reported to the school because of its stigma to the family. Instead they prefer to have the child's problems 'hidden' by diagnoses such as ADHD or Asperger's Disorder or ASD.

Thus in many countries such as Ireland, Stigma can 'cast a long shadow' and pervade personal, family, community and general social interactions (Sartorious 2007, Stuart and Sartorius 2013).

Ireland, unfortunately, has a particular problem with the stigma and the shame of mental illness. Whether this is because of the centuries old patriarchal repressive influence of the Catholic Church is hard to know. There are some historical antecedents. About 30 to 35 years ago Ireland was reputed to have one of the lowest suicide rates in the world, next to Malta. At that time it was considered a 'mortal sin' in the eyes of the Catholic church to have committed suicide and so doctors and coroners in particular were encouraged to write 'death by misadventure' on the death certificates. Families were shamed and further traumatized by a loved one's suicide as it was unholy and the shame was a stain on the family. This 'stain' was amplified by the authoritarian church's stance regarding burial in sacred ground. The sacred ground could not hold the body of the person who had committed the mortal sin of suicide. Now, many years later, suicide has come out of the closet, so to speak, and Ireland recognizes and is recognized as having one of the highest per capita suicide rates in the world, especially in the 15 to 14 year old age bracket.

In the Irish context the fear of stigma to the birth mother is so ingrained in physicians that the diagnosis of ARND, dysmorphic or ARND non dysmorphic is not uncommonly made in the medical chart, but is minimized and so not communicated outside the bounds of the medical institution.

THE EFFECT OF STIGMATIZATION IN THE IRISH CONTEXT IS MANIFOLD

1) There are psychosocial consequences of shame and self-blame which lead to a wish for secrecy and social withdrawal.

2) There are family consequences in which this blame is seen as a flawed genetic trait. Also there is a fear that the person, and family, are harboring potentially dangerous individuals.
3) There are health system outcomes which in the Irish context lead to a health policy vacuum in respect to appropriate mental health initiatives for the transgenerational alcohol problems.
   a. This in turn inevitably leads to inadequate mental and alcohol counseling health care for individuals with transgenerational alcohol related neurodevelopmental disorder (ARND).
4) There are professional consequences such that psychiatrists who work in this vague field of developmental psychiatry with alcohol at its roots are seen as not really true doctors, but 'social doomsayers'.
5) There are implications for recovery in this complex area of transgenerational alcohol problems as the stigmatized conditions such as ARND are not diagnosed, not managed and continue through succeeding generations. So morbidity, medical and psychiatric increase, level of functional disability increases and unique mortality risks increases from such areas as impulsive suicide. (Stuart and Sartorius 2013).

Example 1

This is more than typical of the medical dilemma. An infant is born in a well-known city Canadian maternity hospital. There are many documented notes of the birth mother's heavy alcohol consumption in pregnancy. The infant is examined by one medical specialist, who notes the dysmorphic and growth features consistent with FAS (ARND dysmorphic). The patient is referred to a second medical specialist in the maternity hospital. He agrees with the first doctor's findings and writes the same diagnosis in the medical records.

The birth mother is unable to cope with parenting due to continued alcohol addiction after delivery and the infant is placed in an emergency, then long term foster placement, at 4 months of age. The foster mother brings the infant in follow –up to the specialist, and is not given any diagnosis. The specialist, then discharges the infant from active medical follow up at 12 months of age.

The foster mother is overwhelmed by many unusual difficult behaviors in her foster child but has no medical follow up in place, so she ends up being parent and manager of her unseen brain damaged infant, without the knowledge of the brain damage and the fact that 2 specialists had already diagnosed the specific alcohol related neurodevelopmental disorder (ARND) with classic facial features. This diagnosis is well recognized as chronic and posing many problems through the lifespan.

At 7 years of age the foster mother receives a diagnosis of ARND dysmorphic or FAS in her foster child. At this stage he is out of school because of severe hyperactive behavior and unexplained explosive episodes. As well the birth mother has died at 35 years of age, of alcohol related liver problems in the last year. She also hears that there are 2 other older children of the birth mother's in care with no diagnosis. Both were delivered in the same city maternity hospital. The social service want to institute sibling visits and the foster mother is fearful that these could be disturbing for her son, especially if the other 2 children have behavioral/mood problems because of ARND. The maternity hospital is contacted by the social service regarding the records of the 2 other children, especially pertaining to maternal alcohol consumption in pregnancy, and are told the records are missing.

This is clinical case scenario repeats itself too often in Ireland. It seems to offer an interface between fears of stigmatizing the birth mother leading to professional behavior on the boundaries of ethics. Far from 'proceeding slowly to do no harm'.

Thinking positively, the diagnosis made by the two medical specialists, offer a real opportunity to acknowledge the serious alcohol addiction in the mother and make sure she had active alcohol counseling treatment as well as a plan put in place to delay next pregnancy (using birth control), or to monitor subsequent pregnancies such that another alcohol effected infant was not born.

What would have been the parent and child outcome if the severe alcohol addiction affecting the infant had been acknowledged at the birth of the first child?

This is another clinical example and it serves to illustrate another problem with stigma attached to a diagnosis in the infant or young child (or even older child) immobilizing clinicians as it feeds into their pre-conceived notions of 'nothing to be done'. Psychiatry and Pediatrics have extensively moved into a marriage of our scientific understanding of developmental psychological milestones and process, to incorporating the developmental stages of the brain, including anomalies in that development. The truth is that many child and adolescent specialists (especially in the UK and Ireland) loathe giving a diagnosis of brain injury, damage/dysfunction; as this is seen as permanent and so incurable. Thus ARND, dysmorphic or non-dysmorphic is not diagnosed in order to protect the child from the 'stigma' of a permanent brain damage.

Does this help the child?

Does this help management either to the child or to the caregivers whether birth, foster or adoptive?

Does this avoidance of stigmatization in the child in fact inadvertently lead to further societal stigmatizations as the child's behaviors are misunderstood?

Example 2

Not infrequently children with ARND are labeled as Oppositional Defiant Disorder or Conduct Disorder because of their level of behavioral irritability. This actually labels the victim, stigmatizes the victim, and avoids an understanding of the role of true cognitive disconnections and emotional communication disconnections in the patient's developmental psychiatric presentation.

The 'incurable' thesis become quickly a self-fulfilling prophesy.

It is somewhat ironic as Psychiatry has been home to so-called incurable diseases such as Schizophrenia. Furthermore, there is a long standing mantra in psychiatry which speaks of the 'quality of life' as being the important treatment element in patients with chronic mental illnesses.

Quality of life sometimes like holding water, as for stressed, demoralized foster or adoptive parents who have been stigmatized as' not good enough' parents' and have been subjected to years of attachment work, A diagnosis of ARND releases some of their psychic pain.

Does it cure the child? No, but it offers the opportunity to begin new conversations and actually bring the child and his/her developmental psychiatric problems to the table for a more studied evaluation.

Management of Ethical Dilemmas

These exist in many shapes and sizes when applied to transgenerational alcohol and approaches to management.

A reflection on the changing landscape of public health disease can put this into a perspective.

In the 19th and early 20th century it was infectious disease that ravaged populations of all social classes and ethnic groups. The advances of medicine heralded more specific diagnosis and treatment, mycobacterium blood assay analysis, vaccines, immunizations, antibiotics all played their part in changing the overwhelming morbidity and mortality from these diseases. The natural history of infectious disease changed dramatically to make them not the source of the previous century.

In the mid-20th century another plague arrived AIDS. The concentration of medical minds in Europe and the USA created a viable treatment regime for a hitherto incurable disease.

Now in the early 21st century people live longer, but is the scourge of self-inflicted illnesses that have become the major public health battle ground. Transgenerational alcohol is one such battle ground. One wonders how the self-inflicted ethical dilemmas often intermingled with stigma issues have immobilized therapists to attempt to enter into this murky field. Needless to say industry do not have a keen interest in testing the efficacy and effectiveness of psychotropic drugs in ARND as they generally dismiss these patients as intellectual disability and choose to not see that over 75% have a normal IQ and the patients present developmental psychiatric profiles which are amenable, and do respond, to carefully chosen medications (Byrne 2008, O'Malley 2010, 2013).

When reviewed dispassionately from a distance it is strange that no specific psychological or medical/psychiatric management strategies have resulted from the minute multitudinous neuropsychological mapping of ARND. Techniques such as CBT have a firm place in depression and now are a panacea for PTSD and many other disorders, DBT has a role for Borderline Personality Disorder. Psychoanalytic therapy is well established for complex genetically rooted interpersonal problems, but no accepted therapies have surfaced for ARND. Coaching in mathematics has its role for education in the short term, and parent support indirectly helps but both do not really address the essence of the transgenerational problem. It is the proverbial elephant in the room that no-one sees or hears or smells. Maybe in the future it is in the area of Trauma Centered therapy that a certain core non- threatening approach can build to connect with ARND patients.

Why?

Is it because there is no entry point into to a circular transgenerational alcohol addiction?

Is any entry point too froth with complex mixtures of perceived ethical and stigma inducing dilemmas?

Motivation Interviewing and alcohol counseling such as Alcoholics Anonymous are well established approaches but they do not address the transgenerational issues inherent to alcohol and especially transgenerational ARND.

If you begin with the pregnant substance abusing woman then you have to establish a relationship to elicit the history of alcohol abuse in pregnancy. Many practitioners feel that type of questioning is too intrusive, too much like policing. So avoidance becomes the norm.

Then an alcohol exposed infant is delivered which offers an opportunity for recognition, but avoidance is the norm because of the introduction of stigma to the birth mother. However there is a unique programs started in Washington State called the Parent Child Assistance Program (PCAP) (Grant et al., 2008), which does intervene when an alcohol exposed infant is delivered and for 3 years offers a wrap-around support for mother and baby. It's strength is in the normal developing substance abusing mother with a normal or ARND infant, but the program struggles when it enters into the true transgenerational ARND world as the paraprofessional advocates do not have specialized skills to deal with two generations of organically brain damaged individuals with their resulting unpredictable disorganized attachment nurturing pattern. But it is important to remember that the mother/infant intervention are being done and the entry point is acceptance of substance abuse in the pregnant mother. This is a major breakthrough for all concerned and the fact that the program is replicated in different States in USA, and some provinces in Canada speaks volumes for its utility, and ability to break both ethical and stigma barriers.

Countries such as Ireland are still unable to grasp the nettle and plunge into the murky waters of the primary mother/infant bond, especially when alcohol is the story and they are most needed.

Total annual cost to the U.S. economy for ARND dysmorphic or, FAS alone is estimated at $3.6 billion, and annual lifetime cost per affected individual due to health, social, and justice system costs plus indirect costs (lost productivity due to mortality, morbidity, disability, and/or incarceration/career crime) is estimated at $2 million or more. Reports suggest that individuals with ARND, dysmorphic or non-dysmorphic, are over-represented in psychiatric samples and in juvenile detention and correctional settings (Novick Brown et al., 2011).

Sometimes happenchance and opportunity are chance bedfellows. In Canada a Minister of Indian (Native) Affairs adopted a First Nations child. Later he discovered the child had dysmorphic ARND (FAS). When he became Minister of Finance he released significant Government (Federal) funding to study the effects of prenatal alcohol exposure. Canada quickly became an International Research leader in the field. Although the subtle stigmatization of First Nations people as being the sole victims of maternal alcohol drinking quietly crept into Canadian national consciousness. Money in this case was a 'double-edged sword.'

Maybe it is not an accident that 25 years after this pool of money the well-respected International Meeting on Fetal Alcohol in Vancouver, British Columbia, spring 2014 has Ethics as its Conference Topic?

Can continued stigmatization be that far behind?

This book has been influenced in its own way by fear of stigmatization.

1) The families and patients did not want their photographs in the book as it was too stigmatizing and embarrassing for them (the only photographs that will appear will be of patients and families that I had previously treated in Canada). One Irish foster family did agree to have their photographs inserted.
2) All the clinical examples are real, but the names, ages, ethnic groups, hospitals, physicians have been changed or made anonymous to protect the identity and prevent stigmatization.

The Stigma of Transgenerational Alcohol. An Update, 2020

This 2020 update is approached from an international perspective and not the narrow world of Ireland.

Stigma is clearly a universal issue and not limited to this small island. It is one of those concepts that can diminish with time, but may sometimes become more entrenched.

a) Alcohol continues to create contradictory statements. It's good for your heart, your blood, but too much of it is not good for you.
b) Countries throughout the world continue to study the minutiae of the prenatal alcohol effect on the developing face. Vast sums of money are contributed to facial recognition research, which has quickly become incorporated into the worldwide forensic services. One wonders if the obsession with facial recognition is only another way of 'stigmatizing' an already vulnerable group of individuals.
People are becoming reduced to 'faces'. It is as if the breath of science research on prenatal alcohol exposure has not progressed during the last 50 years.

I was taught in medical school in the late 1960's to look out for the 'FLK', funny looking kid in pediatric training.

Has this crude labelling and stigmatization fundamentally changed in 2020?

c) The societal attitudes to mothers to not drink alcohol in pregnancy has in many ways hardened and is becoming more judgmental, blaming and stigmatizing. This was demonstrated in a study from Berlin (Wessel et al., 2002). Even more supposedly FASD/NDPAE enlightened progressive countries, such as USA and Canada, have introduced legislation in different states and provinces to incarcerate women if they drink alcohol during pregnancy, as this action is seen as a willful abuse of the developing fetus.

The children adopted from places including Russia and Romania engender mixed welcomes in many countries because of their prevalence of prenatal alcohol exposure. In some countries, such as USA, children from Russia are now not accepted for international adoptions. Whereas in other countries, Ireland for example, the adoption agencies and perspective parents are 'persuaded' by the society to deny or minimize the potential risk of neurodevelopmental disorder problems in the adoptive child. So, medical/psychiatric services are not sought and the adoptive, potentially brain-injured, child's problems are solely seen in an 'attachment disorder' frame. The adoptive parents thus receiving most of the blame and shouldering the guilt for their child's unmanageable or misunderstood problems.

Reflexive Questions

1) Which is more stigmatizing and demoralizing for a mother, or father for that matter, than to be told that they are 'unfit parents'?
2) Which is more stigmatizing and demoralizing for a child than to be told that there is no solution or even diagnosis for his/her problems?

3) Which is more stigmatizing and invalidating for an ethnic minority group than to be told that 'they are the problem' and the epigenetically acquired vulnerability to neurotoxin alcohol is minimized or dismissed as just a product of multiple years of trauma and poverty chaos?

Entering the world of transgenerational alcohol stigma.

As much as international science progresses the realities of confronting the societal, ethnic, family and personal stigmatization of transgenerational alcohol continues. No medical specialty service takes responsibility and thus it is an 'orphan condition'. So it continues to be isolated, unknown, unheralded, and of course globally stigmatized.

There is a consistent unconscious negative theme that pervades all discussions of approaches to diagnosing and managing children, adolescents and adults with NDPAE (or FASD). This is society's implicit permissive attitude of passive acceptance of alcohol and in some ways alcoholism:

- prohibition did not work,
- raising alcohol taxes worked in the short term,
- abstinence worked at times in different western societies, but was not sustained.

Alcohol is widely accepted and celebrated until you, the individual, begin to behave irrationally. At the time alcohol takes over your life society quickly stigmatizes and shuns you. Naturally a mother learns the stigmatic risk of exposing her alcohol use in pregnancy. Many midwives and obstetricians are still ambivalent, and so the double stigma of personal alcohol problems and acquired alcohol problems in your infant are avoided for yet another generation. Who wins?

Children born exposed to alcohol enter a world with a probable biological vulnerability, but as well, a fundamental social vulnerability/stigma. These children are shunned, not wanted, not recognized (except as a face), not diagnosed, not managed. They, not uncommonly, enter state care and a double blame or jeopardy ensues. They are damaged children ('Damaged Angels'), and their parents, are damaged parents. as children age and are confronted with clinicians who are often reluctant to acknowledge the potential role of acquired brain injury in their complex challenged development. Gradually they become more isolated, stigmatized as they have become truly 'orphans' in the society.

Social History tells us that the alcohol affected children come from Aboriginal/Indigenous communities in Australia, New Zealand, Canada, USA, South Africa, Ireland. So, they are not 'us', but separate from us.

The stigmatization and devaluation of the condition rationalizes societies inability to see the Faustian Demon within their midst.

Denial and minimization throughout many diverse societies maintains the unseen transgenerational alcohol legacy. We still create adults who have an epigenetically kindled alcohol craving which may become an addiction, and can then result in the adults being more vulnerable to life's stresses. The biological roots of their addiction misunderstood or even ignored.

It is, again, as if 50 years of animal and later human research are lying forgotten, or maybe never learned.

Chapter 4

THE ETHICAL DILEMMA OF DIAGNOSING AND MANAGING ARND

THE KNOTTED CORD. (2014 BOOK)

"Sure what's the point of diagnosing ARND there's nothin' you can do anyways."

For five years I taught a credit course at the University of Washington, Henry M Jackson School of International Studies. The course was entitled Comparative Health Care Practices and compared and contrasted the USA, UK and Canadian health systems. The 1st module was called 'The Politics and Ethics of health care delivery' and the students had to write an essay; Health Care as a Commodity. No problem for USA students which has the highest number of medical patents waiting to be licensed to create wealth for their medical inventors and drug industry drives many so called 'evidence based guidelines'. Much to the chagrin of Canada and UK health care boosters the exponential rise in private health care in both countries spoke silent volumes about consumer attitudes to waiting for service provision and quality of service provision. (O'Malley 2007).

Ironically, I had a paper published on 'The Politics and Ethics of Health Care Delivery' in a national Political Science Journal in the USA, but the editor commenting on the long paper said, it was interesting but *a narrow interest topic in the USA*. As you watch the machinations of the visceral rage over Obamacare in 2013, you really begin to wonder.

Ireland of post Celtic Tiger fame is a small country with overarching fiscal problems. It makes sense at one level that the revenue from alcohol taxes could not be diminished as they are essential part of the GNP.

Is it possible to create an equation that places the health care costs of alcohol related disorders on one side of the page and the revenue from alcohol on the other side of the ledger?

How do you quantify the financial and societal cots of transgenerational alcohol, and more specifically transgenerational ARND a currently hidden disorder in Ireland?

Is it ethical for a society to deny and minimize a toxin in their society which creates wealth and jobs and in equal measure chronic morbidity and mortality?

Is Mammon the God of government or is there another path?

The death of the egalitarian mother and child scheme for free health care delivery 60 years ago spoke of not just financial interests but religious interests and control of health care in the new emerging Republic of Ireland. (Browne 1952, Mc Cord 2013).

There continues to be a pervasive level of therapeutic nihilism which pervades the approach to transgenerational alcohol disorders. It is as if the centuries old experience of intractable alcoholism has desensitized professionals to utilize even minimal interventions. The challenge of acknowledging the collateral damage of alcohol through time visited on each new generation's arrival of prenatally brain damaged infants.

Over 20 years ago working in Western Canada I encountered numbers of physicians who felt it was a waste of time diagnosing FAS or ARND (called Fetal Alcohol Effects, FAE, in those days). They reasoned that the condition was chronic and incurable so why waste your energy dealing with it. Not unlike the therapeutic negativity experienced by many professionals working with Intellectual Disability. The quandary of the clinical understanding of ARND is that over 75% have a normal IQ, and so it is the complex developmental psychiatric presentations through the life span that are the challenge in diagnosis and management.

Compounding the negativity to the perceived chronic incurable intellectual disability component to ARND was an unsaid, implicit professional understanding that the ARND patients were not 'our' patients. No, they belonged to the minority populations of disadvantaged, the First Nations and Native Americans. Wasn't it the 'firewater' that had destroyed their communities and continued to destroy them, and there was nothing to be done. International parallels for the socially convenient understanding of ARND exist in Australia, New Zealand and South Africa, where the aboriginal communities, and Cape Colored are, in many ways conveniently, seen as the source and root of the transgenerational alcohol, ARND, problem.

Nothing could be further from the truth. As far back as 1993 George Steimitz a photographer with the National Geographic Magazine went around the world photographing patients with dysmorphic ARND from Finland to Chicago to make this point. Ironically the cover picture on this photographic essay on transgenerational alcohol was an Irish mother and her child. Returning to work in Ireland in 2006 it was as if history was discontinuous (to use Jerome Kagan's 1999, phrase).

A number of authors including myself have for many years described ARND, both dysmorphic and non-dysmorphic, as 'orphan conditions'. They are orphans from society and as well general medical care as their problems are seen as too vague or complicated.

Naturally in Ireland the professional resistance to diagnosis and management was widespread and quite reminiscent of North America 25 years ago. However, in this case the indigenous population was everyone, not just the so called Travelers, Ireland's own disadvantaged community. Another hidden population in Ireland were the inter country adopted children from Russia and Romania. Only now, very slowly in 2013, are adoptive parents and adoptive organizations facing up to a certain 'inconvenient truth' (Al Gore) about many of the children adopted into Ireland. They did not only have emotional dysregulation from their institutional upbringing alone but also from, sometimes hard to unravel, prenatal alcohol exposure.

Although the clinical examples that follow may seem a bit harsh it has been amazing to witness the professional and service system disconnection over the last 25 years working in North America and the UK and Ireland. You only have to consider the diagnostic and management service for Autistic Spectrum Disorder, ADHD, Down's Syndrome, Fragile X syndrome, Schizophrenia, Bipolar Disorder to have an understanding of the void when it comes to ARND. The fact that it is a transgenerational condition makes this void all the more startling.

Clinical vignettes abound of the disconnection from diagnosis and treatment, but a few key examples will suffice.

1) Once a teenage girl with ARND was sent to an inner city hospital because of active suicidal ideation, impulsivity and pervasive hopelessness. The Native American was assessed by an adult psychiatrist, who discharged the patient home telling her Native American foster mother there was nothing to do as she had brain damage due to alcohol. This naturally sent the adoptive family into crisis but fortunately she was contained within the Native American community by simple nurturing and careful attention to impulsivity.
2) More recently in Ireland a teenage Boy with ARND was sent home after a series of impulsive suicide acts in the school setting precipitated by verbal and phone text bullying. The triage psychiatric nurse felt that the patient with ARND did not have serious enough intent, and the adoptive mother was too anxious with her anxiety making him anxious. The impulsive risk related to the brain damage was not seen as relevant to the assessment. He ended up being admitted to a psychiatric day hospital because he could not be managed safely by the adoptive parents in the home environment.
3) A psychiatrist was reluctant to diagnose ARND on his inpatient who was acutely ill with severe disruptive mood dysregulation and intermittent suicidal and psychotic features needing a complicated medication regime. She did not want to

diagnose ARND as this would upset the birth mother and her family and they would be upset with the psychiatric inpatient team.

4) Another time a senior pediatrician refused to make the diagnosis as he said there was nothing he could do. So he 'hid' the diagnosis under the label ADHD which was more comfortable to him and avoided any discussions with the middle class birth family. This class/ethnic blindness in diagnosis and thinking did not do a good service to many children in North America. It had quickly become apparent that ARND became a diagnosis of disadvantage and so naturally only occurred in disadvantaged populations of ethnic minorities, the First Nations or Native Americans. One senior pediatrician in Canada over 20 years ago honestly acknowledged that the introduction of ARND, dysmorphic or non-dysmorphic, as a diagnosis had challenged his natural tendency to diagnosis by social class and ethnic group.
5) Finally a number of pediatricians and psychiatrists in Canada, UK, USA and Ireland had refused to support a diagnosis of ARND, dysmorphic or non-dysmorphic, as they felt the diagnosis made no difference to the patient and it was better to code the diagnosis under the catch all Autistic Spectrum Disorder or ADHD. This would satisfy the often middle class parents, avoid any discussions about prenatal history, and serve to support school support in the short term.
6) A 10 year old girl is given methylphenidate for ADHD. She does not get better and her attention and concentration does not improve. The pediatrician increases her medication to over 2 mgs per kilogram and she continues to pose school and home problems with increased aggression and moodiness. A diagnosis of ARND invites change of medication and fluoxetine is prescribed which works well. The patient has had decreased linear growth since starting methylphenidate and growth hormone levels are low. As well X ray of bone age shows it to be 3 years behind chronological age. The differential response and risks with medication (especially methylphenidate) in ADHD with an ARND etiology have become more acknowledged but offer just one example of a therapeutic rigidity in stance which was not in the patient' s best interest.

THE 'LARGER SYSTEM' ETHICAL ISSUES IN RECOGNIZING, AND MANAGING ARND

1. The *Commercial Drug Industry* continues to show little interest in studying medication efficacy and effectiveness in ARND, as this population are lumped into the Intellectual Disability arena, and so seen as more likely to have side effects and be more complicated to manage. This would in other circumstances be a motivation for

psychopharmacological science, but not so in ARND. At one stage a drug industry representative informed me in Canada that there was 'nothing to be gained' by testing his psychostimulant against another one in ARND as his company had so much of the pediatric market share already. This study he informed me could run the risk of losing market share by exposing safety or medical problems. A strange logic if you are in the business of helping patients, but understandable if your corporate goals lie elsewhere.

2. The *Alcohol Industry* has theoretically a vested interest in producing a product that makes a profit but causes minimum harm. The aptly named term collateral damage of alcohol through generations is seen in succeeding children, adolescents, parents, grandparents but ARND seems too big a step to make. (Matthew et al., 2013).

The expenditure on alcohol in Ireland, a country of under 5 million, was 6.3 billion Euro (7.5 to 8 billion US dollars) in 2013, which was up for the second year in a row whereas 3.7 billion Euro (or 4.5 to 5 billion US dollars) was spent on alcohol related harm costs. Currently in Ireland alcohol accounts for 7.7% of personal income expenditure. (Evening Herald, 23rd August 2013).

In the UK equivalent figures are 21 billion pounds sterling estimated cost of alcohol misuse each year, and 2.7 billion pounds sterling cost to the National Health Service of alcohol misuse annually.(The Sunday Times Magazine, December 29th 2013).

It is fascinating to see that the medical costs estimated in the UK related to alcohol misuse are about the same as the figures in Ireland, but the UK population is at least 12 times greater!

It is no accident that organizations such as MotherRisk in Canada (which alert women to the risks of substances in pregnancy), funded by the alcohol/brewers industry initially did not subscribe to ARND as a diagnosis as it is too vague, not real and seemingly understudied. As 75 to 80% of infants and young children exposed to prenatal alcohol do not show dysmorphic features there exclusion would be a simple way to not acknowledge risk, but continue to marginalize and minimize the true extent of the problem.

In Ireland the public health consultants for a recent maternity hospital alcohol in pregnancy study were 'educated' by the alcohol industry into the complexity of alcohol teratology and so 17 categories of alcohol intake were proposed for this study. Needless to say this was not unlike the 256 diagnostic categories from the dysmorphology University of Washington 4 digit code diagnosis, and it amply served to de-rail the alcohol in pregnancy study as there would be too many variables and too many study group cells with small numbers which would make the statistical analysis impossible.

At the same time as the general awareness of the harm of alcohol in pregnancy is increasing worldwide there has been a planned systematic targeting of young professional women with more disposable income. New products such as wine coolers, sweet alcohol laden drinks of all varieties, sweet beers, i.e., banana! and the explosion of cheap available wines. The alcohol industry has done their homework and for some reason knows the sweet drinks will entice the women. How responsible is this marketing ploy when ARND is described as having a prevalence of 1 in 100 live births worldwide?

> Another one of modern society's quandaries, as the scientists are beginning to show, is the possible fetal programming link between sugar craving as predating alcohol craving. A phenomenon that the Native Americans and First Nations have recognized for years as witnessed in their high prevalence of diabetes compared with the Caucasian populations in North America.

3. One of *the Larger System Clinical Service Disconnections* in managing ARND comes from the interaction with addiction service providers both in North America and Ireland/UK. For some reason addiction medical or psychiatric providers are reluctant or just plain refuse to manage patients with an addictive disorder when it is co-occurring with organic brain dysfunction especially ARND. It appears that the ARND patients are seen a solely Intellectual Disability so do not 'fit' the addiction model of management. This is unfortunate and denies patients interventions such as naltrexone or acamposate which could be, and are, useful.

This addictive service disconnect is even more destructive when placed in the liaison between child providers and adult providers about the continuing addictive disorder in a birth mother which impedes her ability to parent her alcohol effected child. As well there are few if any conversations about helping her to be off alcohol for her next pregnancy.(The Parent Child Assistance Program pioneered in Seattle and replicated in various centers in USA and Canada is one shining exemption to the general rule, Grant et al., 2008, 2009). This type of collaborative work seems to be a proverbial bridge too far for the adult alcohol providers, and is delegated to social workers who are then blamed by 'the system' when inevitable crisis arises between the management of the complex alcohol brain damaged child and the continuing addiction in the birth mother which seems to be managed in a certain vacuum which does not include her as a parent. Needless to say the addictive disorder in the teenage or young adult father with ARND does not get 'on the radar', and often becomes managed by the family court system in assessing the stress of access on a vulnerable child with an alcohol addicted brain damaged parent. The courts doing the medical work as necessity breeds one temporary solution to an ongoing transgenerational problem. This clinical disconnection poses ethical questions at many levels, not the least the exclusion of biologically vulnerable patients with co-occurring addiction to basic medical and psychiatric services, because they 'do not fit'.

4. *The general systemic minimization, misinformation and denial in the maternity hospitals* are still rife. (This is much more of an issue in Ireland and the UK than in Canada or the USA). Maybe it is because there is a feeling that midwives do not want to so-called 'police' the pregnant women. In Ireland and the UK there is a lot of press given to the safety of low dose alcohol in pregnancy. Still not proven. (Laufer 2013 2013a). But the

realistic problems of significant alcohol maternal intake by pregnancy mothers still is not considered a priority. The standard questions by midwives do not routinely inquire about current and continued alcohol intake in pregnancy, especially binge drinking, and if documented this information does not seem to be communicated on a routine basis to the pediatricians or GPS.

It is not unlike a systemic 'conspiracy of silence', and this silence brings no comfort or suitable diagnostic or treatment services to the continuing generations of alcohol effected infants and young children. Here 'the system' is again blamed for the brain damaged infants passing through the so called cracks. Cracks which include no identification of an at risk baby being born with prenatal biological vulnerability exposed to alcohol, and now exposed to postnatal vulnerability due to being brought up in a home with active alcohol or substance abuse in one or both birth parents. The silence is only interrupted when a crisis arises and then no-one can be found who had responsibility for the abused, malnourished, or even dead child. 'The System' is the cause but cannot be identified. Orwell would be proud.

5. *Inter-country adoptions* become a breeding ground for placements of undiagnosed infants and young children with ARND. The private contracts are often 'rather loose ' when subjected to medical scrutiny and the unfortunate perspective parents are not uncommonly traumatized by experiencing failed fertilization treatments which makes them more vulnerable in the placement process. These adoptive parents then find themselves 'blamed 'as poor/inadequate parents as their adoptive child is labeled Reactive Attachment Disorder, rather than considering that he/she may be more challenging to manage because of undiagnosed biological emotional and or sensory dysregulation problems due to ARND.

6. *Cultural competency and cultural sensitivity:* The USA and Canada are light years away from Ireland and to a lesser extent the UK in incorporating these principles into the practice of child psychiatry. In fact they are one of the core competencies needed to be a child psychiatrist in the USA. In the management of ARND they include an ethical approach to the sensitivity of alcohol stigmatization, but not avoidance, in the mother, the child and the adolescent. (Pumariega 2003).

They also, borrowing from the principles of ethno- pharmacology, behoove doctor's child psychiatrists and medical alcohol specialists to be aware and trained in the management of the complicated drug interactions that may occur when a patient has an underlying organic brain dysfunction related to ARND.

7. *Therapeutic residential or group home care centers*: This is a complicated, underserviced area of high need. It is unfortunately not uncommon to have privately funded residential care or group home centers servicing high risk children or adolescents with complex misunderstood behavioral problems, including undiagnosed ARND. In Canada, the USA, and especially in Ireland and the UK it is not uncommon to have medical/psychiatric consultations done on a 2 or 4 weekly basis with outside consultants flying in from cities out of town or even countries, such as the UK into Ireland. This is a

continuing ethical and risk dilemma for the service managers of these private, but essential, care centers. Developmental Psychiatric disorders such as ARND highlight the need for more manpower training in the medical and nursing areas of developmental psychiatry and developmental pediatrics.

8. *Scientific Research questions:* There are a number of fundamental ethical questions that need to be considered when considering research in vulnerable patient populations such as those with ARND.

a) "What are the special considerations around informed consent for vulnerable populations such as ARND?
b) How does the researcher maintain the highest ethical standards when performing vitally needed research on vulnerable children with ARND embedded in high risk families?
c) How may the ethical principles of justice and beneficence be considered in the light of these constraints? "(Edelsohn 2012.)

The area of informed consent is the most problematic as the children, parents and grandparents with ARND often have problems in cognitive understanding, which is not just a product of IQ under 70. In the USA there is a concept called Assent for younger children. However the use of an advocate who is trained in developmental disability or a legal representative such as a guardian ad litem (if the child is in state care) are both useful monitors for proposed research.

A Brief Historical Perspective on Alcohol in Pregnancy

It is worth considering the medical history of the discovery of the link between maternal alcohol, consumption in pregnancy and effects on the developing fetus and infant. To shed light on today's ethical problems in diagnosis and management.

The facial dysmorphic and Alcohol Related Neurodevelopmental Disorder, Fetal Alcohol Syndrome (FAS) was initially described by pediatrician Paul Lemoine and his colleagues in Nantes, France in 1968, and published in a small regional French medical publication. They based their clinical findings on the similar dysmorphic facial features in 127 infants born to mothers who had drunk wine in pregnancy (Lemoine 1968). Subsequently it was re-discovered in Seattle, Washington, USA, by an independent team of medical researchers at the University of Washington, Seattle, USA. This group reported similar physical and growth anomalies and central nervous system (CNS) disorders in a small group (8) of children born to alcoholic mothers. (Jones & Smith 1973a, 1973b). The early diagnoses in the USA were made by dysmorphologists, experts in birth defects and physical anomalies. Historically these facial and other physical anomalies were attributed to genetic causes and the possibility of environmental cause was less likely to be considered. (Smith 1970). It was only when the science of teratology expanded that the environmental etiologies of such anomalies were considered. (Novick Brown et al., 2011).

Even though the early American clinical descriptions were dominated by the dysmorphological clinical frame it became quickly evident to the primary researcher David W. Smith that there were a spectrum of alcohol induced neurodevelopmental brain damage present which did not depend on the presence of facial dysmorphology. Thus Smith coined the initial term Fetal Alcohol Effects (FAE) for those infants and young children with prenatal alcohol exposure but no facial dysmorphology. (Smith 1981).

Twenty years later in 1996, the Institute of Medicine (IOM) studied the effect of prenatal alcohol exposure on the developing fetus and young child. A significant change in clinical thinking about the effect of prenatal alcohol on the developing fetus came with their publication of a multiple medical specialty academic review and diagnostic manual on Fetal Alcohol Syndrome. This seminal book introduced with equal importance specified neurodevelopmental and neurocognitive deficits which accompanied the previously well documented familiar physical abnormalities, They came up with a new term Alcohol Related Neurodevelopmental Disorder (ARND) to describe persons who did not have the full dysmorphic FAS, but had neurodevelopmental problems already shown to be associated with prenatal alcohol exposure (Stratton et al., 1996). Historically, to that point, the diagnosis of the clinical effects of prenatal alcohol exposure had been left to dysmorphologists and so naturally skewed to the dysmorphic ARND, i.e., FAS, with the identifiable facial features.

The current and recurring ethical dilemma in the scientific field of ARND has been its refusal to leave the clinical teratology/dysmorpholgy past. The original findings of facial dysmorphology linked to the mother taking alcohol in pregnancy have in many ways unbalanced the diagnostic process. What it did not do is improve the quality of thought and service to alcohol dependent women in pregnancy, and their subsequent brain damaged infants.

In fact the clinical field became so complex that a diagnostic schema from the University of Washington, a tertiary care medical institution in the USA, unveiled a protocol that gave the clinician *256 diagnostic categories!* No wonder this did not reach the common man/woman physician, working in a small community, rural hospital or even city hospital. In many ways it became a proverbial 'kiss of death' for the following generations of general practitioners, developmental pediatricians and child psychiatrists who were maybe tentatively interested and/or actively managing patients with ARND. However this impossibly complex diagnostic matrix did not give them the useful language to describe infants and young children exposed to alcohol prenatally. This complex matrix of dysmorphology driven diagnostic categories did not address the long term neurodevelopmental problems that the patients posed and offered no way to describe their specific developmental psychiatric problems.

Predictably, if you have 256 categories for any medical condition it will drive away all but the most obsessive of doctors, and was only really viable in a tertiary care center removed from the nuts and bolts of day to day management with families. Imagine of autistic spectrum disorder had 253 categories? How many physicians' specialists and non-specialists would venture to attempt a diagnosis?

The intimidation of finding the small dysmorphological features now pursued in 2D and 3D is never ending. The dysmorphic ARND has in many ways created an exponential field of imaging pursuit, and so practical transgenerational management of the epigenetic effect of alcohol can never really begin. There should be public health questions posed about the ethics of expensively pursuing three dimensional facial images at ever increasing costs.

What benefit does the patient and his or her family receive from these sophisticated facial pictures?

Do they inform management strategies of the developmental psychiatric problems?

Does the face tell the clinician about the severity of the brain damage?

Does the Face tell us anything new about transgenerational alcohol related neurodevelopmental disorder?

These are the type of questions that federal and national research funding agencies should be asking the continuing crop of ever more obsessive epidemiology driven dysmorphologists.

At so the continued research money poured into three dimensional image finding is directly inhibiting and creating more disadvantages to the already socially and medically disadvantaged.

It is indeed true that Astley and Clarren did sterling clinical work in developing their diagnostic schema which introduced a more objective set of diagnostic criteria, commonly referred to forever as the "4-Digit Code." Their source material being from a formulation of the reviews of the medical records of 1014 children with dysmorphic ARND i.e., FAS in the Washington State Fetal Alcohol Syndrome Diagnostic and Prevention Network, Seattle, USA. But in truth this was, and still is unworkable, intimidating, and placed management outside its remit.

The process became about the process and the effect of transgenerational alcohol abuse passed from one generation to the next got lost somewhere between the next set of 3D images and discussions about 'Is this Full FAS or Partial FAS? The functional impact of the ARND on the patient, his or her family seemed to disappear in a dysmorphological fog. In the meantime new generations of alcohol exposed infants were being born, not identified, growing up with an alcohol craving risk, procreating with or without alcohol use in pregnancy and continuing the roundabout that has become worldwide ARND.

Although '4 Digit code' paid lip service to other adverse prenatal and postnatal factors they did not form a practical part of the diagnostic or prognostic resolution of the case. Therefore they were in many ways 'hidden' from diagnostic or initial management discussions or plan. This is plainly unrealistic in a patient population which comes from transgenerational alcohol abuse, and features commonly domestic violence, abandonment and disorganized transgenerational parenting.

Unfortunately, even as I write worldwide training in the minutiae of dysmorphological measurements is occurring in diverse countries whereas the schools and family systems that harbor these dysmorphological ARND children are not receiving the same quality of attention and follow up. In countries such as Africa and Italy and Russia screening methods have been developed using an experienced dysmorphologist to train local pediatricians in diagnosing children using a more traditional exam including hands, arms, ears, and heart as well as face. (Cicennti et al., 2007, May et al., 2006, 2007, 2009). This apparently is successful in obtaining concordance over the physical features associated with prenatal alcohol exposure and traditionally the more problematic alcohol related neurodevelopmental disorder is either minimized or not mentioned. It's a kin to the denial and minimization of the very cause of the transgenerational problem which occurs especially in countries such as Ireland, and to a lesser extent the UK.

It would seem to me that the alcohol industry would not be unhappy with the continued avoidance of dealing or acknowledging transgenerational alcohol problems, specifically ARND. The endless pre-occupation with dysmorphology consumes new and older researchers and clinicians, so they are much less likely to wade into the muddy waters of actual management. This current never-ending situation with the use of depleting research money resources would be highly satisfying for alcohol industry lobbyists as it continues to delay the true recognition, scope and management challenges of the worldwide transgenerational alcohol problem.

This is a thorny ethical dilemma for the coming pool of researchers, university academic departments and funders who are more easily seduced by 'real evidence-based science' and discouraged from the suspect world of social science and the vague world of public health. The ethical problems in transgenerational ARND lie in the vulnerability and lack of ability of each generation to articulate and advocate for services. This continuum of disadvantage starts from the developing fetus exposed to alcohol, to the birth mother who has acquired an alcohol craving addiction and cognitive/executive decision making problems embedded in her own ARND. Then, to the grandparents, or aunts and uncles, who become involved with raising their grandchildren as the birth parents cannot cope, thereby enabling their continued alcohol addiction. And so the cycle runs.

No professional organization has claimed ownership of transgenerational alcohol or ARND, and so the perception that ARND is a truly an 'orphan' condition living often in an unclaimed orphaned world remains the societal norm.

Logically the medical profession would understand the societal ravages of a, not uncommon, transgenerational neurodevelopmental disorder which is eminently, if challengingly preventable.

An Ethical approach to diagnosis and management becomes part of the Gordian knot that is ARND.

For example, the Times of Malta recently reported a study by the *British Medical Journal* which exposed the fact that the UK government had met with the Drinks Industry 130 times from 2010 to 2013. Did these meetings decrease the problems and cost of transgenerational alcohol abuse? If not, what was their ethical purpose? (Times of Malta, Reuters, February 11th 2014).

The Ethical Dilemma of Diagnosis and Managing ARND (Now NDPAE). An Update. 2020

Five years have passed since I wrote this chapter. But nothing has fundamentally changed. This update expands its remit to an international perspective, and again leaves the confines of the small island of Ireland behind, entering the global stage.

At this stage I have now worked 30 years in total with patients with NDPAE, or FASDs in 4 different countries: Canada, USA, UK and Ireland, and this experience has made me both sadder, but also wiser, as the Ancient Mariner of old.

When I approached this Chapter a second time my thoughts became more coalesced around attempting to understand the motivations that lie behind ethical behavior.

Introduction to the Chapter Update

I agree with Stalcup, (2000), that this is not only an academic, philosophical debate. The theories that underpin ethical behavior can bear an influence on societies adopting certain measures to encourage ethical behavior on their citizens, or to persuade them to introduce measures addressing chronic unethical behavior in both individuals or institutions.

It is within the world of ethical principles such as Justice and Human Rights that societies must decide if they are independent of human experience, or are they solely a human invention? The choices between these two fundamental understandings makes all the difference in the way we see ourselves as a species. In many ways they become the touchstone to measure our individual and collective values, and also determine the conduct of our moral discourse or reasoning, see Wilson, (2000) and Flynn, (2001).

"No professional organization has clinical ownership of transgenerational alcohol or ARND, (now called NDPAE), and so the perception that ARND, now NDPAE, is truly an 'orphan condition' living in an often unclaimed orphan world remains the norm." A harsh commentary in the 2014 book on the lack of empathy and ethical responsibility for this vulnerable population. No different now, as I sit and write once more in 2020.

What Has Happened in World Societies in the Last Five Years?

1. Commercial Drug Industry

In 2001, I approached the Centers for Disease Control (CDC) in the USA with a project proposal to see if they would be interested in a study on the use of neuroprotective agents in pregnant alcohol –abusing women. I was told that this would enable the women's alcohol addiction. Although somewhat biased because I was a child psychiatrist it still surprised me that the heath of the brain-injured child was not in the equation.

Now embryonic studies are assessing the neuroprotective role of prenatal choline and folate in alcohol abusing pregnant mothers and other international scientists are considering the neural tube prevention model utilizing iron, folic acid, vitamin B12, choline.

A Healthy Positive Start

Still, no medical specialty worldwide, locally or internationally, has entered into the area of medical responsibility for diagnosis and medical management of patients with potential NDPAE. Therefore, this alcohol-acquired brain injury, non-IQ, non-face-driven global neurodevelopmental disorder receives little organized scientific pharmacological assessments, or proposed protocols of management. The common mantra is that this patient population of brain-injured children and adolescents are too complicated to treat so you don't treat. This form of therapeutic nihilism remains unfortunately quite prevalent when a physician is invited to deal with complex patients in the developmental disability world who most commonly present co-morbid neuropsychiatric issues.

Roots have however sprouted in the UK as a consensus report on the treatment of ADHD and FASD (known as NDPAE in this updated book) was published. A follow-up NICE guideline process is planned in 2020, but as it stands no major international drug company or medical specialty has committed finance, manpower or confirmed interest in the topic (Young, et al., 2016).

2. Influence of the Alcohol Industry

Is it the overarching smothering influence of the alcohol industry which continues to deny the extent of this transgenerational alcohol problem?

Now we are bombarded by TV, Internet, and Billboard advertisements, as during the recent Rugby World Cup in Japan 2019, which told us that the 'Black Brew' makes us "made of more." Old newsreels of great sporting achievements are recruited which show us how "the Black Brew can make us to be made of more, as our heroes of old."

Time has been re-defined as "Black Brew Time," slow down and savor the ambrosia, and live in the sublime moment, with no hint of consequences.

Politically savvy pictures of Japanese female rugby players fill the TV screens with toothless smiles as they crash over the try line to score, and show us that "they, too are made of more." Manna for the new generation of sporting, ambitious, fearless, millennium women, with no hint of consequences.

The Black Brew is global now and celebrating its influence on the global arena, (ironically it reminded me of being involved with Professor Ann Streissguth 20 years ago in a TV Documentary on FAS, done in Seattle by Korean Television!).

Alcohol lobbying of governments continues to be the rule. The Irish Times reported on January 26th 2016 that more than 40 lobbying meetings with the Irish Government had occurred over a 3-month period. The lobbying was aimed to curtail proposed legislation combating alcohol abuse. Now the alcohol industry had the "bit between their teeth" and were bent on banishing the ancient catholic rite of no alcohol on one day of the year, namely Good Friday. Rapidly Ireland was joining the capitalist secular society of the western world. So these old customs of abstinence had to go.

In the UK the shift in alcohol marketing is currently targeting women - with the growth of the new Gin Industry becoming exponential. It was as if we were 'going back to the future'. The Gin palaces of Hogarth's engravings metamorphosed into the Facebook maps of our modern world.

Nevertheless, All Is Not Lost

Legislation in Scotland has approached alcohol abuse and addiction proportionately, with the introduction of a minimum price on alcohol. Already in October 2019 its positive effects on lowering the rates of alcohol-related medical problems are being reported.

Ireland introduced a legislation on minimum pricing of alcohol, but as always in Irish society "the divil is in the small print." Thus, when you peruse this Alcohol Bill you begin to notice certain brands are exempt from this minimum pricing. They include: The Black Brew, the country's favorite rugby lager, the country's favorite Irish cider, and naturally the country's favorite Irish whiskies. (The Irish Times reported on Dec 30th 2019, that the Irish Government would NOT be implementing a minimal price for alcohol until at least 2020).

In my 2014 book I had ended the chapter on Ethics by quoting the number of lobbying meetings that the alcohol industry had with the UK government.

Five years later nothing has changed, and the 'fake news' created from alcohol industry lobby groups continues unabated. For example; in November 2019 it was reported by the Organization of Economic Co-operation and Development (OECD) that the UK consumes 9.7 liters of alcohol per year per person - nearly a liter more than the average of 8.9 liters for the 36 countries of OECD.

Although the alcohol consumption in the UK has gone down it is still more than countries such as Australia, New Zealand and the USA - the good news is that the UK drink less than France (11.7 liters a year) and Germany (10.9 liters a year).

Health concerns in the UK were elucidated by the OECD report:

i. Dr. Richard Piper, Chief Executive of Alcohol Change UK, in response to this report stated "our drinking habits are causing more and more harm," i.e., Hospital admissions related to alcohol and alcohol-related deaths are both on the rise.
ii. Dr. Tony Rao, Addictions Faculty at the Royal College of Psychiatrists, in response to the OECD report, stated that "it is alarming that we are not addressing the harm being caused by alcohol."
iii. Richard Fernandez, Head of Policy at the Institute of Alcohol Studies, was equally concerned and stated "it's time for the UK Government to take this seriously, with a strategy that includes minimum unit pricing (of alcohol)."
iv. In the meantime, the Industry-Funded Alcohol Information Partnership said:
v. "the amount of alcohol people is drinking in the UK has been falling for more than a decade. People are leading more balanced lifestyles, especially among the younger generations."

So, obviously, problems such as transgenerational alcohol, NDPAE are not problems. Plus, ca change... (Daily Mail November 8th 2019).

Larger System Clinical. Service Disconnections

These service disconnections continue to abound throughout the world in 2019. Historical medical silos appear to be unbreakable.

The Addiction services still unfortunately seem to be unable to truly incorporate a model of care that runs through child, adolescent and adult services needing working, active co-operation. They also seem ambivalent and resistant when it comes to embracing a fully organic basis for alcohol addiction, and its implication for addiction service management through the lifespan.

Finally, the leap to incorporating a prenatal epigenetic link to alcohol craving and alcohol dependence disorder continues to be an enigma.

Mothers with alcohol addiction who are pregnant and have co-occurring psychiatric disorders are inadvertently abandoned by both specialist service providers, not individually, but collectively. It seems that you can only have Dual Diagnosis as a pregnant woman if you enter one door first, and then rarely could this door open to two providers simultaneously.

The Family Court System continues to perpetuate this medical system disconnect as adult service providers continue to be disconnected from the child service providers.

Example: A young adult mother who has alcohol addiction and bipolar disorder has her young infant removed into care because she cannot manage his complex neurodevelopmental disorder, NDPAE, due to prenatal alcohol exposure.

This medically and psychiatrically ill birth mother continues to have access to her growing child as the management system cannot seem to incorporate regular consultation between the adult providers for the birth mother and child/family providers for the child and foster care-providers. The birth mother's continued illness and her in ability to control her alcohol addiction effect the quality of the access visits to her child.

The inability of adult service providers to be involved in the family court system to report on the impact of the birth mother's illness on her ability to parent impedes progress in management, and is not in the best interests of the vulnerable child.

This continued impasse is really an ethical service neglect dilemma for both the birth mother and the child with foster care-providers. It, as well, impacts the social services who have no control over the access of the vulnerable child to a potentially emotionally, toxic, impaired birth parent.

Foster parents are subtly devalued as they attempt to set predictable structural boundaries for the child with NDPAE which are constantly undermined in access visits and create ongoing attachment disruption.

Larger health care systems become ethically compromised when they receive seed money for training in alcohol education from the alcohol industry.

1) This has been an issue for a well-known adoption agency involved in school public health teaching on alcohol. The alcohol-based funding has obviously influenced the public health message about transgenerational alcohol risk, under-age drinking and dangers of any alcohol in pregnancy.
2) Also, an equally well-known FASD advocacy agency which trains midwives in safety of alcohol. This is in many ways a subtler undermining of the science. The midwives are at the 'coal face' of alcohol at risk pregnancies, and so it is not surprising that the carefully controlled 'disinformation' diminishes the potential existence of a non-face, non-IQ driven global neurodevelopmental disorder caused by prenatal alcohol. Thus, midwives are trained to look for 'the face', which only presents in 10 to15% of the individuals with NDPAE. Not unpredictably many midwives are unsure of a safe level of alcohol in pregnancy and communicate this uncertainty to pregnant mothers.

The General Systemic Minimization and Denial in the Maternity Hospitals

Five years later this has not changed substantially in the Irish and UK settings.

Only recently an updated book on Perinatal Psychiatry (Henshaw et al., 2019) may in some ways have missed the opportunity to acknowledge the complexities presented by alcohol-affected children and their birth parents with alcohol addiction, co-morbid psychiatric and sometimes developmental issues. It is as if there has been no fundamental evolution in perinatal psychiatry, which in some ways is trapped in the mantra of vulnerable pregnant mothers, as solely the victims. This continues to pay little attention to the challenges in the perinatal period of parenting a neurodevelopmental-challenged infant.

This is even more apparent when you, yourself, may have chronic psychiatric disorder, transgenerational alcohol neurodevelopmental challenges or alcohol dependence which all impair basic parenting. These differing examples all show that the problems are firmly rooted in the mother/infant dyad perinatal but also antenatal periods. Nothing will change globally until this fact is recognized (O'Malley, 2003).

At the basic level of mother/infant care this inadvertent 'conspiracy of silence' remains subtly but also critically present.

It is easier to blame either ethic origins of the disenfranchised birth mother, who is in evidently in the 'born to fail' (Davie et a.,1972) rather than shine the mirror on the collective maternity, neonatal, addiction, psychiatric and developmental services.

Ironically it is the so-called financially socially advantaged parent who is just as disadvantaged by this collective medical system blindness. These women may find themselves as hidden 'functioning alcoholics' delivering infants with normal birth weight infants, normal developmental milestones, except language, and later discover the cracks of this unique global neurodevelopmental disorder appearing.

Who is there to validate the anxious, well-meaning birth mother of the true nature of the difficulties in parenting that she is experiencing? She is not always depressed, as the Pavlovian diagnosticians believe, but is managed in a shared system that perpetuates the denial of the influence of alcohol on her and her developing child's life. Not every child is Autistic and/or ADHD; the services need to ethically appreciate this to be the case and begin the painful job of acknowledging transgenerational alcohol effected parents and children by providing culturally sensitive services nested at the mother/infant dyad level.

A Fundamental Schism in Rights

At the heart of the continued ethical dilemmas in acknowledging and managing patients with NDPAE is the disconnection in the rights between the fetus/infant and the mother.

At this moment in time, 5 years later, it is not uncommon to be unable to obtain antenatal birth and neonatal records of an alcohol-exposed 'at risk' infant as the maternity hospitals are guarding the confidentiality and stigma to the adult/mother. Therefore, the adult/parent right has the priority more than understanding the unborn child's needs.

Many Years Ago the Well-Respected Pediatrician and Psychoanalyst Donald Winnicott

(Winnicott, 1984) coined the phrase that there is no such separate entity of a mother and a child, they function as one unit. Words and sentiments which ring through in 2019, and if remembered could inform an ethically different maternity and post-natal care system.

5. Intercountry Adoptions

In the last 5 years there have been a number of changes in this, well recognized, population of at-risk infants. In the USA for example, children born in Russia have been banned from private adoption because of concerns about undisclosed amounts of exposure to alcohol in the prenatal period. Other countries such as Romania have, as well, been implicated in having unrecognized infants set up for adoption with exposure to alcohol in pregnancy.

Ireland, nevertheless, has continued to receive these infants through private adoption agencies and the fees charges range from 30,000 to 40,000 euro, a significant amount of money. As this country still does not fully accept the concept of NDPAE these infants are not uncommonly 'missed' in screening medical/pediatric examination. Later in life, they invariably present a multitude of neurological, psychiatric and learning problems when they enter the school system. The adoptive parents in this country, are frequently perceived 'as the problem', and so are routinely subjected to attachment therapy which does not cure the un-diagnosed neurodevelopmental disorder.

Despite the historical problems, in the last 5 years the complexity of intercountry adoption has been addressed more systematically at an international level. Now the potential challenges of adopting an undiagnosed infant with an alcohol-acquired neurodevelopmental disorder, NDPAE, are very much considered in the process of the formal adoption and clinical follow-up.

6. Cultural Competency and Cultural Sensitivity

In the last 5 years both the USA and UK have entered into the world of *pharmaco-genomics,* and so there is a greater sensitivity to the individual's response to medication depending on genetic background, tests, such as HLA typing and Cytochrome P450 analysis of liver metabolism, are quietly coming into psychiatric management practice (Ernak, 2015, Rowland et al., 2011, MC Donnell et al., 2013).

Scientific studies on adoption have shown *the challenges for children adopted under 5 years of age or adopted after 5 years old* (Calarusso 1987). The issues of cultural adaptation, language development and identity have all been clearly identified as longer term clinical/psychological issues to be addressed. This is an area of specific relevance for children with NDPAE adopted from other countries or social class/ethnic groups.

There are many examples of *casual racism* that exist unrecognized in the lives of these vulnerable children and adolescents, who do not always have the social communication skills to confront their various subtle and unsubtle denigrations, and may react by angry or regressive behaviors, such as overt defiance, encopresis and enuresis. In chapters 9-11 of their book Offer and Sabshin (1991) provide a salutary lesson in the diversity of normal behavior.

7. Social Competence and Social Communication

This is an area of clinical importance that is often at the kernel of life struggles and challenges for individuals with NDPAE. There has been a wealth of research showing that social skills are critically linked with neurological and cognitive functions (Adolphs, 2001, 2009). However, it is in the disruption of early brain development that prenatal alcohol influences vital social competence and social communication and competency. Clear models of the importance of brain regions, such as the prefrontal cortex, temporoparietal junction, insula and amygdala in overall social competence have been studied in the context of brain insults or damage (Anderson et al., 2012). This scientific understanding is part of the world of social neuroscience and its application to patients with NDPAE is still very much in embryonic form. This conceptual frame is an important distinction from the overarching preoccupation with ASD, and lately the relationship between NDPAE or FASD and ASD has been established.

NDPAE is not ASD and ASD is not NDPAE, so it is of clinical importance to bring the injured brain to the table when analyzing deficits in social competence or communication. Alexithymia, the inability to read emotions in others or to have words to express one' s personal feelings, is a critically misunderstood concept in NDPAE needing further investigation (Sullivan, 2008, in O'Malley (ed.), 2008). This social deficit includes a limitation in reflective function (Hobson, 1993).

8. Therapeutic Residential or Group Home Centers

The last 5 years have not been kind to these specialized facilities. In the UK there was an expose on TV which prompted a later formal investigation of the maltreatment of residents in W (a residential center dealing with adults who have Learning or Developmental Disabilities). Similarly, In Ireland, A, a residential center and M, a hospital have unfortunately had scathing investigations revealing the extent of the abusive treatment of adult residents with Learning or Developmental Disabilities.

The ethically unacceptable management of this vulnerable population speaks volumes about societies' value system regarding dependent individuals.

Now, this is often the world that patients with NDPAE will inherit; it can be a world of devaluation, stigmatization and complete lack of tolerance and basic understanding of neurodevelopmental and neuropsychiatric disorders.

The ethical management of these patients/clients comes, not just from a lack of manpower, but from a general lack of fundamental training in Neurodevelopmental Disorders which cuts across all health care professionals, medical, nursing, social work and care professions, naming but a a few.

9. Scientific Research Questions

These questions posed in the 2014 book bear repeating and updating 5 years later.

a) What are the special considerations around informed consent for vulnerable populations such as ARND, now known as NDPAE? (Some of the clinical and research challenges of this unique patient population were discussed in the 2014 book).

To date the almost complete absence of FDA, NICE or European therapeutic guidelines, driven by research, have continued to create a void for the understanding of the complexity of informed consent in this dependent population. This is necessary as they can be easily suggestible and/or manipulated, and sometimes spoken-for by caring but emotionally exhausted and frustrated parents or care providers.

The lack of systematic social science/psychological and neuropsychiatric collaboration on research protocols for intervention continues. At this juncture it is really a fundamental block to any quality intervention, especially pharmacological, which has shown clear efficacy in on-going clinical management.

Therefore, 5 years later, there are no evidence-based guidelines for pharmacological management of FASD or NDPAE, and the majority of medication used, even if effective, is give in an 'off label, 'off license' context.

b) How does the researcher maintain the highest ethical standards when performing vitally needed research on vulnerable children with FASD, now NDPAE, who are embedded in high risk families?

When I read this now, 5 years later, it highlights the simple truth that this is at the heart of this clinically challenged population, and poses the essence of the management of transgenerational alcohol and its sequelae.

If society, especially medical specialties, cannot understand the critical need to communicate across their historical adult/child service silos then nothing will continue to happen.

Case Example:

A 6-year-old girl with NDPAE is in a foster home placement and continues to have access visits to her alcohol dependent mother and father. The addiction counsellor and adult psychiatrist do not share information with the family services social worker on the rate of progress of their clients including their emotional suitability for access visits with the 6-year-old, because of confidentiality and protection of adult rights.

The foster parents feel undermined as the 6-year-old is chronically anxious about family visits but has no voice in saying so.

The social worker, foster parents and child with NDPAE feel abandoned by the adult system, but must try to work within it as a larger care system.

Invariably the child becomes more distressed, needs more therapy including medication, and even hospitalization is considered. There is no systematic acknowledgement of the high-risk birth family environment, and its influence on the brain-injured child well-being.

> Into this arena steps a conscientious researcher.
> Where do they begin? Can they begin?

At the moment no starting point in the health care system exists. Then absence of any collaborative care for NDPAE children between these differing adult/child specialties precludes the thought of holistic ethical treatment. Similarly, the entry into holistic ethical research still remains an anathema.

c) How may the ethical principles of justice and beneficence be considered in the light of these constraints?

These are overarching principles which 5 years after seem almost impossible to achieve in the management of NDPAE.

But there are positive changes ahead.

The European Charter of Rights for Children and The European Charter of Rights for Persons with Learning Disabilities are all well-intentioned aspirations. It is how to make them functional that is the question.

Children in care are not infrequently coming from families at risk because of alcohol/substance abuse, violence and abuse. These children may have acquired brain injury due to alcohol which presents clinical challenges from infancy. They need to be diagnosed, acknowledged, not denied, stigmatized and marginalized.

Only a systems of care approach can suffice to solve this dilemma. The American Academy of Child and Adolescent Psychiatry has shown the value of this type of approach in their new care management plan for teenagers with Substance Abuse. (AACAP 2019).

Unfortunately, scientific literature continues to invalidate and marginalize the patient population of FASD or NDPAE, For example Helgeson and colleagues in Sweden in 2018 stated "the value for the individual of obtaining a FASD (or NDPAE)-related description of their condition- for instance in terms of wellbeing-is not well established, nor is it established that allocating resources based on whether individuals fulfill FASD (or NDPAE) –related criteria is justified, compared to allocations directed to the most prominent needs."

The Alcohol Industry would quietly applaud them, but there is a rather disturbing demeaning and un-ethical side to their biased conclusions which will of course, be used to further stigmatize reduce and invalidate this transgenerational alcohol effected population.

Denying the very existence of NDPAE does not uphold justice and beneficence, and will not make the problem disappear.

d) An ethical holistic approach to diagnosis and management is complicated but possible.

Notwithstanding the pervasive negativity of the professional and scientific community, the logistical and ethical complexities of multi-professional research into this specific complex clinical area have been well and long evaluated.
(Ciccetti et al. 1991, 1997, Cummings et al. 1994, 2000, Rutter 1998)

As Cummings and colleagues stated in their 2000 book the:

> "risk of developmental psychopathology in a child exposed to parental psychopathology does not occur in a vacuum."

Many factors are involved:

1) Genetic (parental psychiatric, addictive or developmental disorder)
2) Epigenetic (such as exposure to prenatal alcohol)
3) Pregnancy and birth complications (i.e., toxemia, difficult birth with anoxia and fetal distress)
4) Infant factors: (i.e., difficult to settle, or slow to warm temperament, neurological poor sucking reflex)
5) Parenting impairments (psychiatric, addictive or developmental disorders)
6) Disturbance in parent/child relations (i.e., neglect, abuse, placement out of home in care)
7) Socio-cultural factors (i.e., poverty, lack of community resources or support, cultural isolation)

Many researchers and clinicians have approached the challenges of developmental psychopathology from the parent as well as the child's perspective. (Glick et al. 1992, Nuechterlein et al. 1992, Rutter 1992, Sameroff et al. 1992).

Transgenerational alcohol encompasses all these arenas, and is informed by the previous research experience. The scientific study of this problem needs a combination of adult and child research specialist knowledge as in the developmental psychopathology field has shown for over 20 years. Although needing larger professional teams, this does not negate the need, or indeed the inherent value, of this multi-systemic, respectful, ethical research.

Alcohol in pregnancy research has already benefited from over 50 years of research, starting with the painstaking animal transgenerational teratogenic research. Now is the time to acknowledge this work, and move to new therapeutic horizons (Hannigan 1996).

Questions such as:

Does the pattern of alcohol exposure matter i.e., heavy drinking, binge drinking matter? or both.

Yes, but the important point is both have an epigenetic effect.

This means light drinking is still not safe, although not a message that the general population want to hear,

b. Is there a threshold level of alcohol consumption below which there is no harm to the developing fetus? No

c. Does the timing of alcohol exposure effect the development of the fetus?

Yes, so 1st trimester physical dysmorphic and motor and sensory problems, Whereas, 2nd and 3rd trimester the more complex neurodevelopmental features including language, cognition and psychiatric disorders (Jones et al. 1973).

A recent book by a European expert on FASD, 'Fetal Alcohol Spectrum Disorders. Exploring Prevention and Management', 2014, ends with the statement;

> "the evidence to decide whether there is indeed a large amount of neurodisability linked to prenatal alcohol exposure is currently lacking."

So Much Work Appears to Be Needed to Be Done

Nevertheless, clinical treatment evidence from countries such as Australia, Canada and USA would refute this opinion, as would my personal experience as a child and adolescent psychiatrist, who has treated patients exposed to prenatal alcohol and their family networks for 30 years in 4 countries Canada, USA, UK and Ireland. Naturally, I would fundamentally disagree about the level of neurodisability present, However I fully understand that this rational scientific, but ideological schism, will continue to inhibit any progress, or appreciation of the ethical issues which continue to be minimized or just plainly denied in this population of transgenerational alcohol affected individuals. (Stoller et al. 1999, Barr et al. 2006, Elliot et al. 2008).

10. There is another Question which continues to pose a fundamental change in scientific thinking in psychiatry. The question and hypothesis is that "mental disorders are

more accurately understood as continuously distributed dimensions of psychopathology" (Krieger et al. 2018, Haltigan 2019).

It is the presence of co –morbidity which is at the essence of NDPAE or FASD.

Historically it has been the use of disorder-specific summary scales which has been the primary approach utilized by researchers to measure therapeutic change (i.e., Conner's, Brown, Social Responsiveness Scale, Beck Depression Inventory, Youth Mania scale). We are now on the threshold of creating and testing methodological models to study the true utility of dimensional models for the assessment of change in mental health treatment. (Weyrauch et al. 2017, Haltigan 2019. Constantinou et al. 2019).

Therefore, it is the utility of a single 'general psychopathology' factor called a 'p' factor that has been shown to summarize the co-occurrences among many symptoms of differing types, in addition to more specific factors such as internalizing or externalizing. (Constantinou 2019).

Standardized Neonatal Instruments such as the BAYLEY II are not designed for this particular neurodevelopmental/neuropsychiatric population, so give a false negative picture. The neuropsychiatric scale developed by Max is more relevant for NDPAE patients at an older child/adolescent age but still does not fully bridge the dimensional world in which these children and adolescents exist (Max et al. 1999).

The literature on brain injury can be helpful (in NDPAE it is acquired over the gestational period through prenatal alcohol exposure, rather than of an acute traumatic nature). Nevertheless, it remains the brain injury that is critical part of the clinical problem in NDPAE.

Chapter 5

THE SCIENTIFIC THINKING THAT UNDERPINS TRANSGENERATIONAL ARND (2014 BOOK)

There are General Principles recognized that need to be considered in Developmental or Neurodevelopmental Psychiatry.

The teratogenic effect of alcohol can be seen within this frame.

The developmental psychiatric disorders that appear from infancy to adulthood have their origins in varying levels of central nervous system dysfunction which may be a combination of different genetic and acquired (epigenetic) factors.

I. The association between chromosomal or genetic abnormalities and obstetric hazards.
II. The association between chromosomal or genetic abnormalities and psychosocial adverse events.
III. The association between prenatal and perinatal adverse events or stressors.*
IV. The risks and benefits of medication treatment during pregnancy and the postpartum period.
   (Pasamanick et al., 1956, 1966, Harris 1995, Glazer 2000, Shaw et al., 2008, Haycock 2009, Siegel 2012)
   *Alcohol teratogenic effect would be classified as no (iii), but it is well to acknowledge the synergistic or additive effect of (i), (ii).
V. It is also recognized that medication used in psychiatry and neurology may have their own unique teratogenic effects on the developing fetus i.e., lithium, phenytoin, valproic acid, SSRIs

The Science of Teratology

This is the beginning point for understanding and believing in the science which guides the path of understanding to transgenerational alcohol abuse and ARND.

A *teratogen* is any agent that disrupts the developing fetus i.e., viruses, drugs, heat, toxins, X rays.

The teratogenic effects depend on three basic principles:

I. Dose of the agent,
II. Timing of the exposure
III. Host factors (the pregnant Mother)

There is an extensive history in medicine of the varying effects of teratogens, lethal, sub lethal and chronic. (Sulik, 1981, Stratton et al., 1996, Streissguth, 1997, Weiss, 2000).

1941 Rubella Virus
1961 Fetal Mercury Effects
1961 Thalidomide Embryopathy
1973 FETAL ALCOHOL SYNDROME (*1968)
1975 Fetal Hydration Syndrome
1978 Hyperthermia
1980 Retinoic Acid

Current Evidence is pointing to nicotine, cocaine, marijuana, methamphetamine, depleted uranium, and PCP.

Already medication such as Valproic Acid has been shown to cause a Fetal Valproate Syndrome with facial dysmorphology and a neurodevelopmental disorder akin to alcohol.

SSRIs in pregnancy also run their own still unexplored risk.

Sanz et al. in 2005 published a series of 93 cases describing a Neonatal Withdrawal Syndrome related to maternal use of SSRI in pregnancy.

64 associated with paroxetine
14 associated with fluoxetine
8 associated with sertraline
7 associated with citalopram

This concept has also been pursued in Canada by (Oberlander et al., 2009).

The Mechanisms of Alcohol Teratology (Sulik et al., 1981, Streissguth 1997, Hagerman 1999, Goodlett & Horn 2001, Orakwue 2012)

In alcohol teratology the timing is different than the classic teratogenic principles as it is not only the 1st 3 months of pregnancy that the fetus is vulnerable, but in fact the whole of gestation. The differential effects of alcohol on the central nervous system are the key to unravelling the alcohol related neurodevelopmental disorder. It is these alcohol induced Central nervous system changes that occur throughout pregnancy. In fact many researchers have pointed out that the 3rd trimester is the most critical when it comes to the neurocognitive, executive function and language function areas of brain development and so exposure at this time poses its own unique long lasting neurodevelopmental risk.

Also there is NO safe dosage of alcohol in pregnancy. This is not what the general public and many physicians want to hear. Only this year new and continuing animal research is showing the unpalatable truth seen for years when taking the history in clinical assessments of ARND. (Laufer, 2013, 2013a). Binge drinking exposure, leading to a higher blood alcohol concentration, has been recognized for 40 years in the primary animal teratology research, as the most destructive. This is the drinking pattern of choice in countries such as Ireland and the UK.

Prenatal exposure to the neurotoxin Alcohol which is a classic teratogen and affects the developing fetus throughout the whole of gestation.

(Sulik et al., 1981, Watson 1992, Stratton et al., 1996, Streissguth & O'Malley 2000, Goodlett et al., 2005, Thomas et al., 2011, Boyadjieva et al., 2010, Benke et al., 2013, Mahabin et al., 2013, Learnpediatrics UBC, FASD 2013).

Alcohol causes a range of effects on the developing central nervous system:

- Direct cell death
- reduced cell proliferation
- migration errors in brain development
- inhibition of nerve growth factor
- disruption of developing neurotransmitters
- abnormalities in the neurophysiology of the developing brain
- abnormalities in the structure of the developing brain

Alcohol Effects on Free Radicals Causing Oxidative Stress and Mitochondrial Dysfunction, Which in Turn Causes Cell Death

It is known that oxidative stress resulting from excess free radicals can induce cell apoptosis or necrosis. Free radicals contain oxygen, reactive oxygen series (ROS). The levels of ROS are controlled by antioxidants. Therefore if ROS are produced in excess of antioxidants, or if prenatal alcohol causes a decrease in the number of the antioxidants, then oxidative stress can occur resulting in cell death.

As well, excess ROS can result in oxidative stress by interference with basic mitochondrial function in its effect on calcium which is essential for maintaining normal neuronal function and survival.

The brain 'wiring' is not just a product of brain structure building but is essential to the process of brain development (Watson 1992, Harris 1995, Chudley 2009).

a. An embryo's brain produces many more neurons, or nerve cells, than it needs, and subsequently eliminates the excess.
b. Thereafter, spontaneous bursts of electrical activity strengthen some of these neural connections, while the connections that are not re-enforced by electrical activity will atrophy.
c. The surviving neurons then create axons, which are the long distance transmission lines of the nervous system. At their ends, these axons in turn spin out multiple branches that may temporarily connect with many central nervous system targets.
d. After birth, the brain experiences, what is called a second growth spurt, as the axons (which send nerve transmission signals) and dendrites (which receive them) greatly increase with exploding new neural connections.
e. Thus, electrical activity, triggered by environmental events such as increasing sensory experiences, can fine tune the brain's neural circuitry, and thereby determines which neural connections will be retained and which will be primed.

(Harris 1995, L. Madeline Nash, 1997, Streissguth and O'Malley 2000).

Alcohol Affects Growth Factor

Alcohol interferes with the Growth factors which are needed to regulate cell proliferation and cell survival.

Several growth factors are necessary for cell division including IGF 1 and IGF 2, and they act by binding to protein molecules called IGF 1 receptors.

The alcohol interferes with the IGF-1 receptors by inhibiting IGF -1 mediated cell division and by signaling function.

(Watson 1992, Goodlett et al., 2001, 2005, Benke et al., 2013)

Effect of Alcohol on Glial (Non –Neuronal Cells)

These glial cells (non-neuronal) cells are an essential part of brain development and subsequent function. They are critical in the support and embryological development of neurons

Here Growth factors have a role as alcohol can interfere with the Growth factors which are supporting cells that have reached their final function, thus preventing their survival.

There are different types of glial cells with specialized functions:

Radial Glial Cells: These cells direct the migration of newly formed neurons to their final location in the developing brain by serving as elongated cellular tracks.

Alcohol interrupts radial glial cells and so interferes with neuronal migration. This in turn causes neurons to end up in abnormal positioning. (Example, 10 year old boy with ARND who has heterotopic grey matter in corpus callosum).

Star –Shaped Astrocytes: Radial glial cells change to star –shaped astrocytes once the neurons have reached their final destination. These star-shaped astrocytes then become the structural support for the neurons.

Alcohol equally interferes with astrocyte structure and function.

Research Studies have shown:

Low alcohol exposure (ethanol) DNA, RNA and protein content Increased

High alcohol exposure (ethanol) DNA, RNA and protein content Decreased

(Ferrer et al., 1987, Watson 1992, Benke et al., 2013).

Effect of Alcohol on Development of Neurotransmitters

The science of alcohol teratology continues to advance in leaps and bounds and one of the core findings has been the effect of prenatal alcohol on the dynamic balance of the developing neurotransmitters. Thus alcohol affects both the structure and function of the developing brain by its effect on the neurotransmitters.

In parallel with the more focused autism research on the role of serotoninergic neurotransmitters has been the identified effect of alcohol on the embryological serotoninergic neurotransmitter system (Hannigan et al., 1996).

This research branches into the study of the serotonin transporter gene which has been studied as a potential marker for deleterious effect of prenatal alcohol exposure. (Warren et al., 2005).

But again parallel work on epigenetics in alcohol has begun to unravel probable trans-generational shifts in genetic transcription through effects on DNA methylation (Haycock 2009) are implicated in prenatal alcohol exposure. Authors such as Behnke et al. 2013, Kodituwakku et Kodituwakku (2011) Streissguth and Connor (2001) reviewed animal and human studies over these 25-30 years demonstrating that heavy doses of alcohol administered to a wide range of laboratory animals produced a spectrum of CNS effects starting with the cell death seen in nerve cells. As well the prenatal alcohol has been demonstrated in many animal studies to interfere with the embryological development of most of the neurotransmitters. This has been studied and reported by Manteueffel (1996),

Hannigan (1996, 1997) Stratton et al. (1996); O'Malley and Hagerman (1998) among many others.

Deficits have been found in the dopaminergic, noradrenergic, serotoninergic, GABAergic, cholinergic, glutaminergic, and histaminergic systems. Human studies are progressing replicating the animal study findings.

The deficits in dopaminergic and noradrenergic systems most likely are connected with the attentional deficit hyperactivity disorder (ADHD) presentation of patients with ARND non dysmorphic or dysmorphic. Previous animal research on rats has demonstrated that the D1 receptors of the mesolimbic dopamine system are affected by prenatal alcohol more than the nigrostriatal or tegmental dopamine D1 receptor system.

There has been recent impetus to study the relationship of developing neurotransmitters to later psychiatric disorder. Serotonin receptor genes (5HT) have been shown to increase the risk for major depression as a function of stressful events. However, the serotonin receptor genes HTR 2A have been shown to decrease the risk for depressive symptoms in the context of high maternal nurturance. These findings nicely capture the dynamic equilibrium between environmental neurotoxic suggested a etiological factor prenatal alcohol, and the potential protective effect of the nurturing rearing environment. As can be appreciated this is a challenge in a home where alcohol addiction and domestic violence hold sway. Studies such as Uber et al. 2009 and Jakela et al. 2007 debate the role of the serotonin transporter gene in environmental adversity in the etiology of mental illness, and the impact of childhood nurturance on not just the separate serotonin 2A gene, but as well later adult depressive symptoms.

Further research has studied the central concept of emotional regulation in its generality and postulated the differing influences of either the mother or the father. The core concept of emotional development and regulation includes the ability to adjust internal processes i.e., thoughts, emotions, respiration in co-ordination with social demands and opportunities. This is seen by many as a central tenet in the grounding of child mental health. As well it is regarded as essential for the nursery and school preparedness of the toddler and young child. Thus executive control of emotional regulation is seen to influence the perceptions and interpretations of situations and experiences that modulate emotion. Furthermore, self-regulation does the work of striking the balance between protecting the self from misfortune and promoting opportunity for positive experience. Patients with ARND enter the world, not uncommonly, with biologically induced disconnections in both the critical genes, pathways and neurotransmitters involved with basic emotional regulation. So it is understandable that these infants, young children will readily display disruptive mood dysregulation disorder problems from an early age, irrespective of the containment in the home environment.

As you analyses the concept of emotional regulation further the neurobiological vulnerabilities dovetail with the nurturing vulnerabilities. Therefore, it is realistic to expect a change in the quality of emotion regulation in the infants of clinically depressed mothers compared with non-depressed mothers. (Marian et al., 2009). Within the Irish context this effectively means that the mother's alcohol use in pregnancy is frequently linked to significant familial depression. This mother/infant dyadic dance of fortune and misfortune is acted out through generations, in the synchrony and construction of shared timing, physiological processes, developmental outcomes and risk conditions all interwoven in this delicate balance, not unlike the nurturing of a fragile orchid plant. (O'Malley 2003, Feldman 2007, Tronick 2009).

Current research in epigenetics is beginning to help professionals unravel the contradictory clinical presentations of patients with ARND (Manteuffel 1996, Lattmore et al., 2005,). Animal research has implicated the short allele of the Serotonin Transporter Gene (5HTT) as being affected by prenatal alcohol and influencing the appearance of anxiety disorders through its action in increasing HPA axis (Hypothalamic Pituitary Adrenal Axis) activation (Meewise et al., 2007). Furthermore, animal research has identified the effect of prenatal alcohol exposure on Dopamine 2 Receptors (D2R) as a key biochemical factor in the development of sensory under or over-responsiveness. Furthermore, animal research has identified the effect of prenatal alcohol exposure on Dopamine 2 Receptors (D2R) as a key biochemical factor in the development of sensory under- or over-responsiveness (Screiber et al., 2008).

Also, the effects of prenatal alcohol exposure on inhibitory gamma-aminobutyric acid (GABA) and excitatory N-methyl-D-aspartic acid (NMDA) can kindle seizures. (Hannigan et al., 1991, 1996, Harris 1995, Hagerman 1999). Alcohol can reduce the numbers and function of NMDA (Glutamate) receptors during embryological development. As well withdrawal from high levels of alcohol has been shown to lead to excitotoxicity i.e., exaggerated/NMDA/Glutamate activity which can lead to neuronal death, which is another risk factor in a fetus exposed to alcohol in pregnancy and then experiencing a sudden period of alcohol withdrawal at delivery.

Effects of Alcohol on Glucose Transporter and Uptake

Alcohol exposure has been shown to lead to disruption of the utilization of glucose by the developing brain.

Glucose has many diverse roles:

- It serves as a basic energy source
- It is involved in the nucleic acids, DNA and RNA essential building blocks in the brain function
- It is involved with molecular and hormone growth and development, such as lipids and steroids

Prolonged alcohol exposure as in pregnancy causes reduced cellular glucose uptake, as well as the levels of transporter protein. Finally, there can be an effect on GLUC-1 gene expression.

This alcohol related disruption in brain development function is linked to the decrease in glucose that is necessary to traverse cell membranes utilizing these glucose transporter genes GLUC -1 as well as GLUC-.

In summary the alcohol effect on glucose is seen in growth deficits in the fetus and central nervous system damage at a more global level.

(Singh et al., 1992, Benke et al., 2013, Goodlett & Horn 2001, Learnpediatrics UBC 2013).

Effects of Alcohol on Cell Adhesion

Intact cell adhesion is a basic concept in nerve cell development. It is needed for diverse tasks such as neuronal growth, cellular migration and the development of neural connections with neighboring nerve cells.

Alcohol, especially ethanol, causes decrease in cell adhesion by its effect on the cell adhesion molecules (CAMs).

This effect has been implicated in the global level of functioning reflected in the general intellectual disability seen in ARND, as well as structural deficits in the cerebellum and the corpus callosum. (Manteuffel 1996).

Recently, research studies have analyzed the effect of alcohol on inhibiting L1, an immunoglobulin cell adhesion molecule that promotes cell-cell adhesion, neurite outgrowth, cell migration, and synaptic plasticity (Bearer 2001, Dou et al., 2011).

Effects of Alcohol on Regulation of Gene Expression

Alcohol has been linked with reduced retinoic acid which influences the genes that regulate the craniofacial development genes.

Alternate isoenzyme forms of ADH gene metabolize alcohol differently. It has been discovered that the ADHI B2 allele has a protective effect from alcohol neurotoxicity as it is associated with rapid metabolism of alcohol to acetaldehyde.

Whereas isoenzyme coded by ADHI B's slower metabolism can contribute to ARND.

(Warren et al., 2005, Chudley 2009)

Effect of Alcohol on Developing Brain Structures

The following references give an overview of structural brain anomalies from prenatal alcohol exposure

(Clarren & Astley 1978, Watson 1992, Harris 1995, Astley 2009, O'Leary et al., 2011, Learn pediatrics UBC 2013, Nyugen & Riley 2014).

Alcohol differentially affects the structure of the developing brain

Global Brain

Early research studies using post mortem data demonstrated the presence of microcephaly in infants with heavy prenatal exposure. (Clarren & Smith 1978 a, b).

Continuing research using, not post mortem data, but live MRI scans have confirmed this microcephaly, but as well delineated decreased total brain volume and simultaneous volumetric reductions of the whole cranial vault (Astley et al., 2009).

Cerebral Cortex & Neocortex

Alcohol causes a reduction in all neocortical areas in the neuronal cells. There is a delay in the onset of neurogenesis and proliferation and the redistribution of neocortical neurons. The motor and somatosensory cortices are most affected with the auditory cortex less affected. Also altered synaptic development, dendritic spines and as well altered migration due to abnormal morphology of radial glial fibers. (Watson 1992 Stratton et al., 1996, Hagerman 1999).

Hippocampus

In this area the issue of timing of alcohol exposure to the development of a particular part of the hippocampus and the peak blood alcohol concentration (BAC) were of critical combined importance. The area most affected has been shown to be the dentate gyrus mossy fibers or excitatory efferent granule cells to the pyramidal cells of the hippocampus CA3 region. Many studies have demonstrated a decrease in size and volume in the hippocampus. (Kodituwakku et al., 2011, Nguyen et al., 2013).

Corpus Callosum

The corpus callosum is large bundle of white matter fiber which connects the right and left brain cerebral hemispheres. It has received the most interest, and scientific study in relationship to prenatal alcohol exposure. Now alcohol has been recognized as the commonest acquired cause of agenesis of the corpus callosum.

(Stratton et al., 1996, Streissguth & O'Malley 2000, Bookstein et al., 2001, 2005, Nguyen et al., 2013).

This is the area which was eloquently shown by Norman Gescwind back in the mid 1960s as central to the development of disconnection syndromes (or disconnexion as he called it.). This concept is very much at the essence of clinical presentation in ARND.

Cerebellum

With early alcohol exposure in the gestational period there is impaired cerebellar growth with the purkinje cells particularly affected. The cerebellar lobes I, IX and X have been shown to be most affected. However a maximum blood alcohol concentration of less 160 mg/dl was not associated with impaired development of the purkinje cells. (Stratton et al., 1996, Green 2004, Kodituwakku et al., 2011).

White Matter Microstructure

Initial studies using MRI showed what was called macrostructure abnormalities in the white matter. However, more recently diffusion tensor imaging technology has shown significant micro structural abnormalities when analyzing the integrity of white matter tracts (Watson 1992, Nguyen et al., 2013).

Soft Neurological Symptoms and Signs

Infants exposed to prenatal alcohol may show immediate neurological sequelae, as shown in the 1974/1975 Seattle 500 Longitudinal Study. Streissguth and colleagues demonstrated that on neonate days one and two infants showed problems in habituation, and state regulation, decreased suck reflex and longer latency to suck (Smith 1981, Streissguth et al., 2004). The immediate temperament challenges of these brain damaged infants and neonates may result in abnormal attachment, bonding and dyadic connections. Although this is often attributed to postpartum depression in birth mothers (Murray et al., 2011), it is frequently the temperamental difficulties of the infant from basic feeding to state regulation, habituation and general reactivity that drive the mother/infant dyad and not the other way around.

The 'difficult to settle' or the 'slow to warm' temperaments offer clinical frames for understanding infants with FASD (Chess and Thomas 1977).

As well, researchers such as Benini et al. 2002 have explored the clinical clues to differentiating inherited and non inherited etiologies of specific childhood neurological disorders called ataxias. This gives credence to one aspect of so called soft neurological signs; seen in conditions such as ARND. Developmental Coordination Disorder is a not uncommon feature of ARND and an integral part of this presentation is truncal or gait ataxia. This is part of a general dyspraxia.

Disruption in Developing Neurophysiology

Further neurobiological research is analyzing the clinical effect of the prenatal alcohol disruption of the balance between GABA the inhibitory and Glutamate (NMDA) the excitatory neurotransmitter in the brain. Scientists in the USA have shown the kindling of seizures due to the effect of prenatal alcohol on the GABAergic cells in the hippocampus which leads to a lower seizure threshold (Bonthius et al., 1992).

The following references cover many diverse areas of brain disruption from prenatal alcohol exposure from animal research to human studies.

(Riley et al., 1995, Stratton et al., 1996, Streissguth 1997, Hagerman 1999, Archibald et al., 2001, Goodlett et al., 2001, 2005, British Medical Association 2007, Kraemer et al., 2008, Sowell et al., 2008, O'Malley & Mukarjee 2010, O'Malley 2011, Novick Brown, O'Malley, Streissguth 2011, Mukarjee et al., 2012, Nguyen & Riley 2013).

General Scientific Theories Which Explore the Protective and Risk Factors in Infant and Later Development

1. Genetic influences on birth and subsequent development attest to both protective as well as risk factors for the fetus and the infant in dealing with adverse environmental stressors. So there can be a dynamic equilibrium established as the infant grows. Therefore there is a concept to be considered whereby various adaptations in early life might actually have an immediate positive benefit on the infant or the young child. Conversely they can also make the individual more vulnerable to develop adverse life outcomes if he/she is presented with a different or novel type of environment. Thus a dynamic equilibrium can be established which is mediated by certain genetic protective factors and exposure to stressful environments of varying intensity and duration. (Giarratano G 2006, Anum et al., 2009).

The role of genetic susceptibility for maternal alcohol metabolism in determining pregnancy outcome is one area still being researched (Jones 2006). This type of research dovetails with the work on alcohol metabolism substances such as acetaldehyde and its role in re-enforcement and motor reactivity in newborns with or without a history of prenatal alcohol exposure. (March et al., 2013). Therefore a number of genes which regulate alcohol metabolism have been identified which have been seen as having either risk or protective role in the impact of prenatal alcohol exposure on the fetus. (Chudley 2009).

As is well understood, alcohol is metabolized to acetaldehyde then to acetate and excreted through the kidneys and the circulation. There are two primary enzymes involved Alcohol Dehydrogenase (ADH) and Acetaldehyde Dehydrogenase (ALDH). Al Chudley, among others have pointed out that these two enzymes function at variable rates depending on the genes that control them.

Acetaldehyde build up in alcohol metabolism creates toxicity due to its production of a reactive oxygen radical which causes cell death. So individuals with a fast acting ADH variant or a slow acting ALDH variant have metabolic problems in handling alcohol (Densmore 2011).

In ARND it is the phenotype which leads to clinical understanding of the developmental psychiatric disorder.

2. The challenges of delivery have long been identified as stressors for the developing infant. (Pasamanick & Knoblock & Lilienfield 1956, 1966).

The early researchers documented the impact of difficult labor and delivery with resulting hypoxia to the infant. They described a Continuum of Reproductive Wastage with lethal, sub lethal outcomes.

There was also a Continuum of Reproductive Casualty with minor motor, perceptual, learning and behavioral disabilities. The latter became called 'minimum brain dysfunction'. This formed the basis for the a etiological theories on Hyperkinetic Disorder, the forerunner of ADHD.

Current ongoing research on these stressors offers an epigenetic entry into changing gene expression as Wright and colleagues in 2009, showed in their study of the role of oxygen. They specifically identified hypoxia as a phenomenon capable of manipulating gene expression. As they described, in rather dense detail, "the hypoxia activates a small proportion of NF-KB and Nef -2 regulated genes and drives expression of antioxidants, glutathione, perixodase, catalyse, superoxide dismutase detoxifying genes glutathione -5 – transferase and stress response gene heme-oxygenase 1 (HO-1). This HO-1 gene in turn incorporates antioxidant enzymes which are important in the detoxification of electrophiles as well as genes involved in cell cycle regulation and the inflammatory response." The authors conclude that "it appears that the overall effects of the hypoxia on gene expression depended on the maturational stage of organogenesis."

3. Nutrition both in the prenatal and the postnatal period has a critical role not to be ignored.

Lessons learned from animal studies include the understanding that differential periods of a peri-conceptional under-nutrition have different effects on growth, metabolic and endocrine status in fetal sheep. This also alters the fetal growth response to stress. Early work was done on fetal programming and serum cholesterol and nutrition effects in adult life by Barker and colleagues in 1993.

A scientific conceptual underpinning not a mile away from understanding differential fetal growth effects in the infants of alcoholic, poorly nourished pregnant women enduring stressful or violent relationships during pregnancy. (Dreosti 1993, Bell et al., 2002, Rumbull et al., 2009, O'Malley 20011b).

As far back as 2003 Waterland and colleagues had analyzed the early nutrition effects on adult metabolism in humans and other mammals which they felt were mediated by persistent alterations in DNA methylation. The researchers showed "that dietary methyl supplementation of a/a dams with extra folic acid, vitamin B12, choline and betaine alter the phenotype of the Axy/a offspring via increased CpG methylation at the Axy locus."

They further extrapolated that "the epigenetic metastability which confers this liability is due to the Axy transposable element."

Other work has looked at the epigenetic role of folate (Padmunabhan et al., 2013)

4. Biomarkers of CNS activity continue to be explored and tested.

Alpha amylase (AA) which is produced locally in the oral mucosa is showing some promise. It appears to be unrelated to cortisol influences.

There are also no consistent biochemical tests such as GGT, MCV, Folate, which relate to alcohol usage in pregnancy as they do not fit into the general protocol, are too expensive, or seen as too intrusive. As long ago as 1996, these types of biochemical tests were recommended by the Institute of Medicine in the USA (Stratton et al., 1996).

Biomarkers are also being tested in pregnancy and delivery such as FAEE in meconium or fetal movement under ultrasound, but are still not robust enough to be part of clinical practice, and have too many confounding variables (Bearer 2001).

Fetal movement and postnatal startle reflex continues to be studied as it pertains to indenting fetal risk of prenatal alcohol but appears to have little practical utility and is subject to too many confounding variables i.e., exercise, diet or emotional state of mother (Little et al., 2002).

Alcohol teratology researchers have postulated that dysmorphic ARND and/or Alcohol Related Birth Defects (ARBD) could be useful as biomarkers for heavy binge exposure early in pregnancy. Maybe researchers claim it could predict a worse neurodevelopmental prognosis (Riley and McGee, 2005, Coles et al., 2011). This is however not verified by clinicians and the likelihood of facial dysmorphology and a cardiac structural defect such as ventricular septal defect predicting the course of an ARND patient with for example Disruptive Mood Dysregulation and Alexithymia is unlikely.

5. The concept of Fetal Programming and its relationship to ARND

There is an epigenetic Fetal Programming embedded with prenatal alcohol exposure which leads to one conceptual frame for the clinical understanding of the developmental psychiatric presentations of ARND from infancy through childhood.

a. Emotional Development:

Science has explored and continues to establish that emotional development is inevitably built into the architecture of the infant and young child and reflects genetic and epigenetic (environmental) risk and protective factors. The concept of 'brain plasticity' has enabled an understanding that the growing interconnections among brain circuits, especially in the first 3 years of life, serve to support the emergence of increasingly mature emotional behavior. Hence the critical importance of the stable nurturing environment for this period, especially if the fetus/infant is 'programmed' by prenatal alcohol for certain developmental vulnerabilities. (LeDoux 2000). The long standing research on attachment and bonding does not negate the biological fetal programming effects of prenatal alcohol. It is the confluence of the infant entering the world into a supportive or non-supportive environment that ultimately mediates the critical difference in the developmental psychiatric presentation of the emotional regulation.

The central features of emotional development are generally accepted to include:

- the ability to identify and understand one's own feelings.
- to accurately read and comprehend varying emotional states in others.
- to manage strong emotions and express them in a constructive manner.
- to regulate one's own behavior.
- to develop empathy for others.
- to establish and sustain relationships

(Denham 1998, Lewis 2000, National Scientific Council on the Developing Child. 2004, Thompson et al., 2005).

Patients with ARND have immediate challenges in the arenas of emotion development which span two quite different extremes.

On the one had the child is overwhelmed by a Disruptive Mood Dysregulation Disorder (now a category in itself in the newly arrived DSM V psychiatric classification) which pervades and dominates all social interactions. This may include the rather puzzling phenomenon of 'emotional incontinence' in which the patient cries and laughs with no clear provocation (not unlike what can be seen in traumatic brain injury, except in this case it is an acquired brain injury).

Conversely the patient may exhibit 'Alexithymia', having no words for emotion and unable to read or comprehend emotions in others. (This latter category has been misdiagnosed as Autistic Spectrum Disorder or Asperger's Disorder, whereas it is a unique, but not uncommon, part of the ARND). (Sifneos, 1973, Sullivan 2008). The arrival of the DSM V psychiatric classification from the American Psychiatric Association in 2013 has also included a category Social Communication Disorder which aptly describes this clinical aspect of a disorder emotional development seen in ARND.

b. Alcohol Craving:

Animal research going back over 35 years has shown the relationship between prenatal alcohol exposure and postnatal alcohol craving. (Bond & Di Gusto 1976, Reyes et al., 1985, Dominquez et al., 1993, Sinha et al., 1999, Abate et al., 2008).

This also leads to clinical questions such as: Could sugar craving be related to prenatal alcohol exposure and predate alcohol craving?

Therefore prenatal alcohol exposure can lead to a genetic susceptibility to alcohol craving in the succeeding generations. As well it forms the template for early onset alcohol addiction and transgenerational alcohol addiction. The alcohol craving/addiction is not just a product of family history, but is kindled by the effect of alcohol on the developing nucleus accumbens, delta B fos cells. For example a scientific study analysing enzymes involved in alcohol metabolism in 3 groups

1) Mothers who have children with FAS
2) Children with FAS
3) Controls, this study showed a variability of these enzymes thus emphasizing the importance of alcohol metabolism in ARND.

In the USA there are higher rates of ARND in African Americans and Native Americans than non-Hispanic Whites which lends credence to this work. (Li &Warren 2008, May 2011).

Studies abound across many disciplines and professions that attest to the importance and complexity of taking gene structure expression and epigenetic influences from the bench to the clinical office.

The epigenetic concept that alcohol craving and subsequent alcohol abuse or dependence in adolescents and adults with ARND may have their origins in prenatal alcohol exposure has been demonstrated by animal researchers going back 40 years, and later human researchers. (Dominquez, Bond, Baer et al. 2001).

Alcohol use during pregnancy is at the very heart of ARND, and so conceptual frame for effective management should involve general acceptance that maternal drinking may not be just an inherited genetic condition, but may reflect a biochemical craving for alcohol due to the effect of prenatal exposure on the developing brain, especially the Nucleus Accumbens.

Already, longitudinal studies using standardized psychiatric assessment instruments such as the SCID I and II have shown the prevalence of alcohol dependence and abuse in young adults prenatally exposed to alcohol. Alcohol counseling for birth mothers is a key therapeutic approach, but it needs to be acknowledged that this form of psychotherapy and motivational interviewing does not always connect with patients who have cognitive impairment in fundamental cause and effect reasoning. At least with cocaine addiction, psychopharmacology has been used successfully (O'Malley & Sinha 1995) in blocking the central nervous system craving.

Agents such as Naltrexone or Acamprasate also have been used successfully in patients with FASD but still require rigorous scientific testing, especially for use during pregnancy (Prof. Lingford Hughes, Plenary Talk, All Ireland Psychiatrists meeting, Malahide, Dublin. November 8th 2013).

c. The effect of prenatal alcohol on DNA methylation and genetic transcription and its role in the *fetal programming of the introduction of new developmental psychiatric disorders* into the familial line, i.e., ADHD, ASD or Social Communication Disorder.

(Driscoll et al., 1990, Nanson 1991, O'Malley & Nanson 2002, Mukarjee et al., 2006, O'Malley 2008, O'Malley & Rich 2013).

The field of Intellectual Disability is indebted to the pioneers of syndrome identification and description which continue to give a template of clinical and scientific grounding to the genotype/phenotype link in expression. The longstanding concept of 'behavioral phenotype' has given clinicians an entry into rare disorders and the ever expanding genetic lab research has married the behavioral phenotypes with specific genetic disorders.

Witness some well-known examples, Down's syndrome, Fragile X Syndrome, Angelman Syndrome, Prader- Willi Syndrome, Noonan Syndrome, Lesh Nyhan syndrome, Velo –Cardio Facial syndrome to mention just a few.

The Knotted Cord. Summary (2014 Book)

The science of alcohol teratology brings a clear understanding to the multi- facetted effect of prenatal alcohol on the totality of brain development, from the cellular, neurochemical, electrical to the structural levels.

Although there are well identified protective and risk factors it is the absence of alcohol during pregnancy that is the only true preventive measure for discontinuation of ARND. Therefore the best biomarker still remains the mother's history of alcohol consumption in pregnancy. This is where the science and the art of diagnosing ARND meet, and the challenge to intervene in this transgenerational condition goes back to the basic mother/infant dyad.

Factors such as genetic vulnerability, pregnancy and delivery complications, nutritional factors, epigenetic programming are beginning to complete the scientific picture of the ARND risk and vulnerability paradigm.

There are many imaging techniques available to quantify the suspected organic brain dysfunction from,

Cranial ultrasound,
CAT scan of the head with contrast,
MRI of the Brain,
FMRI,
Spect scan of the brain,
Diffusion Tensor technique
and PET scans of the brain.

Sleep deprived EEG is also an useful method of quantifying a possible seizure disorder, especially complex partial or absence seizure disorder both seen in ARND.

The scientific unraveling of fetal programming and alcohol's uncanny ability to 'sow the seeds of the next generations' individuals who will crave alcohol, become pregnant, or become the father of a child, and so continue the ARND cycle.

There is a crying need for a transgenerational management approach to alcohol abuse and dependence which requires health and social service systems to collaborate across traditional age-divides (e.g., child/adolescent/adult).

For example:

1) Obstetricians, GPs and midwives and maternity hospital social workers need to become sensitive to the implicit risks in the developing fetus from alcohol use in any trimester of pregnancy.
2) Although teenage pregnancy has been acknowledged as a risk for pregnancy and delivery, co-occurring alcohol or substance abuse is too often simply accepted as expected and almost normalized, rather than seen as a warning sign for the health of the infant.
3) The 'perfect storm' of mixing early onset alcohol drinking with unprotected SI creates a sure recipe for the following generation of fetally programmed, alcohol craving, impulsive, with so called executive decision making lacunae.
4) Until such time that all of the professionals managing and delivering pregnant women who drink really believe that any amount of alcohol is unsafe, the ongoing clinical management of ARND will remain with us.
5) There needs to be a way that the ever increasing sophisticated science regarding the pervasive effects of prenatal alcohol become communicated to active practicing clinicians, and do not continue to be sequestered away only for presentation in academic scientific meetings removed from the cut and thrust of transgenerational alcohol abuse, dependence and intervention.

The Scientific Thinking That Underpins Transgenerational NDPAE (Previously ARND), an Update 2020

In the last 5 years the wealth of scientific papers involved with analyzing the science of this unique epigenetic- created global neurodevelopmental disorder has increased in leaps and bounds.

No longer hidden in the back waters of scientific research journals the consciousness and truth of the long-term legacy of prenatal alcohol exposure existing through generations is becoming more widely appreciated. (Streissguth & O'Malley 2000).

This update chapter builds on the science and structure of the 2014 chapter and ideally should be read in tandem with the 2104 chapter, as it essentially introduces new research re- enforcing the previous studies and discoveries.

Alcohol Teratology Re-Visited

Summary

It is fascinating to review the literature, in an unhurried manner, on this subject some 5 year later.

The 1970s, 80s, 90s and early 2000 period were full of major studies animal and human on this topic but the last 10 to 15 years this well has run dry.

Do the international researchers know something about the veracity of alcohol teratology that the normal population do not?

> "alcohol effects on the developing human brain appear to be a continuum without threshold when dose and behavior are quantified appropriately" (Sampson et al., 1990).

> "no clear threshold," "definite effects in animal and human studies"
> (Rennick et al., 1983, Emhart et al., 1987, Coles 1994)

> "a safe level of alcohol use in pregnancy has not been established" (Streissguth et al., 1980)

> "complete abstinence" was advocated to eliminate risk (Martinez et al. 2004)

Moderate prenatal alcohol consumption:

> maternal effect: "increases risk of spontaneous abortion in 1st trimester, but also in in 2nd trimester" (Windham et al. 1997)
> child effect: "effects child IQ and learning problems" (Streissguth et al., 1997)

Current International research is now pursuing the minutiae of alcohol teratogenic effects and mechanisms, coupled with the understanding that alcohol has a true epigenetic effect which can span generations.

Alcohol Effects on Free Radicals Causing Oxidative Stress and Mitochondrial Dysfunction, Which in Turn Cause Cell Death

The involvement of free radicals has been shown to have a dual role in both diseases but also in health. Therefore, free radicals have been demonstrated to be both toxic and beneficial compounds since they may be harmful or helpful to the body systems. As research has shown that low or moderate concentrations of ROS*/RNS are necessary for maturation process of cellular structures and may act as defensive weapons for the host defense systems. However, when in excess free radicals and oxidants generate the process of oxidative stress which can seriously alter cell membranes and other structures, such as proteins, lipids, lipoproteins and DNA itself. (Pham-Huy et al., 2008).

* ROS = Reactive Oxygen Species which is increased by prenatal exposure to alcohol.

Recent research has postulated that a subset of children may be genetically predisposed to oxidative stress damage to their DNA. This process then mediates subsequent birth defects and postnatal neurodevelopmental abnormalities. These genetic and/or environmental mechanisms can include enhanced pathways for ROS formation and as well deficient pathways for ROS detoxification or DNA repair (Bhatia et al., 2019).

The mechanism of oxidative stress and its relationship as one of the teratogenic effects of prenatal alcohol, continues to stimulate new research. This has, as well, created opportunities for use as biomarkers of alcohol exposure (Mancincelli et al. 2011, Patten et al., 2014).

Lastly, the utility of antioxidants such as Vitamin E, Vitamin C, B Carotene, Lycopene, Selenium, Flavomide, Melatonin, Omega 3 Omega or Omega 6 Fatty Acids is being explored for patients with fetal alcohol spectrums disorders or neurodevelopmental disorder prenatal alcohol exposure (Pham-Huy et al. 2008, Patten et al. 2014).

Effect of Alcohol on Glial (Non-Neuronal Cells)

Continued research pinpoints this as an area of concern for the teratogenic effect of prenatal alcohol. For many years the animal studies have shown that damage to radial glial cells may be one of the underlying factors in alcohol exposure resulting in abnormal neural and glial formation. Further exploration has postulated that delayed oligodendrocyte development and/or increased oligodendrocyte precursor optosis may be linked to altered myelination and white matter integrity which has been demonstrated in children prenatally exposed to alcohol. (Wilhelm et al., 2015).

It has been demonstrated that cell death also changes developmental plasticity, and in fact there is a reciprocal interaction between cell death and maladaptive plasticity which has been seen as underwriting the main pathogenic mechanism of prenatal alcohol induced damage.to the developing brain in utero (Granato et al., 2018). The clinical correlation between disruptions in early infant and childhood motor and sensory development seen in NDPAE which are seen as Regulatory Disorders fits nicely into this concept of maladaptive plasticity.

Furthermore, new evidence has brought to light the alcohol teratogenic effect on neuro-inflammation and neurodevelopment which is medicated by developmental glial cell disruption (Densmore 2011, Kinada et al. 2017).

Effects of Alcohol on Cell Adhesion

The variability in the effects of alcohol teratology have been governed by a wide range of issues in which effects on cell adhesion form a key role. The dosage and timing of alcohol exposure influences the inhibition of cell adhesion mediated by L1 neural cell adhesion molecule. It is in this area that the modulation of mitogen-activated protein kinase has its role. (Eberhart et al., 2013).

Many researchers continue to identify the toxic role of alcohol, in inhibiting the L1 mediated neurite growth. (Bearer et al. 1999, Ramanthan et al., 1996).

The L1 cell adhesion molecule has as well been isolated as a potential neuroprotective factor in alcohol induced cell death which speaks to its unique position in the world of alcohol, teratology. (Gubitosi et al., 2007).

Effects of Alcohol on Developing Glucose Transporter and Uptake

Continuing research analyses, the teratogenic effect of alcohol on the Glucose mediated metabolic systems, including its effect on the Serotonin transporter system. (Ngai et al., 2015).

This work further probes the effect of alcohol on HPA axis, lowering Nr 3C-1 mRNA, Nerve Growth Factor, NGF. The implications include a long- term brain effect gene expression, which is one of the entries into understanding the potential hidden transgenerational alcohol legacy.

Effects of Alcohol on Developing Growth Factor

Growth is controversial in NDPAE as the infants are not generally low birth weight but can exhibit growth trajectory problems growth throughout early life. Often mis-diagnosed as failure to thrive or faltering growth due to emotional environmental factors rather than teratogenic effect of alcohol (O'Neill 2010).

Other research studies have investigated the effect of prenatal alcohol on nerve growth factor (NGF) and brain derived neurotropic factor (NDNF) as w well as postnatal growth (Aros et al., 2011, Corito et al., 2019).

Effects of Alcohol on Developing Brain Structures

The burgeoning research on brain imaging has continued, and is offering new horizons to explore, as well as helping in our understanding of the neurological impact of prenatal alcohol.

This is not just a neurobehavioral legacy, but a brain injury –derived neurological and neuropsychiatric neurodevelopmental disorder.

This prenatal acquired brain injury is more and more showing unique alcohol related deficits on the structures of the developing brain.

7. Effect on Developing Body Organ Systems

Alcohol exposure usually in the 1st trimester.

Prenatal alcohol effects development of Kidney, Heart, Eye, Ear, Skeletal system. (initially described as Alcohol Related Birth Defects (ARBD) in Institute of Medicine, USA, book (Stratton et al. 1996)

See Table 7 The Knotted Cord 2014.

8. Effects of Alcohol on Developing Brain Neurophysiology and Neurotransmitters

The interest in the effects of prenatal alcohol on the developing brain neurophysiology and neurotransmitters continues over the last 5 years. Alcohol is a false neurochemical which competes for site in the developing brain and has a particular influence on the balance between excitatory and inhibitory neurotransmitters Glutamate and GABA.

The neurological underpinning of Seizure Disorders in NDPAE or FASD commonly lies in alcohol effect on neurotransmitters. Particular attention has been shown to alcohol exposure in 1st and 2nd Trimesters (Duke University, USA, 2016).

Studies over the last 10 years has shown a prevalence of Seizure Disorder ranging from 3 to 21% in patients with NDPAE or FASD. (Bell et al., 2010, Nicita et al., 2014, Boronat et al., 2017). Unlike other Developmental Disorders the seizure disorder in NDPAE is not related to level of IQ i.e., the lower IQ the higher rate of Seizure. This makes the unravelling of potential seizure disorder more challenging as the patients are commonly seen as deliberately oppositional and defiant, or willfully explosive, rather than having an alcohol- brain injury derived seizure disorder. The studies have involved 425 patients (254 males, 171 females, aged 2 to 49 years) in one sample series, and 61patients in another sample series.

Further research has highlighted the risk of sudden death from Seizure Disorder and indicated that the population of patients with Intellectual Disability and Seizure Disorder are at particular risk. Not uncommonly because the Seizure Disorder has not been diagnosed, A real factor in NDPAE (Young et al., 2016a, Shantar et al., 2019).

Table 7. Summary: Brain areas effected by prenatal exposure, and neuropsychiatric & neurological consequences

Whole Brain:
Microcephaly, usually associated with full dysmorphic syndrome Fetal Alcohol Syndrome (Jones et al., 1973).

Corpus Callosum:
Most common brain area effected by alcohol.
1st Trimester alcohol exposure prevents its Formation
2nd/3rd Trimester alcohol exposure Alters the Shape.
This major bundle of nerve white matter microstructure fibers is of critical, they connect the Right and Left Brain in important arenas such as:
Timing,
Motor and Co-ordination Tasks
Disorders in Verbal learning ability
General Executive Function disorders in organization, planning, problem solving.

Cortex:
Disorders in motor and sensory control, with effects on cortical thickness
Cognitive disorders

Prefrontal Cortex:
3rd Trimester Alcohol exposure;
Executive Function Disorders,
Disorders in Inhibition,
Problem solving and planning problems,
Time perception problems,
Disinhibited sexual urges.

Cerebellum:
2nd and 3rd trimester alcohol exposure, but has not completed the organ development at birth so postnatal exposure to alcohol a further risk as cerebellum circuitry still being developed.
Disorders in balance, truncal and gait ataxias.
Cognitive functioning disorders,
Disorders in development of language fluency.
Time perception and Time sequencing problems

Hippocampus:
3rd Trimester alcohol exposure
Learning and memory problems, especially working memory.
Amygdala/Hypothalamus/Hippocampus:
Form Limbic System,
Emotional dysregulation problems,
Social interaction and sexualized disinhibition boundary problems.

Amygdala alone:
Disorders in emotional regulation with specific deficits in overreaction to anxiety and fear/danger provoking situations.
Exaggerations in fear/flight response to situations.
Disorders in empathy, over or under-reactive.

(Kellerman 2010, Densmore 2011, O'Malley 2014, Zieff et al. 2016, Rae et al. 2018., Treit et al. 2018., FASD.HUB. Australia, 2019).

Research on the modulation effect of prenatal alcohol exposure on the developing neurotransmitter system continues to produce new information relevant to clinical understanding of the clinical phenotype of NDPAE, but also informing possible avenues of targeted medication intervention.

Alcohol has been shown to bind directly and also modulate various specific neurotransmitter systems i.e., (5HT, GABA, NMDA or N- Methyl- D- aspartate, which ae located in the brain reward pathways. As well Alcohol indirectly modulates the mesolimbic dopamine neurotransmitter system via a mechanism of increasing VTA (ventral tegmental area) by decreasing the suppressant/inhibitory effect which GABA exerts on them (Goodlet et al., 2000, Tomkins et al., 2001, Ngai et al., 2015).

Table 8. Role of neurotransmitters relevant to NDPAE or FASD

GABA	learning, working memory and general/reactive anxiety
	As well, GABRA -2 has been implicated in increasing the risk for alcoholism in the next generation
Glutamate	general cognitive processing, learning, working memory. and excitation/reactivity
Serotonin	general moodiness and anxiety,
Noradrenaline	general moodiness, anxiety, attention and concentration
Dopamine	motor control, attention, impulsivity, general cognition and judgement
	Alcohol has been shown to increase dopamine 2 receptors (DCD2) in the nucleus accumbens which links to a reward feed- back and craving of alcohol.

(Hannigan 1996, Goodlet 2000, Le Strat et al., 2008, O'Malley 2008, 2014, Kellerman 2010, Collaborative Study of Genetics of Alcoholism, Densmore, 2011).

Genetics and Epigenetics in Development of FASD or NDPAE: Effects of Alcohol on Regulation of Gene Expression

Epigenetic principles:

1) Predetermined: Development is scripted and predictable
2) Probalistic: Development is a bi-directional structure-function with experiences and external molding of development.

Inspiration

Dr. Christine Loock an internationally well- respected Pediatrician from Vancouver, Canada, has coined this phrase which lies at the heart of understanding the challenges to diagnosis and management in FASD now NDPAE.

"The egg that made you was developing in your mother when she was a 6-week old fetus in your grandmother."

a) There is a dynamic relationship between genetic vulnerability, epigenetic changes to the developing brain, and the inherent risk that the alcohol –induced epigenetic changes to the DNA methylation and the developing brain structure, kindle the alcohol craving in subsequent generations (Bond et al., 1976, Mead et al., 2014). The biology of Addiction, specifically alcohol, is mediated by prenatal alcohol exposure modulating the neurotransmitters in the mesolimbic dopaminergic, which in turn impacts the developing nucleus accumbens (Carelli et al., 2004).
b) The teratogenic effect of alcohol continues to be the central core to NDPAE or FASD, but scientists and clinicians are beginning to see and acknowledge the transgenerational nature of this teratogenic, epigenetic condition.
   The studies on epigenetics continue unabated, revealing new potential transgenerational mechanisms of transmission of NDPAE. (Haycock 2009, Chudley 2010).
c) One problem elucidated has been the tendency for most studies to be done on males nor females (Lussier et al., 2017), but this does not negate specific issues, such as the male germ line transmitting the fetal alcohol effect on hypothalamic propiomelonocortin (Govorko et al., 2012).
d) Previous studies have shown that prenatal alcohol's impact on reducing retinoic acid synthesis could be one method of developing the dysmorphic neurodevelopmental disorder Fetal Alcohol Syndrome itself (Deltour et al., 1996).
e) The father's role is often misunderstood. Therefore, a binge alcohol drinking father at the time of conception does not cause a teratogenic effect on the developing fetus. Alcohol effect is on the male spermatozoa and mRNA which contributes to impaired protein synthesis. It is probably no accident that nature created blighted ovum's in pregnancies with high exposure to both male and female alcohol drinking as the additive effects of alcohol on the developing fetus can compromise the progress of the pregnancy.

A controversial concept (suggested to me by First Nations communities many years ago) relates to the transgenerational transfer of NDPAE phenotypic traits through a birth father who has been diagnosed with NDPAE, does not drink alcohol, and a birth mother who does not drink alcohol in pregnancy. In this situation clinical observation has noted the clear traits of ADHD or ASD which are NDPAE, not familial related, which appear in the new born infant. Food for further thought along the transgenerational alcohol pathway.

Biomarkers of Alcohol Use in Pregnancy

Continued research in this area is expanding and becoming tentatively incorporated into clinical practice.

Further research is pursuing the feasibility of fatty acid esterase in meconium as a marker for alcohol exposure in pregnancy, including detection and quantification of ethyl glucuride in placental tissue and placental perfusate (Matlow et al., 2012, Peterson et al., 2008).

However, newer areas are opening such as the quantification of micro RNAS and their role in brain de elopement when compromised by prenatal exposure to alcohol (Miranda et al., 2012).

More detailed brain imaging techniques are beginning to identify areas of the brain which are central to level, of emotional responsivity. Research which is not just relevant for Bipolar Disorder but as well NDPAE (Ladouceur 2012).

Chapter 6

WHERE DO YOU BEGIN IN THE DIAGNOSTIC PROCESS? THAT'S THE QUESTION!

It is no mean feat to recognize the width and breathe of the transgenerational alcohol problem. The first stage is to decide at what clinical point you can begin to identify, diagnose and begin a holistic management plan?

INFANTS AND FAMILIES

The 'at risk' infant comes from an at risk pregnancy, and will continue to be a clinical challenge until there is a more consistent monitoring of substance use in pregnancy, but more especially alcohol. There is a current reluctance in countries such as the UK or Ireland to ask pregnant mothers about alcohol use in pregnancy as this is seen as policing them. In Ireland unfortunately an infant can be delivered with little or no antenatal care and little or no post-natal follow up when there is a clear history of alcohol abuse or addiction in the pregnant mother but for some reason the infant is not identified as 'at risk'.

In these cases the risk is two-fold:

a) Organic brain dysfunction as well as physical birth defects due to prenatal alcohol exposure.
b) The probability of entering a toxic and possibly violent rearing environment.

The disconnection between the obstetric services, public health, social service and addiction services are critical factors in the continuation of brain damaged infants entering the world only to be further traumatized in the world that they enter.

A scenario develops whereby the infant is abandoned or comes into the social service arena because of neglect and has to be placed in emergency foster care. It is not long before a new foster career is involved and the label 'attachment disorder' becomes the working hypothesis with the memory of toxic exposure to the fetus in pregnancy being lost.

Prenatal alcohol exposure does not necessarily lead to prematurity. It can cause intra uterine growth retardation and many studies have shown increased miscarriage and spontaneous abortion. Recent studies of women with in vitro fertilization have highlighted the level of emotional distress in these pregnant women which includes a certain level of alcohol abuse. Sadly this will have an untoward effect on the developing fetus that has been so long expected. Personally I have diagnosed Fetal Alcohol Syndrome in a number of children born after in vitro fertilization with, as one can imagine, the doubly devastating effect. Alcohol use in pregnancy continues to be a subject of much disinformation. However if you talked with a mother or father of a child with dysmorphic ARND or FAS after a little alcohol in pregnancy, maybe you would not be as cavalier about alcohol's obvious *uncertain* safety in low amounts. (Laufer et al., 2013, 2013a).

There has been a clinical conundrum since the initial descriptions of Fetal Alcohol Syndrome. The emphasis on facial dysmorphology skewed the early diagnosticians to pursue this as the 'sine qua non', and the pervasive and much more relevant neurodevelopmental disorder was relegated to a lesser category of Fetal Alcohol Effects a lesser condition which merited little attention or clinical interest, as it was too vague. Needless to say the neurodevelopmental disorder remained in limbo and attracted very little if any interest from pediatricians, psychiatrists or neurologists. In truth the Alcohol Related Neurodevelopmental Disorder, dysmorphic type, or non dysmorphic type are the conceptual developmental psychiatric frames of the phenotype of ARND.

This being said it does not in any way remove the continuing conundrum over developmental psychiatric diagnosis in ARND. (See chapter on Ethics).

There has been a host of research measuring the physical manifestations of ARND (i.e., 2-D and 3-D facial modeling, brain imaging), itemizing neuropsychological deficits, and continuing research trying to identify clinically useful biomarkers of alcohol use in pregnancy. However, relatively little effort has focused on refining diagnostics, the developmental psychiatric diagnostic assessment of the co-occurring psychiatric conditions that frequently mask the ARND.

The diagnostic process for ARND is hampered as well by history of alcohol related problems. The 50 year or so history of Children of Alcoholics (COA) or Adult Children of Alcoholics (ACOA) has degraded the complex learning and behavioral/psychiatric problems in these children and young adults as being solely due to their chaotic home environments. The COA or ACOA present symptoms which are merely reflections of the chaotic environments in which they were reared. They are insecurely attached and so emotionally upset and they are exposed to domestic violence and so have early onset PTSD. A coded social class laden message that it is only heavy drinking alcoholics have problem children and it is the home environment of the addicted, neglectful alcoholic that is the root source of the child's clinical problems. The fact is that you do not have to be an alcoholic or live a marginal life just above the poverty line to have an alcohol effected child. No wonder countries such as Ireland are frozen in the 'stigma' of the condition. As ARND means that "you, the birth mother, are a severe alcoholic''. Thus the diagnosis is avoided for fear of a derogatory label, or stain, that does not by any means run true.

> In many ways the absence of physical dysmorphic features has reduced ARND to a 'non condition' or a 'Not It' condition.

The continued minimization and lack of understanding of this unique Alcohol Related Neurodevelopmental Disorder relegates many patients to labels such as Oppositional Defiant Disorder', Antisocial Personality or Passive Aggressive or Borderline personality disorder. A true 'blaming' of the victim.

The Phenotype of ARND is contained within the 6 Dimensions of the Developmental Psychiatric Disorder frame presented in previous chapter.

This captures the varied clinical Dimensional areas of the Disorder which are played out in the developmental psychiatric arena and developmental disability arena. So the ARND 'masquerades' as recognized conditions, ADHD, ASD, Disruptive Mood Dysregulation Disorder, Social Communication Disorder, Intermittent Explosive Disorder with little credence given to possible etiology.

The general lack of clinical understanding, and in some ways clinical resistance to understanding, was shown recently in a rather chastening study which identified the reluctance of pediatricians to even identify and diagnose the dysmorphic ARND, i.e., FAS The previous 40 or more years of animal and then human research did not seem to have a lasting impact on these specialist clinicians.

One study showed that only 62 percent of pediatricians felt capable and prepared to identify the condition, 50 percent felt prepared to diagnose it, and only 34 percent felt prepared to manage and coordinate the treatment of children with ARND (Gahagan et al., 2006). If you repeated this study in Ireland or the UK what percentage of pediatricians would you hazard a guess would feel comfortable in identifying the dysmorphic ARND, let alone the non dysmorphic ARND. (Orakwue et al., 2012).

Would modern day obstetricians in USA/Canada, UK or Ireland be any more comfortable with acknowledging an 'alcohol at risk pregnancy' and subsequent 'at risk for ARND infant'? Even midwives in the UK have voiced a reluctance to 'police' women in pregnancy and so are not keen to inquire about alcohol use in the pregnant mother.

Could this in one way be a denial of alcohol's transgenerational impact which continues to pass through generations of pregnant women and their prenatal alcohol exposed children?

Thereby one crucial part of the health care delivery system effectively colluding, even if inadvertently, with the lack of acknowledgement of alcohol exposed and effected children. This naturally diminishes an understanding of alcohol's epigenetic and social impact effect, and continues to make ARND basically unchecked, undiagnosed, and so unmonitored.

Among the most common misdiagnoses and co-occurring mental conditions in children with ARND are the following:

- Attention-Deficit/Hyperactivity Disorder
- Reactive Attachment Disorder
- Posttraumatic Stress Disorder
- Intermittent Explosive Disorder
- Major Depressive Disorder (*now in DSM V, Disruptive Mood Dysregulation Disorder)
- Autistic Spectrum Disorder (*now in DSM V Social Communication Disorder)
- Asperger's Disorder
- Generalized Anxiety Disorder
- Separation Anxiety Disorder
- Conduct Disorder
- Oppositional Defiant Disorder.
- Substance Use disorders (*No acknowledgement of alcohol craving fetal programming risk due to prenatal alcohol exposure)
- Bipolar Disorder, Rapid Cycling

The USA Institute of Medicine book, published in 1996 was helpful but no developmental psychiatric research was suggested or instigated in defining the parameters of ARND and so the minute pursuit of dysmorphological features continued unabated.

In 2004, the diagnostic process for FAS was refined by the Center for Diseases Control (CDC) In the USA which published precise criteria and recommended multidisciplinary assessment. Unfortunately the CDC chose to exclude diagnostic specifications in this publication for conditions that did not meet the full facial and growth criteria for the dysmorphic ARND, namely FAS, and so ARND was diminished and degraded much like the Fetal Alcohol Effects concept mooted by the early dysmorphologists as a sort of secondary 'catch all'. These omissions left the Institute of Medicine publication in 1996 as the only government-endorsed guidelines in the United States that specifically mentioned ARND.

As a well-respected and experienced multi-medical specialty group it was not surprising, as well as most valuable, that the Institute of Medicine also introduced the clinically useful term Alcohol Related Birth Defects, (ARBD). This term, category, acknowledged the widespread and varied physical sequelae of prenatal alcohol on the developing fetus. Therefore ARBD delineated the already proven specific effects of alcohol on the developing heart, eyes, ears, kidney, liver and skeletal systems. This set the stage for an opening up of diagnosis to developmental pediatricians, child psychiatrists and GPs, making it clearly evident that the diagnosis of ARND dysmorphic, i.e., FAS, or ARND non dysmorphic, could be in their purvey and not only the, limited in numbers, super specialized child dysmorphologists. It was common sense that a physician would be necessary to assess the physical manifestations of ARND (including structural brain damage and associated neurological dysfunction as well as facial abnormalities and growth deficit). This medical triage approach would begin a standard differential diagnostic hierarchy of conditions, ruling out other medical or genetic diagnostic possibilities. The added complexities of prenatal alcohol on neurodevelopment and neurocognition would necessitate the recruitment of psychiatric or mental health expertise trained in the diagnosis and investigation of central nervous system dysfunction (i.e., the lasting functional deficits).

Later in Canada another set of guidelines was published in 2005 (Chudley et al., 2005), but again the developmental psychiatric component to ARND was minimized. Although multidisciplinary team assessments were advocated for diagnosis the developmental psychiatric essence of the ARND remained essentially concealed, and this document served to perpetuate the continued removal of ARND from psychiatric diagnosis and management. The Canadian document basically ignored the specter of transgenerational alcohol abuse/addiction, at the heart of ARND, or, in many ways worse, reduced management to simple platitudes about the need to prevent alcohol addiction in general. No mean task….

At the moment both the USA and Canada, influencing Australia and the UK, continue to propagate a diagnostic process skewed to physical/dysmorphology and quite inconsistent on the developmental psychiatric side of the ARND. As yet, no medical specialty has taken a clear role in coupling diagnosis with management and stepping into the murky area of trans-generational alcohol abuse wherein ARND is embedded. Canada and the USA espouse the multidisciplinary professional management but most of the diagnostic clinics have little if any connection to child or developmental psychiatry for active management. The model seems still to be more of quantifying the disorder driven by the physical dysmorphology presentation rather than function ability or clinical problem presentation. School programs have recognized FAS or ARND as special needs disorders needing specialized education which has been a big positive factor in remediation. Nevertheless the dearth of mental health professionals involved has kept the condition un-quantified regarding morbidity and response to active therapy.

In the UK the British Medical Association produced a guide in 2007. They again were emphasizing the dymorphology and placed management in the realm of the GP and Health Visitor. One flow chart indicated the role of the pediatrician and Child and Adolescent

Mental Health service (CAMHS) but this seemed more discretionary. There is a GP FASD (Fetal Alcohol Spectrum Disorder) Tool kit now available, but again the dysmorphology is the entry point and central emphasis to make this a real medical disorder.

However there are definite winds of change in the UK lead by Dr Raja Mukarjee, Adult Learning Disability Psychiatrist in co-ordination with FASD Trust, NOFAS UK and community pediatrics, a series of expert management strategies have been developed and are in the early stage of dissemination.

In parallel with the medical/psychiatric thrust to management the Education System in the UK has embraced the concept of FASDs, dysmorphic ARND or FAS and non-dysmorphic ARND, and the neurocognitive and psychiatric challenges that these children present within the school system which require a new way of teaching and understanding academic challenges not only based on level of IQ below or over 70. A recent interdisciplinary academic and lay book, Fetal Alcohol Spectrum Disorders, edited by Carpenter, Blackburn and Egerton, 2013, sets the stage for the next phase in educational management.

It is nevertheless a critical issue in the clinical diagnosis of ARND to understand that the severity of the acquired brain injury is not correlated with the presence of facial dysmorphology (and these facial dysmorphic features commonly change significantly in adolescence and adulthood).

Therefore facial features are minimally useful to assess and then to come to treat the neurocognitive and developmental psychiatric problems associated with prenatal alcohol exposure. (Streissguth, et al., 1991; Steinhausen, et al., 1993, Novick Brown et al., 2011, Kodituwakku et al., 2011, O'Malley 2011, Rich & O'Malley 2012).

Two diagnostic treatises are commonly used to communicate diagnostic findings as they relate to Developmental Psychiatric disorders and they had categories that can be used for shoe -horning the diagnosis of ARND, dysmorphic or non dysmorphic:

1. International Classification of Diseases (ICD), published by the World Health Organization. The ICD-10, published in 1992, The *ICD is now in its tenth edition (ICD-10*), lists 'Fetal Alcohol Syndrome' (dysmorphic ARND)' (Q86.0) as a specific medical diagnosis under a section on congenital malformations. Thus, there is no dispute that an, ARND dysmorphic or FAS diagnosis is a medical condition that belongs with other medical conditions on Axis IV in a complete diagnostic formulation.

However, the ICD-10 has no acknowledgement of the far more common ARND. Since both ARND dysmorphic (FAS) and ARND are of course also associated with brain damage and CNS structural, neurological, and functional problems, it is common practice to diagnose these conditions on Axis IV (Physical/neurological problems) as with dysmorphic ARND, namely FAS.

The most prevalent diagnosis in ARND is Hyperkinetic Disorder can be listed on AXIS I with prenatal alcohol exposure as an etiological factor and clinical evidence of ARND dysmorphic or non dysmorphic added to the diagnosis.

ICD 10 does offer the advantage of: AXIS II for specific Learning disabilities and AXIS III for the quantified cognitive Testing WPPSSI or WISC IV to be noted.

This helps bring out the complex learning disability which is NOT just a property of Intellectual Disability i.e., IQ under 70.

This international manual is used for both medical and mental health diagnoses. ICD-10 includes Fetus and newborn affected by maternal use of alcohol (P04.3) but excludes FAS, Dysmorphic ARND (Q86.0)

2. The Diagnostic and Statistical Manual (DSM), published by the American Psychiatric Association and the DSM is now in its fifth edition with a Text Revision (DSM-V), 2013.

It is instructive to reflect on the DSM-IV-TR which immediately precedes the DSM V. It gives an insight into the longstanding non developmental psychiatric view of diagnosis. ARND whether dysmorphic (i.e., FAS) or non dysmorphic were considered are medical conditions. So ARND was not included in the DSM-IV-TR, and since ARND conditions were not listed as psychiatric diagnoses, they were often ignored by child or adult psychiatrists and mental health professionals. Moreover, the symptom presentations of individuals with ARND appear similar to what is seen in a number of psychiatric disorders. Compounding these structural diagnostic category problems was the fact that there was, and is, a high prevalence of psychiatric disorders in the ARND population as well 75 to 80% of the ARND population had an IQ over 70, and so did not fit into the Intellectual Disability or old fashioned Mental Retardation (MR) categories. It was only in the noting of the importance of underlying General Medical Conditions in differential psychiatric diagnosis that the DSM-IV-TR was of some help. Nevertheless, it did not specifically note prenatal alcohol exposure as a general medical condition which could be an etiological possibility for many of the psychiatric disorders associated with ARND. The one exception was except for Learning Disorders. FAS, the leading non-hereditary cause of mental retardation and preventable birth defects, is sequestered away in Appendix G of the DSM-IV TR as a congenital malformation (760.71).

This omission of the psychiatric sequelae of ARND in the DSM IV-TR did not serve the patients or the variety of psychiatric and/or mental health professionals invariably involved with their care, but with no language category to describe what they were seeing. In the USA where health care is governed by health insurance companies, the absence of a DSM IV –TR code (and possibly DSM V Code) meant that many patients continued to be faceless, hidden, or orphaned from society and general and specialist psychiatric care, as the professional treating them would not be reimbursed without a relevant billing/diagnostic code.

It is particularly noteworthy that the DSM-IV-TR's differential diagnostic guidelines omit specific reference to prenatal alcohol exposure as an etiological possibility in 'Cognitive Disorder Not Otherwise Specified (NOS),' which other than learning disorders and Attention-Deficit Hyperactivity Disorder is the condition that best captures some of the core co-occurring psychiatric disorders, often associated with ARND. Thus, the only way to achieve diagnostic clarity with respect to psychiatric disorders, associated with prenatal alcohol exposure is for well-trained diagnosticians to note specifically the underlying medical condition if an ARND has been diagnosed (e.g., Cognitive Disorder NOS, secondary to FAS) or confirmed exposure itself if an ARND has not been diagnosed (e.g., Cognitive Disorder NOS, alcohol exposed). Although the DSM-IV-TR does not provide explicit decision-tree guidelines for each and every psychiatric diagnosis, in the manual, it does clarify a differential diagnosis process to be used prior to making any mental health diagnosis from the DSM-IV-TR when an underlying medical condition may account for the mental health symptoms:

'When a Mental Disorder Due to a General Medical Condition or a Substance-Abuse Induced Disorder is responsible for the symptoms, it preempts the diagnosis of the corresponding primary disorder with the same symptoms' (p.6). So in DSM IV-TR you could say ADHD, Mood Disorder, Intermittent Explosive Disorder due to general medical condition of prenatal alcohol exposure with clinical evidence of ARND, a mouthful! But a code existed so you could be reimbursed. (Kapp & O'Malley 2001, Novick Brown et al., 2011, Rich & O'Malley 2012).

The new classification DSM-V continues to be used solely for mental health diagnoses. The recent introduction of the DSM V psychiatric classification has helped and not helped. A condition Alcohol Related Neurobiological Disorder is introduced (taken from the Dysmorphology, not the neuropsychological or neuropsychiatric worlds), but the 40+ years of animal and human research in prenatal alcohol are considered not sufficient to merit a code diagnosis. There is however a category Neurodevelopmental Disorder with prenatal alcohol exposure, ND-PAE, code 315.8 which can be used. This is much more helpful and places the long term clinical developmental psychiatric legacy of prenatal alcohol in an appropriate frame. Maybe this will offer the opening for scientific research in intervention across the systems of care spectrum which will begin to show the unique clinical trajectory and intertwined transgenerational alcohol use/addiction issues attached to this diagnosis in an infant, child or adolescent.

We are now in the embryonic era of DSM V. Has this helped?

DSM V has not been of much substantive help except in the introduction of two useful co-occurring diagnostic categories:

Disruptive Mood Dysregulation Disorder

Social Communication Disorder.

AND

A Category Neurodevelopmental Disorder, prenatal alcohol exposed (ND. PAE. 315.8)

Both ICD -10 and DSM V are necessary for communicating the complex cognitive deficits and psychiatric conditions associated with ARND but these classification systems present problems with respect to ARND diagnosis because they are out of sync with current thinking in developmental psychiatry and epigenetics.

DSM V makes the situation, one step forward and two steps backward, by introducing a category Intellectual Developmental Disability which harks back to the old the Mental Retardation (MR) days and specifically excludes the 75% or more patients with ARND who have complex developmental psychiatric disorders BUT have IQ over 70.

(DSM IV-TR, 2000, DSM –V, 2013, Novick Brown et al., 2011, O'Malley 2011a,c, Rich & O'Malley 2012, O'Malley 2013).

3. There is nevertheless a not widely known diagnostic system which is eminently useful in ARND.

It is the Diagnostic *Classification of Mental Health and Developmental Disorders of Infancy and Early Childhood (DC: 0-3) (Zero to Three 2005, O'Malley & Streissguth 2006).*

Zero to Three's DC: 0-3 (2005) is an essential validated instrument which can describe the initial presentation of ARND. The three most common presentations of psychiatric disorder in infants or young children with either FAS or ARND come under the 'regulatory disorders of sensory processing' category, and capture quite accurately the range of sensory integration problems caused by the prenatal neurotoxic impact of alcohol. They are:

1) Hypersensitive (subtypes: Type A – fearful/cautious; Type B: negative/defiant)
2) Hyposensitive/underresponsive
3) Sensory stimulation seeking/impulsive.

The Bread and Butter of Clinical Diagnosis Begins with History Taking and the Gathering of Collateral Information:

Therefore a current developmental psychiatric approach to diagnosis in ARND, whether dysmorphic (i.e., FAS) or non dysmorphic ARND.

1) *Review obstetric, birth, history records.*

The initial step in establishing a diagnostic ARND hypothesis is to acquire a detailed drinking and drug use history from every pregnant or recently delivered woman, which is still not routinely done in many places despite the relative ease of adding quick screens to pre- and postnatal examinations. It is important to mention that, while some women may acknowledge cocaine or other drug use, use of drugs seldom occurs without alcohol use as well.

In Ireland it is nigh impossible to obtain an accurate history of alcohol in pregnancy because the mother is 'suspicious' of the question, and the midwife does not want to engender stigma.

Several simple alcohol screening questions measures have been found to be effective, including BARC, TWEAK, and T-ACE, and these should be routinely administered upon admission to delivering women in the USA hospitals, especially in Washington State, which has a long history of acknowledgement of the risks of prenatal alcohol, and much less overt stigma.

2) *Biological Markers*: Although various international scientists are testing biochemical markers for alcohol abuse in pregnancy

- MCV and GGT (first explored by the Institute of Medicine, USA, in 1996 book. (Need folate levels and in Ireland only 1 blood test done in pregnancy, Iron, so another one would arouse anxiety in the pregnant mothers. May have utility in the UK, NHS system however.).
- Fatty Acid Ethyl Esterase (FAEE) in meconium, (always controversial. Is it either early or late meconium that is the best marker?)
- acetaldehyde adduct in the mother's blood, (initial studies not replicated)
- fetal movement (too nonspecific with too many confounding variables, stress, diet, heat, cold etc.).
- Cranial ultrasound, (not sensitive enough, but can identify structural anomalies in corpus callosum, cerebellum and hippocampus),

No definitive marker has yet been established. (Dreosti 1993, Bearer et al., 1991, O'Malley 2008, Novick Brown et al., 2011.

1. In addition, *Genetic testing* in newborns and young infants presenting with dysmorphic and growth features is recommended in cases involving confirmed prenatal alcohol exposure to rule out an ARND. This will eliminate genetic syndrome such as Downs, Fragile X, Velo Cardio Facial, Noonan's to mention just a few.

2. Review of early developmental problems in the infant (e.g., poor suck, long latency to suck, coupled with feeding problems, difficult temperament, attachment issues, slow motor development, ht. and wt. growth deficits.

Later in early childhood, records of delayed motor milestones, sensory over or under reactivity, sleep problems, feeding or eating problems, persistent failure to thrive, delayed language development, and childhood medical records, especially public health nurse or health visitor (in UK).

3. School Records at whatever level the child or adolescent is enrolled, including previous school records can be very helpful. The core subjects' achievement levels are particularly useful, i.e., reading, writing, English, mathematics, science, which are essential academic building blocks for a general education.

As well behavioral problems, especially, so called oppositional defiant behavior, school suspension or even school expulsion, as they can highlight academic or social disconnection frustrations.

4. Social Service Care history records. These are critical in the Irish context, as many children with ARND are undiagnosed and because of their range of complex behaviors are passed into different foster home placements as they cannot be managed.

Records also are more likely than the maternity hospital to document maternal alcohol (or drug) use by the birth mother prior to placement.

There as well be other legal issues that may increase concerns about the 'goodness of fit' of the home environment especially any indications of domestic violence, i.e., traffic violations; drunken driving charges, violence charges, alcohol treatment programs) in Ireland the Court appoints a Guardian ad Litem for all children taken into care by the State, and this person is commonly a good early advocate for the infant or young child to receive early diagnostic and early treatment services.

5. Examine for dysmorphic features; facial, hands, teeth in early photographs, or maternity hospital records if available, which are brought to the child psychiatrist, or developmental pediatrician, for complete diagnosis of the Developmental Psychiatric Disorder.

6. Administer, Retrieve or organize standardized age appropriate *Cognitive Testing* i.e., WPPSSI, WISC IV, WIAT II, WRAT. These will give an initial window into the Cognitive Dimension of ARND.

7. Clarify if previous *Language Testing* has been done. The CELF 4 is the most useful for assessing the pragmatics and social use of language. A key to assess the Language Disorder Dimension of the ARND.

8. For children under 5 years of age a formal *Sensory Assessment* using Dunn Sensory Profile or the University of Washington Sensory Profile is essential to quantify the sensory integration issues affecting behavior. This aids the Motor and Sensory Disorder Dimension assessment

9. Often after the clinical examination of the Developmental Psychiatric Disorder, a further assessment of adaptive function assessment could be utilized, i.e., standardized scales such as the Vineland Adaptive Behavior Scale (VABS) or ABAS.

This is very helpful in the holistic prognostic overview of a newly diagnosed patient with ARND. It is also helpful for advocating for school special education services when IQ is normal.

(Streissguth et al., 1996, O'Malley 2008, 20011a, Novick Brown et al., 2011).

Where Do You Begin the Diagnostic Process? That's the Question. An Update. Chapter 6

The intervening 5 years work in Ireland and some in UK has crystallized the necessity for medical clinicians to approach diagnosis with a different lens.

The Principle of Seeing NDPAE (or FASD) as Part of a Transgenerational Alcohol Problem Is an Essential Starting Point

This means that the traditional medical silos of child medicine and adult medicine are not good enough. There needs to be an implicit acknowledgement that the clinician must intervene with the birth mother at the same time as diagnosing and treating the affected infant/child with NDPAE. Many years of psychiatric consultation practice have taught me that when the state takes a child away from a birth mother who is alcohol –dependent, the first thing she does is to become pregnant again. Thus continuing the cycle of brain injury disadvantage. Sadly, I have been involved with more than one family in which there have been 5 to 8 children born all exposed to alcohol, alcohol brain-injured, and all placed into state care, both in Canada and Ireland.

Therefore, diagnosis and intervention are processes which cut across infant/child & adult medicine, nursing and social service provision.

Women and Alcohol

The steady work of Professor Moira Plant in Edinburgh has shone a constant light on the importance of trying to understand the seminal area of woman and alcohol.

Gender and global health issues are an essential avenue of research (Hawkes 2013, Mc Hugh et al., 2014, Plant 1987, 2018).

It has been shown that the rate of 'drunkenness 'is about the same in girls as in boys, confounding many common on beliefs. Other studies have unraveled the increasing rates of alcohol/substance abuse in women as reflecting social shifts in females with economic empowerment, as well as marketing practices. (Hibeil et al., 2009, Darlington et al., 2011).

The continued prevalence of transgenerational NDPAE is not social-class related, but crosses both social classes, ethnic and cultural groups. Over 50 years of research has shown that there is no safe amount of alcohol in pregnancy, no threshold level to alcohol for risk, and binge drinking is the most destructive type of alcohol consumption achieving the highest blood alcohol concentrations in a short period of time.

These Facts Remain Despite the Alcohol Industry Generated 'Fake News'

The role of women in alcohol is further complicated by the plethora of alcohol disinformation. Thus, some women drink during pregnancy as they feel that alcohol has no effect on the developing fetus. The other subtle issue relates to solid feminist values, in which 'a woman's body is her sole responsibility, and so she has the right to do with it what she desires'. Telling women not to drink alcohol in pregnancy is seen as 'patriarchal/controlling', and so not valid information.

As it turns out the infant exposed to alcohol during pregnancy becomes the child and adolescent with a complex neurological and neurodevelopmental acquired brain injury, called Neurodevelopmental Disorder Prenatal Alcohol Exposure. (NDPAE).

More recently a book by Ann Dorset Johnston (2013) has analyzed the new alcoholic woman. She sites examples such as entitlement, empowerment, or as she says "the modern woman's steroid, enabling her to wear her many hats in life."

a) The book gives facts such as the lowered alcohol dehydrogenase metabolism enzyme in women which leads to higher blood levels of alcohol because of lower metabolism.
b) She also states that excessive drinking in women is the 3rd leading cause of death in the USA. Of the 23,00 female deaths, more than 50% are related to binge alcohol drinking.
c) Finally, she quotes statistics which attest to the fact that alcohol-dependent women are 4.8 times more likely to have shorter lives. On average, she states, alcohol – dependent women lived 20 years shorter than non-alcohol-dependent women. This is quite consistent with recent research highlighting this self-destructive behavior, in which the birth of a child with NDPAE is a marker for premature death in the birth mother due to alcohol related medical conditions (Owens and O'Malley 2018).

Sobering Thoughts

Interestingly, Johnston does not mention the new generations of women who continue to drink alcohol, during pregnancy, and beget the future alcohol brain- injured children with NDPAE. now disguised as atypical ADHD, or atypical ASD.

TV Comedy shows such as Catastrophe, British TV since 2015 and Working Moms, Canada since 2017celebrate the emancipation of women through alcohol, and negative story lines about the risks of transgenerational alcohol are not convenient. However, there are new stories which are beginning to offer 'news of difference' (to use a Michael White term), such as the recent book 'We are the luckiest. The surprising magic of sober life' (Mc Kowen, USA, 2020).

The Importance of the Mother/Infant Dyad

The intervening 5 years has made it clearer that the mother/infant, mother/child dyad relationship is the key nodal point for diagnosis and management.

The impact of development psychopathology in the parent is a key issue in assessing the clinical risk/impact to the developing infant/child. Astley, Clarren and colleagues in Seattle were among the first to acknowledge the vulnerabilities and psychopathology in birth parents of children with dysmorphic FAS (Astley et al. 2000).

Continued Research has highlighted factors in the birth mother such as:

- Parental substance abuse./alcohol
- Parental mental illness, bipolar disorder, depression
- Parental developmental disorder,
- Exposure to domestic physical abuse, sexual abuse or neglect, in both parent's life and child's life
- Disruption in state care-providers lives i.e., foster parents
- Multiple care/residential placements

(O'Malley 2003, Kannabiran et al., 2007, Rasmussen et al., 2012).

This acknowledges the presence of Perinatal Psychiatry which is generally orientated to the psychiatric/psychological well –being of the mother post-delivery with postpartum depression a major concern. However, in the NDPAE population the concerns are more complex and incorporate psychiatric, developmental and addictive disorder challenges to parenting. Neonatology has a key role.

Furthermore, the impact of developmental psychopathology on family and child health and developmental trajectory is being studied in different populations i.e., Parental Depression Parental Bipolar Disorder. (Beardslee 2019, Shalev et al. 2019).

The Essence of Medical/Psychiatric Assessment of the Alcohol-Affected Individual Outlined in the 2014 Book Has Not Changed

However, there are newer approaches being developed described internationally.

(Burd 2012, Ellsoff 2014, Hagan et al., 2015, Olson 2015, Cook et al., 2016, SIGN 2019)

There is still, unfortunately, a schism in diagnostic formulation and assessment which continues to hamper progress in the field, and impairs scientific research on measured therapeutic approaches.

a) The legacy of teratology research and dysmorphology still validates the minute pursuit of facial features as an entry to diagnosis and spawns the diagnostic term Fetal Alcohol Spectrum Disorder, singular, which is predicated on the presence or absence of facial features. Now expensive facial recognition technology increases exponentially, but one wonders what true help has this technology been to individuals suffering the acquired brain injury caused by prenatal alcohol exposure. The sophisticated facial recognition technology belongs in tertiary care centers, and not in the average hospital or medical community. (witness the complete lack of progress in intervention research that has resulted in the use of this technology to map prevalence of the condition in the Western Cape population of South Africa).

   It is important to recognize that only 10 to 15% of patients with alcohol effect have dysmorphic facial features, and that the face does not tell the clinician about the level of brain injury or complexity of the global neurodevelopmental disorder.

b) The introduction of the diagnosis Neurobehavioral Disorder associated with prenatal alcohol exposure (NDPAE), now in DSM 5, harks to the neurobehavioral profile in animal studies of alcohol teratology, which were mainly limited to behavioral sequelae analysis because of the nature of the subjects studied.

   The broad categories of neurocognitive deficits, self -regulation deficits and adaptive function deficits are too psychologically reductionist, and ignore/minimize the much more complex neurological as well as the global neurodevelopmental legacy of prenatal alcohol exposure.

   Although much recent research has supported the idea of a neurobehavioral disorder as result of prenatal alcohol it is not the whole clinical story. It, as well, undermines response to intervention, especially medication, as it minimizes the alcohol impact of brain neurological function and the multi-organ system global neurodevelopmental disorder legacy. (Coles 2019, Olson 2019).

c) The third diagnostic category Neurodevelopmental Disorder Prenatal Alcohol Exposure, NDPAE, code 315.8, in DSM 5 captures the truer essence of the condition related to prenatal alcohol exposure, which is not face- related, or IQ - related but a global neurodevelopmental disorder encompassing many hidden complex neurological and neuropsychiatric deficits.

   Although as a child neuropsychiatrist I am obviously biased, this diagnosis is the only one with lasting common sense when it comes to clinical understanding and management.

The Continued Problem with the Diagnosis Being Actualized

Neurodevelopmental Disorder Prenatal Alcohol Exposure five years later, unfortunately remains an 'orphan condition', with no medical specialty wanting to take ownership. Logically it belongs in the world of acquired brain injury (not unlike traumatic brain injury), so should reside in the shared world of developmental pediatrics, child psychiatry, child neurology and child neuropsychology.

The role of Obstetrics including Midwifery in which the at- risk birth mothers should be identified. This is not only an identification of a vulnerable mother post-delivery but also a vulnerable infant.

But life is not that simple and the unfortunate bias of the historical dysmorphological and/or genetic diagnostic professionals diminishes the acknowledgement of brain-derived neurological and neuropsychiatric sequelae, and so maintains this diagnostic and ultimately therapeutic void (Nasser 1995).

Of course it does not help that 'NDPAE' also is the signature for the neuro-behavioral disorder.

Nevertheless, just as multi-organ system disorders such as AIDS, tuberculosis, diabetes and syphilis entered into mainstream medicine with following natural positive effects on management and prognosis.

This structural change in approach to diagnosis will, I am sure, change the climate for transgenerational alcohol and NDPAE in particular from the longstanding and still current pervasive therapeutic nihilism.

Chapter 7

THE PHENOTYPE OF ALCOHOL-RELATED NEURODEVELOPMENTAL DISORDER (ARND) (2014)

DEFINITIONS

Fetal Alcohol Spectrum Disorder(s) is an umbrella term used to describe the two conditions arising in the infant, child and, later, adult, resulting from a confirmed range of prenatal alcohol exposure be it acute or chronic or low, high, or binge dose variety. (Streissguth & O'Malley 2000).

There are two diagnostic conditions:

a) The more common (85-90%) Alcohol-Related Neurodevelopmental Disorder, ARND, non dysmorphic.
b) The far less common (10-15%) condition. Alcohol Related Neurodevelopmental Disorder, the facial dysmorphic and growth delay type (also known as Fetal Alcohol Syndrome, FAS)

Historically just as Autistic Spectrum Disorders, the term Fetal Alcohol Spectrum Disorders (FASDs) was introduced, and described, by Streissguth & O'Malley in 2000 as an umbrella term to acknowledge the continuum of complex lifelong neuropsychiatric, cognitive, behavioral, social, language, communication and other multi-sensory deficits attributable to prenatal alcohol exposure. This term FASDs was never intended for use as a clinical diagnosis, as was stated in the Consensus Statement on FASD (April 7, 2004) which was agreed upon by representatives of key agencies in the alcohol research field i.e., National Institute on Alcohol Abuse & Alcoholism (NIAAA), Centers for Disease Control and Prevention (CDC), National Organization on Fetal Alcohol Syndrome (NOFAS),

Substance Abuse and Mental Health Services Administration (SAMHSA), and also included the Center for Substance Abuse Prevention (CSAP), and several FAS scientists).

For the purpose of this book and in the appreciation of the true essence of the effect of prenatal alcohol exposure Alcohol Related Neurodevelopmental Disorder dysmorphic (also Fetal Alcohol Syndrome) and non dysmorphic Alcohol Related Neurodevelopmental Disorder are being use as they unambiguously capture the specific long term problem of fetal exposure in utero to alcohol. Namely a lifelong specific Neurodevelopmental disorder and not only syndrome linked to fleeting physical facial features which tell you very little about the developmental psychiatric disorder.

However it is critical to remember within ARND there are physical sequelae aside from the facial dysmorphology, which are associated with all levels of prenatal alcohol exposure (Stratton et al., 1996). This Alcohol Related Birth Defects (ARBD), as they are called, can occur as early as the first few weeks post conception. Thus, unfortunately before most women know they are pregnant (Sulik, et al., 1981).

Table 9. Alcohol Related Birth Defects (ARBD)

FROM: *ADHD and Fetal Alcohol Spectrum Disorders*, Nova Science Publishers, 2008, O'Malley KD, editor.
EYE: Visual impairment Strabismus Ptsosis Optic nerve hypoplasia Refractive problems, secondary to small eye globes Tortuosity of the retinal arteries
EAR: Conductive hearing loss, secondary to recurrent otitis media Neuro-sensory hearing loss Central auditory processing abnormalities related to acquired brain damage in the brain stem and/or cortical areas which process auditory information
TEETH: orthodontic problems related to mid face developmental abnormalities.
SKELETAL: Clinodactyly Hypoplastic nails Shortened fifth digits Radio-ulnar synostosis Pectus excavatum and pectus carinatum Hemiverebrae Scolosis Kippel-Feil syndrome

HEART: Atrial septal defects Ventricular septal defects Teratology of Fallot Aberrant great vessels
KIDNEY: Aplastic or dysplastic kidneys Horseshoe kidneys Hydronephrosis Hypoplatic kidneys Ureteral duplications

Stratton et al., 1996, Streissguth 1997, Hagerman 1999, Chudley et al., 2005, O'Malley 2008.

The central nervous system (CNS) and the brain structure are the most sensitive and vulnerable structures to the effects of alcohol and can be affected by low, moderate and heavy alcohol use, especially binge drinking, at any point in gestation.

Although not widely appreciated, due a plethora of disinformation from various biased sources, there is no safe amount of alcohol (threshold) during pregnancy and the Surgeon General of the United States currently recommends all childbearing age women to avoid alcohol if there is a potential for pregnancy (US Surgeon General, 2005).

Therefore early, frequent, and/or binge alcohol exposures with moderate to high blood alcohol concentrations can lead to a range of reproductive outcomes including infertility, miscarriage (spontaneous fetal loss), still birth, sudden infant death syndrome, and a wide range of physical and neurodevelopmental (functional) birth defects. Varying degrees of dysmorphic ARND or Fetal Alcohol Syndrome (FAS) may be seen clinically at different ranges and times of exposure.

(Jones & Smith 1973a, b, Streissguth et al., 1987, 1991, Manueffel 1996, Stratton et al., 1996).

Alcohol Related Neurodevelopmental Disorder; it was first described and named by the Institute of Medicine in the USA. (Stratton et al., 1996) and were immediately seen as the neurodevelopmental and functional birth defects that manifest in individuals without the previously named, dysmorphic syndrome, FAS. The Institute of Medicine researchers and clinicians recognized an early need to name and document the many patients exposed to alcohol without the facial features. It is a sound lesson in history repeating itself to read the initial descriptions that the Institute of Medicine delineated. Thus they documented ' ARND can be associated with inattention, poor decision making, impulsivity, processing and working memory issues, other areas of executive dysfunction, mood instability, social communication deficits, and difficulties understanding consequences of their actions.' (Jones & Smith 1973 a.b, Stratton et al., 1996).

Both ARND, dysmorphic (FAS), and ARND, non-dysmorphic conditions can be associated with physical sequelae resulting from alcohol exposure in pregnancy. The Institute of Medicine again in a timely fashion described these physical manifestations collectively as Alcohol Related Birth Defects (ARBD), including abnormalities in the developing eye, ear, teeth, heart, kidney, and skeletal system (Stratton et al., 1996; O'Malley & Streissguth, 2000; Chudley et al., 2005; BMA, 2007). As with the typical dysmorphic ARND (or FAS facial features), ARBD occur in the first 8 weeks of embryonic development (organogenesis). Many of these conditions may not be diagnosed or evident at the time of a patient's psychiatric evaluation (Rich 2005, Streissguth 1997, Nowick Brown et al., 2011).

The major difference thus between dysmorphic ARND (i.e., FAS) and non dysmorphic (ARND) Phenotypes is whether or not the dysmorphic facial features are present. These facial features have been shown to correlate to heavy maternal blood alcohol concentration during the earliest points in gestation (late 3rd week to early 4th week of embryonic development) (Sulik 1981). Many researchers in alcohol teratology have shown that both the dysmorphic facial features and ARBD are due to early embryonic changes, disruptions in cell migration, and cell death (apoptosis).

It is well recognized worldwide that dysmorphic ARND (FAS) is the far less common condition, accounting for only 10 to 15% of the affected infants and children exposed to all levels of alcohol exposure. On the other hand, the non-dysmorphic ARND is known to be the much more common clinical presentation of prenatal alcohol effected infants and children, accounting for 75 to 80% of the effected infants exposed to all levels of alcohol during all trimesters of pregnancy.

While maternal alcohol use is the leading known preventable cause of mental retardation and birth defects, only 20-25% of patients with either dysmorphic ARND (FAS), or non-dysmorphic ARND have a total IQ below 70. In other words, 75 to 80% of patients with ARND are estimated to have an Intellectual Developmental Disorder (See new DSM V), or other CNS impairment (acquired brain injury) but are not mentally retarded (Streissguth et al., 1996; Mukarjee et al., 2006, Nowick Brown et al., 2011). Hence ARND is NOT an Intellectual Disability or mental retardation condition, but show complex Developmental Psychiatric Disorders with impairments in possibly Six Dimensions, motor and sensory, disruptive mood dysregulation, language, cognitive, growth and facial dysmorphology.

The dysmorphic facial appearance of an individual is much less an impact than these multi-Dimensional Disorders namely the deficits caused by the neurotoxic effect of alcohol in utero. Therefore, an individual's level of functioning is affected more by motor and sensory dysregulation, temperament, mood and behavioral regulation, cognitive ability, social communication abilities, social relatedness, and growth delays or failure to thrive, than what his or her face looks like. The dysmorphic presentation of ARND, (FAS) has been shown to be an actual a protective factor as it is a visible, recognizable, sign of a developmental disorder (Streissguth et al., 1996, Streissguth and Kanter 1997, Novick Brown et al., 2011).

Current neuroimaging studies suggest that alcohol exposure may be specific rather than global, as was initially described in post mortem studies, in its teratogenicity, but this is still controversial. This includes specific vulnerability in the cerebellum, basal ganglia, corpus callosum and hippocampus. As well, studies have shown deficits in cognitive functions such as learning and memory, visual-spatial functioning, executive functioning, attention, sequencing, processing and motor control. (Mattson et al., 2011, Nygugen et al., 2013). These functional birth defects are related to the alcohol induced impairment in the brain structure and the central nervous system. Riley et al., have shown that functional birth defects are present in children with moderate to heavy prenatal alcohol exposure, even in absence of characteristic (dysmorphic) facial features (Bookstein et al., 2001, Riley and McGee, 2005, Coles et al., 2011).

The first 35 to 40 years of research in prenatal alcohol exposure has been driven by animal teratology and the pursuit of minute changes in facial dysmorphology as biological markers for the level of prenatal alcohol exposure. Nevertheless, in this new generation of research it is becoming quite clear that it is the acquired central nervous system brain dysfunction that is the kernel of the problem and the subsequent guide to diagnostic understanding and management. It is not the face that tells the clinician about the underlying brain dysfunction but the complex mixture of Developmental Psychiatric Disorders, whether the patient has dysmorphic ARND (FAS), or non dysmorphic ARND. (Novick Brown et al., 2011).

Further work has been done attempting to find some consensus in diagnostic approach, but the skew to dysmorphology to the detriment of developmental psychiatry and psychology continues unabated (Chudley et al., 2005, BMA 2007).

DIMEMSIONAL ASSESSMENT OF ALCOHOL RELATED NEURODEVELOPMENTAL DISORDER

The essence of the clinical understanding of this specific neurodevelopmental disorder lies in the conceptual understanding that 6 separate Dimensions of clinical presentation and function may be affected.

This type of paradigm shift in developmental psychiatric clinical assessment is better able to identify the large numbers of children or adults with ARND who are missed, or fall through the proverbial cracks in diagnostic coding, and so become stuck in a revolving door through child and adult psychiatric outpatient and inpatient services. (Brown et al., 2011).

They are:

1) Motor and/or Sensory Disorder, with developmental coordination problems or sensory integration problems.
2) Disruptive Mood Dysregulation Disorder, with impulsive suicidal risk.
3) Language Disorder, especially alexithymia with impairment in social cognition and social communication.
4) Cognitive Disorder especially executive function and working memory deficits.
5) Facial dysmorphology Disorder.
6) Growth Delay Disorder.

Motor and/or Sensory Disorders

This is the first area of assessing global development in the infant and small child. There is an Assessment of Growing II which is a useful screening tool.

(i). Motor: General developmental milestones are essential details in assessment i.e., time at sitting, crawling, pushing to a standing position, walking, holding head upright.

Gross Motor Examination:

- Establish laterality,
- Right/left discrimination problems,
- Test tandem gait (includes truncal and gait ataxia assessment), with eyes open and closed,
- Do Romberg test, with eyes open and closed,

Test for Balance problems with standing on alternate legs and hopping on alternate feet

Fine Motor Dysfunction:

- Test motor problems in hand grip,
- Fine motor problems in writing, especially pincer grip of pencil,
- Evidence of constructional apraxia, (use bender Gestalt Test)
- Test hand-eye coordination, intentional tremor or pass pointing,
- Test for fine hand tremor at rest.
- Motorically disorganized in the under 5 years age group

(ii). Sensory: abnormal sensation in upper or lower limbs,

- neurosensory hearing loss,
- Abnormal visual, auditory, gustatory, olfactory, or tactile sensations, including hallucination.
- Sometimes decreased sensation on one side of the body,

The sensations tested clinically are:

- light,
- sharp touch,
- vibration sense
- hot
- cold.

Standardized instruments such as Dunn or University of Washington sensory assessment are useful.

It is important to test upper and lower limbs, both right and left side.

Regulatory disorder, Hypersensitive, Under-responsive, Sensory seeking/Impulsive in the under 5 years age group

Sensory integration issues, including hypo or hypersensitivities to noise, touch; proprioceptive stimuli, smells, tastes, and light may all be seen in children prenatally exposed to alcohol.

This may lead to infants and toddlers seeming to be easily agitated, over-stimulated, and over-aroused. The Zero to 3 classifications has a category called Regulatory Disorders which describes the immediate behavioral phenotype presentations of ARND. Obviously these types of presentations are not influenced by the absence of presence of dysmorphology. It is the prenatal exposure to alcohol and its quantity and timing during gestation which are the key.

Adolescents and adults may cope by avoiding or over-reacting in situations or environments which provoke their sensitivities. Adolescents or adults who misread or misunderstand social cues may result in paranoid behaviors, such as over-reactions to the tone of someone's voice or an otherwise harmless look in their direction. This sensory over-reactivity can also be seen in a heightened reaction to people's facial expressions. Therefore the adolescent or young adult is constantly 'on guard' and hyper-vigilant in their social environment.

The sensory functional and perceptual deficits are commonly' hidden' and included in a generic autistic diagnosis frame. However they are fundamental to understanding the acquired brain damage caused by alcohol, which pervades brain structures, neurotransmitters and electrophysiology (Hagerman 1999, O'Malley 2008, O'Malley & Mukarjee 2010).

These infants may have pervasive sleep problems (with disruptions in the sleep/wake cycle, initial insomnia and decreased non REM sleep). As well they can display a whole range of regulatory problems in hyper or hyposensivity to auditory, visual, olfactory, gustatory or tactile stimuli.

As young children, the sensory integration issues involving sensitivity to sounds, environmental noise, lights, fans, easily irritated by voices, loud music, smells, tastes, even touch continue, and are often misunderstood as deliberate defiance.

This is commonly a clinical arena in which so called 'autistic' features are noticed. In other words, the young child with ARND may either seek out tactile stimulation (touch and/or movement) or may, alternatively, be sensitive to touch and/or easily over-aroused by vigorous proprioceptive stimuli (e.g., movement on swings, roller coasters, etc.).

Generally, transition periods are challenges, not unlike autistic children. These children require intensive one-on-one adult attention being unable to self-soothe easily, and having difficulty in free/creative play. However, self-regulation techniques can be taught and guide play therapy has a role in integration of the child's exploration of self-expression.

The motor regulation and co-ordination are critical areas of neurodevelopment often overlooked in psychiatric assessments. Within the framework of ARND this area can become a major clinical problem needing active rehabilitation, traditionally through Occupational Therapists. Many researchers have shown the effect of alcohol on motor development beginning with the early animal studies. Ongoing work continues to analyze the inherited and non-inherited/acquired deficits in conditions such as childhood ataxia (Benini et al., 2012) which is an essential part of the Developmental Co-ordination Disorder seen in ARND.

Case Example:

A 19 year old previously adopted female Caucasian patient presented with a long history of autism and psychotic features. She had been hospitalized a number of times and had needed restraint because of her reactivity to the environment. She had not responded to high doses of SSRIs (which produced increased suicidal thoughts), and to atypicals, especially risperidone which made her more effectively unmanageable. When she was assessed in the community her clear history of sensory reactivity to tactile, olfactory, gustatory, visual and auditory stimuli was unraveled as was her history of significant prenatal alcohol exposure, which had been ignored in previous assessments. A combined multi-modal approach addressing her sensory reactivity combined with low dose buspirione was much more effective and she did not need psychiatric hospitalization. As well she did not present any facial features as adult or as a young child. She had been labeled as having unusual paranoid features but these were really her correct sensitivity to what she perceived as a hostile challenging environment. Her adoptive parents recounted many stories of her oversensitivity to noise, light, fabrics food when she was growing op and just saw her as 'over fussy'.

This dimension includes what has been called '*soft neurological signs*' and will most likely be a prognostic indicator of response to active treatment, especially medication.

Prenatal alcohol exposure can have very disabling outcomes for alcohol-exposed children and their families due to the interaction between psychosocial risk factors (Mukarjee et al., 2006), cognitive deficits, and neuropsychiatric sequelae (O'Malley 2011b,c). In addition to a higher prevalence of chronic exposure to domestic violence, neglect, child abuse.

Disruptive Mood Dysregulation Disorder

a. This is seen in infants and assessed within the frame of Temperament. Temperaments are divided into 3 groups:

- Easy to Settle,
- Slow to warm
- Difficult to settle.

Infants and young children with ARND are more likely to fit into the Slow to Warm or Difficult to Settle categories.

Scientists are recognizing that the autonomic or involuntary (parasympathetic and sympathetic) nervous system is affected by prenatal alcohol exposure.

Regulatory Disorders are prime clinical examples of this effect of prenatal alcohol exposure. The differential infant temperaments reflect the effect of alcohol on the CNS. Thus clinically pediatricians see the predisposition for a Hyporesponsive infant or child, shy, inhibited, cautious and, anxious or Hypersensitive, a dis-inhibited, impulsive, intense infant or child produces a highly mood dysregulated child, having random or easily provoked episodes of frustration, irritability, aggression, and anger.

These Developmental Psychiatric Disorders presenting from infancy reflect the impact of prenatal alcohol on the developing neurotransmitter system. This teratogenic effect on the serotonin, GABA ergic, Glutaminergic and other neurotransmitter systems can lead to anxiety disorders, mood disorders (such as depression), aggression, and possibly later substance abuse.

The neurobiology linking prenatal alcohol exposure to mood dysregulation come from many sources. Alcohol's effect on the serotonin receptor genes (5HTT) as well as the serotonin transporter gene as well as the serotonin receptor 2A gene have all been implicated as having some role connecting fetal development, nurturance, alcohol exposure to later mood disorders. (Uber et al., 2007, Jakela et al., 2007).

Infants and toddlers with ARND can thus present with Regulatory Disorder Type I, II, or III (DC Zero to Three, 2005). This phenomenon is akin to a faulty thermostat which instead of controlling temperature controls emotional and arousal regulation. Thus the patient is unable to adjust their emotional or arousal state appropriately in response to sometimes minor challenges i.e., failure of examination, break up from boyfriend. This can lead to emotional incontinence with uncontrollable crying or laughing, or maybe intermittent unpredictable explosive episodes. As infants and toddlers, they are often temperamentally, difficult to settle or slow to warm, and do not seem to enjoy/bond with their parents, birth, foster or adoptive. Sometimes this is misunderstood as an attachment disorder driven by the parent, whereas it is an attachment disconnection driven by the infant. A different way at looking at the mother/infant dyad.

b. A poorly understood and/or recognized mood dysregulation is what is called 'Emotional Incontinence'. This has been described in children and young adults with traumatic brain injury and the same phenomenon of crying and laughing with no clear precipitant is seen in patients with the acquired brain injury from prenatal exposure to alcohol. It is a quite unsettling for the parent who can sometimes feel that their child or teenager is mocking them or' playing manipulative head games' with them, however the re- frame of understanding and clinical unraveling of the true phenomenon is invariably helpful to the parents and/or caregivers.

c. Another disruptive mood dysregulation component is the presence of 'Incongruity of Affect' which is equally discombobulating for the parent or caregiver. This presents with either 'la belle indifference' or a silly/disconnected affect which complicates the clinical assessment of the mood.

d. Early onset mood instability may herald a true Bipolar Disorder and in the Irish context this is a real issue as there is such a relatively prevalence of mood disorders in Ireland. Thus children with ARND have a double loading for mood dysregulation with genetic vulnerability and acquired neurotoxic disruption of developing neurotransmitters which modulate mood regulation and circadian rhythm.

e. The presence of Impulsivity which is embedded in ARND makes the management and risk in disruptive mood dysregulation seen in ARND much more problematic than with children or teenagers without organic brain dysfunction. Self harm and suicidal gestures need careful assessment as it is the intent mixed with the impulsive risk that informs acute management (Huggins et al., 2008).

f. *The Disruptive Mood Dysregulation category* has recently been identified as a separate disorder in its own right in the new classification update on psychiatric disorders from the American Psychiatric Association, the DSM V. (code 296.99).

It is important to remember that the mood dysregulation seen in ARND is commonly pervasive and not generally amenable to the standard Cognitive Behavioral Therapy techniques (CBT) because of the organic basis of the mood disorder and co-occurring cognitive disconnections in areas such as processing of information and working memory. As well the embedded Impulsivity makes planned decision making coping skills rather redundant in the; 'here and now' of a highly emotive situation in which the patient with

ARND feels immediately overwhelmed and may have social language deficits such as Alexithymia which make verbal communication of the personal distress nigh impossible. It is a case of action speaking louder than words and within the context of self-harm or self-destruction this is obviously a potential risk to be considered.

Unfortunately as CBT has become a panacea for all psychological ailments the noncompliance of an ARND patient with this therapy can often causes problems for therapists. This can lead to a 'blaming' of the patient with subsequent negative labeling such as Oppositional Defiant Disorder or Borderline Personality, or even Passive Aggressive Personality disorder.

Case Example:

A teenage girl was hospitalized for continuing suicidal ideation with different plans and pervasive anxiety. She had ARND with social anxiety, alexithymia and profound mood regulation. The patient did not understand or respond to CBT and became labeled as borderline personality disorder due to noncompliance. The 25 point difference between verbal and performance IQ with processing and working memory deficits were not considered for some reason. The patient was discharged to another institution where she was treated with a more holistic and interpersonal approach, incorporating an understanding of the processing and language communication challenges, and she became perceptibly happier, less anxious and more self-confident.

g. Impulsive suicidal risk is much more challenging in ARND pts as the standard assessments instruments for risk are static instruments which do not capture the dynamic quality of a patient with an underlying mood dysregulation subject to sensory overload, the Beck Depression Inventory, Hamilton Rating Scale, or Piers Harris. These well-known clinical psychiatric and psychological instruments do not capture the volatility, changeability and impulsive nature to this self-destructive risk (Huggins et al. 2008). The secret is to look for the 'intent 'behind the act not the act itself. Too often so called trivial acts i.e., overdose of 6 to 10 tablets or trying to cut wrist with plastic knife are seen as only attention seeking and not evaluated in the social context of the organically brain damaged person's life.

In the situation of an ARND teenager, or even child, we have a critical mix which makes an impulsive response to a traumatic episode all the more likely. In these situations, it is essential to look at the 'intent' behind the self-destructive act rather than the method.

Other examples suffice to clarify the missed opportunity to assess true risk.

1) A young 8 year old boy tried to hang himself by using a coat hanger in the school locker room. The coat hanger bent, as it was only soft metal and he was too heavy. It was dismissed as just a negative attention seeking act in the context of a Reactive Attachment Disorder due to his relationship with his foster mother. The school

changed their approach when they were told that he had ARND and a MRI of the brain showed hypoplasia of the cerebellum.

2) Another example of a 14-year-old boy who tried to hang himself impulsively in a local city park by putting a belt around a small tree branch which snapped. He intended to kill himself because he did not know how to apologies to his mother for running up a drug debt as he was addicted to drugs and alcohol from 11 years of age, and used as an innocent drug fence or mule by the local drug hoods. In this case the local Garda (Police) was sensitive to his plight and knew the teenager had some sort of communication and mood problem and was not just a 'run of the mill' delinquent.

Cognitive disconnections in executive function and planning do not diminish the real risk of suicide, and must always be considered in ARND.

The wider co-morbid Disruptive Mood Dysregulation Disorder ranges from emotional incontinence (with crying or giggling with no clear precipitant) to intermittent explosive episodes sometimes of quite a violent nature (again not always predictable). It is important to note that the impulsive self-harm/suicidal risk in patient with ARND is not necessarily related to level of physical hyperactivity (in ADHD) but the underlying disruptive mood dysregulation. A core language disorder Dimensional impairment, alexithymia, can compound the mood dysregulation. This presents as an inability to express feelings in words or understand feelings in others (i.e., teachers or caregivers).

These children can be rather pejoratively labeled as having 'callous/unemotional' conduct disorder because of their so called emotional disconnection to destructive acts, but this is a misdiagnosis of a complex developmental psychiatric disorder with cognitive and language impairment dimensional roots in tandem with the disruptive mood disorder.

Language Disorder with Deficits in Higher Level Receptive and Expressive Language Abnormalities

This is an area of clinical assessment which is less comfortable for the traditionally trained psychiatrist. Not every patient with receptive language problems or problems in communication has ASD. In fact ASD has in many ways become a 'catch all' in psychiatry for patients who have normal or above normal cognitive functioning but do not seem to understand the social context of situations.

- Formal standardized speech and language testing
- Concepts and following directions i.e., ability to understand spoken directions with increasing complexity and length.
- Recalling sentences especially of increasing length and complexity

- Formulated sentences formulate complex, semantically and grammatically correct spoken sentences
- Word classes i.e., ability to identify relationships between words and explain those relationships
- Understand spoken vocabulary which really is governed by auditory attention and concentration ability

In ARND there is a clinical disconnection between hearing, seeing and generating words, and also between generating words and speaking words.

This is the clinical area in ARND which is the most misunderstood.

The formal testing and speech development of the child indicate normal acquirement of the building blocks of language the grammar, the rudiments, the syntax, but it is the poetry that is missing! The standard analysis of the Child's language done routinely through the standard cognitive tests WPPSSI or WISC IV offering so called verbal IQ do not really get you far in the game but really not much past 2nd base (to use a Baseball or Rounder's culturally sensitive analogy).

The quandary for the psychiatrist or psychologist is to see and hear the child's language in a social dimension. The child with ARND is not uncommonly labeled as Oppositional Defiant Disorder by previous professionals or the school and he/she is seen as sassy or cheeky in the school environment.

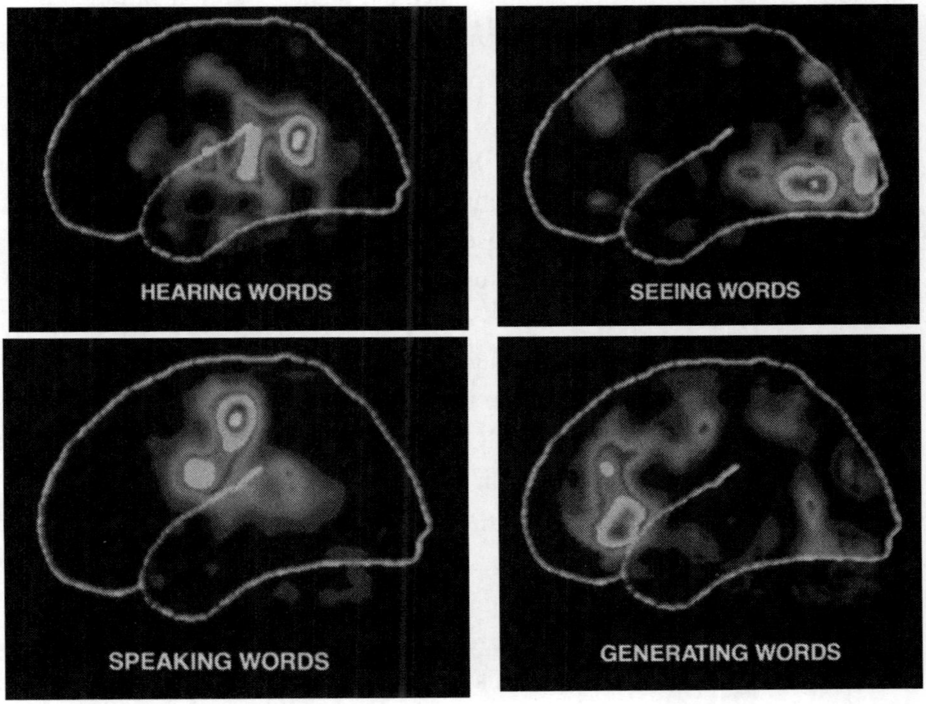

Figure 1. PET SCANS. Permission of Professor Raichle, Washington University School of Medicine.

"His/Her Verbal IQ is at least 80 to 85 so they must know better." Ironically contained within the standard psychological testing are major cues to unravel the unrecognized language disorder. The child's working Memory is at the 1st percentile, the Processing Speed at the 2nd percentile.

Neuropsychology tests add fuel, and information, to the proverbial fire by quantifying executive function deficits. However, in a country such as Ireland where one of the biggest Children's Hospitals in Dublin does not even have 1 neuropsychologist, so you have to use the resources that you have!

What does this mean in the life of a child with ARND?

Well it means they don't remember what they have been taught at the beginning of the class when it comes to the end about 45 minutes later.

It means that they are seen as deliberately slow or avoiding the answer when they have a hard time processing what the actual question means (and that doesn't even include how they process emotional information.)

In essence it is the mixture of a number of well understood and recognized pragmatic language deficits that are the key to assessing and quantifying the language impairment in ARND

They include:

- Sometimes a profound inability to not understand the "gist" of a social situation,
- Subtle, and sometimes unsubtle, impairments in social communication interaction,
- A range of deficits in social cognition,
- the more precise deficits in word and pseudo word decoding and word and sentence recognition,
- the most disabling and in equal measure most misunderstood problems in understanding and expressing emotional feeling i.e., alexithymia. The clinical understanding of the effect of pseudo word decoding and alexithymia in management and understanding is critical to the psychiatrist, psychologist and educator. These children and adolescents can be seen in an 'autistic 'or 'defiant' light but have specific decoding struggles which effect their receptive language). The central alexithymia, (inability to understand others feelings or have words for one's own feelings) irrespective of IQ level is a fundamental clinical construct in FASDs (Greene et al., 1991, Sullivan 2008),
- the ability to confabulate or fill in the blanks can be the most destructive as the children are labeled compulsive liars whereas they are sometimes just attempting to make sense of a no sense situation which they do not fully remember. This is in some ways eerily reminiscent of Wernicke's initial writings in Wernicke's Aphasia related to chronic alcohol usage. It is as if the prenatal alcohol, goes to the same auditory/speech area in utero that it takes many years to achieve as an adult. Unfortunately in the child's situation they enter the world with an inability to

process many of its details and inability to recall these details and recount to various professionals.

To make the clinical assessment of language in ARND even more complex there can be the overlay of traumatic events which have major impacts at many levels on the child. They may, in their PTSD, be seen to 'make up'; stories about other events of victimization which at some level are a cry for help as the child is still traumatized but is unable to fully express this emotional pain due to alexithymia.

In this case the therapist's ability to hear what the behavior is saying is the key to a good trauma centered therapy approach in this ARND child. Whereas the punitive labeling of trouble make or deliberately defiant does no more than punish and restigmatize the victim.

The range of mixed receptive/expressive language impairments are often the heart of the clinical presentation of the developmental psychiatric disorder and, given that 75% or more of patients with ARND have a normal IQ, their communication styles are often misunderstood.

Furthermore, the classic descriptions of this type of presentation were given in Gescwind's 1965 papers, 'Disconnexion syndromes in animals and man'. Here he pointed out the importance of the corpus callosum development in language development and especially social communication. The relevance of Gescwind's original clinical observations was reiterated in an insightful editorial in Brain in 2005, 40 years after the original papers.

The traditional view of language deficits come from the wealth of studies in expressive/articulation problems and the more complicated so called 'receptive' language problems where the person has fundamental problems in the processing of language. These latter deficits were described by Wernicke, as mentioned, as long ago as 1874 in his classic treatise on Sensory Aphasia. It is in this area that patients with ARND truly show their 'autistic type' clinical features. Misuse of language integral to social cognition and communication are quite common problems in adolescents or young adults with ARND. It is important to understand that prenatal alcohol-induced organic brain damage underpins the language deficits. At times, these patients are misdiagnosed with Autistic Spectrum Disorder or Asperger's Disorder.

Now DSM V has come to the rescue! There is a new category, Social Communication Disorder, which aptly captures most of the language impairment integral to understanding ARND. (code 315.39).

It is important to recognize therapy's differing roles as for example the Social Communication Disorder embedded in the ARND does not preclude the fact that medication may engender a positive effect on language functioning, and specifically this very basic social communication. Individuals with ARND suffer from indiscriminate or immature behaviors (e.g., telling inappropriate jokes in the classroom, blurting out what they think of a person even if it is quite insulting, silly or negative). These behavior problems range from silly or irritating socially inappropriate behaviors to sometimes overtly aggressive and even risky behaviors. They can be placed within the ADHD profile of ARND and medication can and does have a positive social communication role in slowly down or even eliminating these inappropriate impulsive language elements.

It is again in this diagnostic arena that the multi –dimensional approach is essential.

The language impairments in ARND are an area of overlap with Autistic Spectrum Disorder (and previously Asperger's Disorder, now for some reason discarded in DSM V). It is not uncommon for patients with ARND to fulfill most of the ADOS criteria, usually missing the stereotypic behaviors, but their etiological history of the autistic type symptoms is rarely considered in either diagnosis or management. (This link between prenatal alcohol exposure and ASD has been made as far back as 1990 by neuropsychologist Jo Nanson in Saskatoon Canada, and extensively examined and reviewed by Mukarjee et al., 2010, and O'Malley and Rich 2013).

Case Examples:

1. This is the clinical arena where the divergence between the classic presentations of Autism Spectrum Disorder and Asperger's Disorder are seen, and understanding a possible epigenetic etiology of prenatal alcohol exposure offers a way to untangle the different etiological routes to these syndromes.

Thus the clinical natural history of the two disorders is instructive. ARND begins at birth and can be seen in infancy. The Mental Health Classification system, Zero to three (DC 0-3R, 2005) has a diagnostic category of Regulatory Disorders which aptly describes the immediate clinical presentations of dysmorphic FAS or non dysmorphic ARND. It is the category of Regulatory Disorder, under responsive type which is the harbinger of Autism Spectrum Disorder or Asperger's Disorder diagnoses in early childhood. So the classic time presentation of Autism Spectrum Disorder or Asperger's Disorder is different in the ARND population.

The stereotypic movements, flapping, posturing are less commonly part of the ARND presentation. However they present more commonly a Developmental Co-ordination Disorder, part of the Motor and Sensory Dysregulation Dimension which is often diagnosed Dyspraxia in countries such as Ireland.

The essence of the overlapping clinical presentations comes in the expressive and receptive language area. The qualitative impairments in social awareness, social cognition, and social communication are not uncommonly very hard to differentiate whether using clinical assessment by an experienced child psychiatrist or psychologist or using standardized instruments such as ADOS among others. In many countries the ambivalence to accept the true prevalence of ARND (in 100 live births) leads school systems and physicians to 'hide' many ARND children under a Autism Spectrum Disorder or

Asperger's Disorder diagnosis because of this will serve the administrative box for receiving school learning disability services.

In Ireland ARND officially does not exist so the children can only receive services under their variety of Developmental Psychiatric Diagnosis, of which ASD, Asperger's Disorder and ADHD are the most common.

As well there is a special needs category in Ireland Dyslexia and Dyspraxia with no etiology given which has a historical acceptance for special education support in Ireland. (part of the ongoing stigmatization and so avoidance of acknowledging transgenerational alcohol problems).

This school education and diagnostic dilemma situation is nevertheless slowly changing, pioneered in countries such as Canada and the USA. Now the UK are acknowledging that FASDs are the current biggest challenge for teaching as these pupils display complex learning disabilities with co–morbid psychiatric disorders for which there is no regular curriculum (Professor Barry Carpenter UK, 2012, Carpenter, Blackburn, Egerton 2013).

Co-morbid ADHD and ASD seems to be a more frequent issue in the ARND population than the ASD population without a history of prenatal alcohol exposure, and this has critical importance in both understanding and management.

For example a successful medication treatment of pervasive distractibility visual and auditory can have a positive effect on the child's social functioning as he/she can now attend sufficiently to read faces and verbal and nonverbal cues in the ARND population of children seen with social disconnection and often diagnosed on ADOS as ASD.

2. Normal I.Q. 14 year old girl with Atypical Autism had a clinical presentation of ASD and ADD and deteriorated with psychostimulant medication which markedly increased her perseveration.

She responded to low dose liquid fluoxetine, and as her attention problems, especially visual, ameliorated, so her 'autistic' features decreased.

3. Another girl 15 years old, with moderate intellectual functioning and ARND with growth and wt. delay from early childhood, had very debilitating social anxiety triggered by oversensitivity to facial cues. She eventually settled for a while with a GABA ergic agent. (Lyrica, pregabulin), but now needs a specialized therapeutic community placement.

She had a history of many unexplained physical problems which were Alcohol Related Birth Defects, i.e., structural cardiac and renal problems.

Cognitive Disorders Which Are a Mixture of Verbal and Non Verbal Learning Disabilities

The ARND is not a mental retardation or intellectual disability condition as research has shown 75 to 80% of patients with the dysmorphic or non dysmorphic ARND have IQ over 70. (Streissguth et al., 1996). Deficits in IQ were, and should be compared with their biological parents.

It is critical to remember that in some cases not all 6 Dimensions will be effected and sometimes only 2 or 3 dimensions. However generally the core piece to the ARND behavioral phenotype is the level of *cognitive impairment*. This is key to understanding the 'developmental' component to the developmental psychiatric disorder as it presents. The cognitive impairment directly relates to the quantity and quality of brain dysfunction acquired through the exposure of the developing fetal central nervous system to alcohol in pregnancy. Hence the term Developmental Psychiatric Disorder(s) to describe the essence of the ARND Phenotype.

Therefore, brain structural, neurophysiological or neurotransmitter abnormalities belie the cognitive deficits in ARND. These include: working memory deficits, difficulty with executive functioning (organization, concentration, auditory processing, processing speed, and problem solving, attention and impulse control.

It is the disruptions in cognitive functioning that commonly lead to an inability to understand consequences, poor judgment, and limited insight into the origins or the impact of one's behaviors on oneself and others. This generally leads to significant and debilitating deficits in basic day to day functional abilities. The child with ARND therefore, rather than thinking through actions, acts either in a disorganized random manner or often impulsively in a rather naïve or primitive manner (as though driven by basic visceral instinct rather than measured, thought out, intellect).

Central Nervous System (CNS) abnormalities:

I. Structural:
   A. Head circumference (OFC) at or below the 10th percentile adjusted for age and sex. (microcephaly lee than 3rd percentile).
   B. Clinically significant brain abnormalities observable through imaging.
II. Neurological problems not due to a postnatal insult or fever, or other soft neurological signs outside normal limits.

This clinical area would be the link to the former Intellectual Disability (Mental Retardation) research and quantification. Unfortunately, patients with ARND in the main do not have Intellectual Disability. So the cognitive testing comes from a premise of another professional generation where ability was solely linked to IQ level.

These multitudinous cognitive deficits in ARND have been mapped going back over 40 years to primary animal research on cognitive functioning including, memory, distractibility and disorganization. In some ways the science has moved forward in more sophisticated tests and functional brain imaging techniques (fMRI, Spect, PET, Diffusion Tensor) but in other ways there is still a fundamental a lack of understanding of the difference between cognitive ability as itemized in a standard test score and the ability to function in life. This split had been shown in the mid 1990's by Ann Streissguth and colleagues in Seattle and published in 1996. Sadly the new clinical diagnostic bible the DSM V harping back, to Intellectual Disability as a key to Developmental Disorders really shows how the classification is out of sync with the clinical reality of patients with the relatively common and lifelong ARND.

These are well studded and documented areas of cognitive dysfunction in ARND:

- Inability to link cause and effect. A capacity for consequential thinking (cause and effect)) is a key requirement for executive decision making. This is an expectation for adolescents or young adults in the school, work legal system, who have been involved in antisocial and/or violent acts. Unfortunately, due to the neurocognitive deficits associated with ARND, these individuals are often mentally and emotionally disconnected from the consequences of their actions, misread social cues, are easily frustrated and provoked, and are unable to navigate logical decision making. So called 'high functioning 'autistic patients fit this neurocognitive profile and have the added challenge of unexpected response to medication because of unrecognized brain damage (Coles et al., 2009, Kodituwakku et al., 2011, Hosenbucus et al., 2012).
- Problems in visual and auditory attention and comprehension. The commonest part of the behavioral phenotype of ARND is in this area. It is now widely accepted that a certain proportion of patients diagnosed with ADHD have prenatal alcohol exposure as an etiological factor and this has implications for management (O'Malley & Nanson 2002, O'Malley & Storoz 2003, and O'Malley 2008).
- A split between verbal and performance IQ if 12 to 15 points at least is one indirect indicator of the ARND. More commonly the Verbal IQ is higher than Performance giving the illusion that the child is more capable than they actually are. On the other hand if it is the other way it can point to strengths based approach for management in which the practical, 'hands on' skill of the child is incorporated in therapy.
- Distractible with lack of concentration. Again these clinical issues are within ADHD presentation and contribute to the cognitive impairment in ARND. Patients may be visually or auditory distractible and the intersecting of sensory integration problems has a role here.

- Poor working memory. This is probably the most disabling, most minimized and chronic cognitive disability. It pervades everyday life and invites confabulation and risk of scapegoating. It colors life's narratives as the individual missed part of their life's journey due to the inability to recall. This is the arena where thinking differently is essential. Using Gardner's ideas from Multiple Intelligence and placing then in a therapeutic arena. Memory is elusive but can be cued by sights, art work, sounds, smells, music, playing with animals. All non-tradition ideas but showing the need for a new paradigm in managing ARND.
- Impulsivity is seen in the cognitive impairment realm but crosses into the dimensions of Disruptive Mood Dysregulation and Motor and Sensory Dysregulation. It is unpredictable and present from infancy where regulatory Disorder, Hyper responsive type or Sensory Seeking type capture this quality.
- Poor processing speed; this incorporates not just the well-known problem seen with ADHD profile, but also the less well recognized problem of delayed processing of emotional information, which coupled with alexithymia leads to complex reactions to loss or disappointment. Most strikingly death of birth mother when patient is not through mid-teens.
- Mathematics disorder with impairment of executive decision- making. This simple disability has profound effects on functioning. It links to deductive reasoning, logic, decision making, and general organization skills all commonly significantly impaired in ARND. Already Claire Coles and team in USA have shown the benefit of an intervention that specifically targets the mathematics disorder.
- Problems in reading, writing and spelling, these are commonly seen and can fulfill the dyslexia criteria which are still used in Ireland and useful for academic school support. Thus specific learning disorders such as, mathematics disorders, reading disorders (e.g., dyslexia), spelling disorders, (may sometimes be grouped under the collective term of nonverbal learning disabilities, used in USA or Canada).
- Problems in judgment and insight. Again a key area which is influenced by the many cognitive disconnections not just mathematics disorder, but attentional and processing issues and impulsivity.
- It is not an intellectual disability/mental retardation condition as 75-80% of patients with ARND have a normal IQ.
- Self-care is another area of concern which is not only a product of cognitive impairment, IQ, but also with the Dimension of Language Impairment especially in the area of social communication and social cognition. So areas, such as able to care for oneself (e.g., hygiene, meal preparation, scheduling appointments), as an adult manage a household (take on responsibilities for chores, balance a checkbook, organize budget for basic shopping.) and perform other activities of daily living may be limited depending on the extent of a person's ARND.

As well time, homework and money management difficulties lead to multitudes of practical daily living problems. Therefore children with ARND can be seen as willful, lazy and showing clear oppositional defiant features. The level of IQ does not offer a guide to these cognitive issues and often suggests a greater capability than is possible, especially if the verbal IQ is higher than the Performance IQ.

Ann Streissguth's group showed as part of their seminal Secondary Disabilities study when data were obtained on 90 adults who were at least 21 years of age (median age: 26 years) at the time of the study. Their results showed that only seven of these 90 lived independently and without employment problems. Adults with FAE (or non dysmorphic ARND) had as high a rate of Dependent Living as those with FAS, (dysmorphic ARND) despite having generally higher IQ scores. However, those with FAE (non dysmorphic ARND) had a lower rate of Problems with Employment, which the study researchers surmised might reflect their typically higher IQ level. Furthermore, caregivers, when questioned, reported that over 80% of these adults with FAS/FAE (ARND dysmorphic and non-dysmorphic) had difficulty managing money, and over 80% had what the caregivers described as poor judgment. Nearly 80% had difficulty making decisions, approximately 80% had poor organizational skills, and around 55% had trouble with interpersonal relations.

All of these impairments served to show the involvement of deficient executive functioning decision making and highlighted this core executive decision making, disconnection disorder, as the developmental heart of the Developmental Psychiatric Disorder in ARND.

- Primitive or rudimentary self-soothing or self-harm behaviors. It has been observed, as in Severe Intellectual disability, that the group of ARND Patients with low IQ under 70 and so more cognitively impaired may have frequent rudimentary behaviors (skin picking, pica, compulsive self-harm or inappropriate/self-stimulating sexual behaviors). These can be a visceral or primitive expression of emotional distress, not unlike what is seen in nonverbal children with Autistic Spectrum disorder.

These cognitive impairments can be related to a mild, moderate, or binge drinking pattern of prenatal alcohol exposure, with binge drinking generally recognized as the most problematic alcohol exposure. (Streissguth 1997, Coles et al., 1997, O'Malley & Stresissguth 2000, Flak et al., 2013).

The brain abnormalities, structural, neurochemical or neurophysiological underpin the changing behavioral cognitive component to the phenotype of ARND from childhood to adulthood.

These include microcephaly, decreased size or agenesis of corpus callosum, decreased size/volume of cerebellum or hippocampus, change in balance of developing excitatory (Glutamate) and inhibitory (GABA, serotonin) or Complex Partial or Absence Seizures.

The Neuropsychological Findings in ARND

It was the science of physical anomaly teratology which drove the research into the link between prenatal alcohol exposure and effects on the developing fetus. Nevertheless, it was not long before Behavioral Teratology entered the scene and began to formulate phenotype profiles for animals exposed to alcohol with or without the signature facial features.

A classic paper by Driscoll et al., in 1990 compared the animal research findings with the human findings as they applied to behavioral effects of prenatal alcohol (Table 10).

Table 10. Animal research findings compared with the human findings as they applied to behavioral effects of prenatal alcohol

Animals	Humans
Poor state regulation	Poor state regulation
Feeding difficulties	Feeding difficulties
Reduced habituation	Reduced habituation
Lack of inhibition	Lack of inhibition
Reactivity	Reactivity
Physical Hyperactivity	Physical Hyperactivity
Attention problems/distractibility	Attention problems/distractibility
Perseveration	Perseveration
Hearing problems	Hearing problems/neurosensory
Global developmental delay	Global developmental delay
Poor gross/fine motor coordination	Poor gross/fine motor coordination

Later Researchers and academics have replicated and added to the initial findings, Hannigan et al., 1996, 1997, Streissguth & O'Malley 2000, Coles et al., 2009, Kodituwaddu et al., 2011).

It was the association with physical hyperactivity that gave the first clinical breakthrough in sifting out the differential presentation of ARND in childhood. This clinical presentation was invariably seen within the context of a certain level of cognitive functioning.

Key areas have been identified in ARND:

1. Cognitive function has been widely tested and the accepted consensus is that ARND, dysmorphic (FAS) and/or ARND non dysmorphic are not a mental retardation (intellectual disability) conditions as only 20 to 25% of the individuals have IQ lower than 70.

2. Difficulty linking cause and effect is a central deficit.
3. Poor working memory.
4. Marked discrepancy between verbal and performance IQ frequently exceeding 12 to 15 points
5. Limited capacity for abstraction
6. Executive function deficits

Many psychologists in Canada and the USA in particular have teased out the neurodevelopmental profile and clearly shown that the presence of facial dysmorphology has no bearing on the psychological profile.

Patients with ARND do not fit into the well-known neuropsychiatric test batteries long used in patients with organic brain dysfunction i.e., Halsted Reitan or Luria Nebraska. Instead a more specific but varied group of tests have proved to be if value.

Information Processing
WPPSI, young child
WISC IV, child/adolescent
WIAS, Adult
WIAT II
WRAT

General Brain Dysfunction
Trail making Test
Rey Ooestterich Complete figure
Bender Gestalt Test

Executive Functioning
Wisconsin card Sorting test
Stroop Color Word test
Consonant Trigram test
Ruff's Figural Fluency test
Behavior Rating Inventory of Executive Functioning (BRIEF) test

Attention and Concentration Tests
Continuous Performance test
Attention Process Training
Tailland Letter Cancellation Test
Stepping Stone Maze
California Verbal Learning Test.

The following references are a broad overview of the neuropsychological deficits in children and adolescents and adult with ARND whether dysmorphic (FAS) or non dysmorphic. They are primarily based in Canada and the USA which have the longest history of clinical assessment work in this population of patients.

(Connor 2004, Stratton et al., 1996, Streissguth 1997, Mattson 1999, Streissguth & O'Malley 2000, Carmichael Olson et al., 1998, Mattson et al., 2001, Riley et al., 2005, Coles, Kerns, Rasmussen et al., 2007, British Medical Association 2007, Mc Gee et al., 2008, O'Malley 2008, Coles 2009, O'Malley & Rich 2012, Mantha et al., 2013, Treit et al., 2013, Flak et al., 2013, Carpenter et al., (UK) 2013).

Characteristic Pattern of Facial Disorder Anomalies

This is the specific dysmorphic phenotype of ARND, called FAS, and requires documentation of all of the following clinical features. This is by far the less common presentation (10 to 15%) of the neurodevelopmental disorder related to prenatal alcohol exposure.

There may, or may not, have a clear history of documented maternal alcohol use in pregnancy;(if the Facial features are present then the diagnosis can include FAS facial dysmorphic phenotype without clear history of alcohol exposure, not uncommon in adoptees from countries from places such as Russia or Romania).

Dysmorphic facial features based on racial norms (including all of the following: small palpebral fissures at or below 10th percentile, smooth philtrum, thin vermillion border) – this requires a physician with an understanding and training in measurement of the facial dysmorphology features

Characteristic pattern of facial abnormalities that include features such as:

- short palpebral fissures and abnormalities in the premaxillary zone,
- flat upper lip,
- flattened philtrum,
- and flat midface.

This has been the pursuit of dysmorphologists and to a lesser extent geneticist for the last 40 years. But in truth it is a clinical identifying entry into only 10 to 15% of patients with the neurodevelopmental disorder associated with prenatal alcohol exposure.

The complete facial abnormalities are only present in ARND, dysmorphic, or fetal alcohol syndrome as historically known. (Jones and Smith 1973, Stratton et al., 1996).

Remember complete facial abnormalities are only present in the dysmorphic ARND (or FAS).

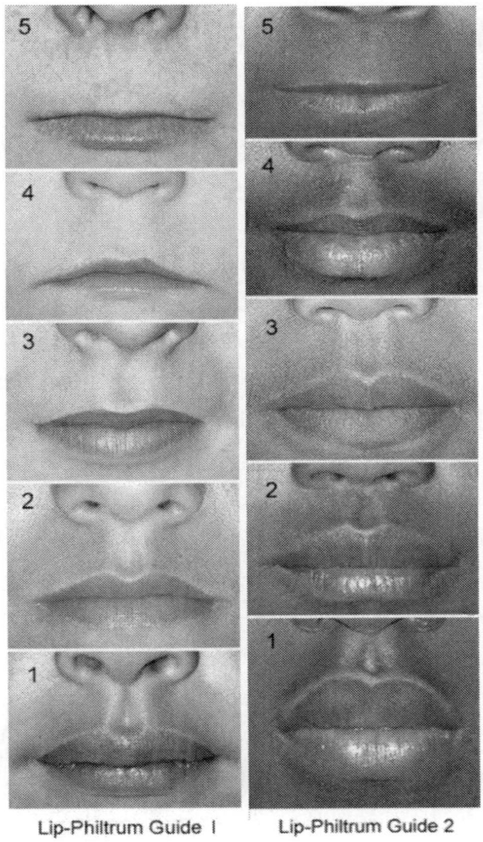

Figure 2. Lip-Philtrum Guides 1 (A) and 2 (B) are used to rank upper lip thinness and philtrum smoothness. The philtrum is the vertical groove between the nose and upper lip. The guides reflect the full range of lip thickness and philtrum depth with Rank 3 representing the population mean. Ranks 4 and 5 reflect the thin lip and smooth philtrum that characterize the FAS facial phenotype. Guide 1 is used for Caucasians and all other races with lips like Caucasians. Guide 2 is used for African Americans and all other races with lips as full as African Americans. Copyright 2014, Susan Astley PhD, University of Washington.

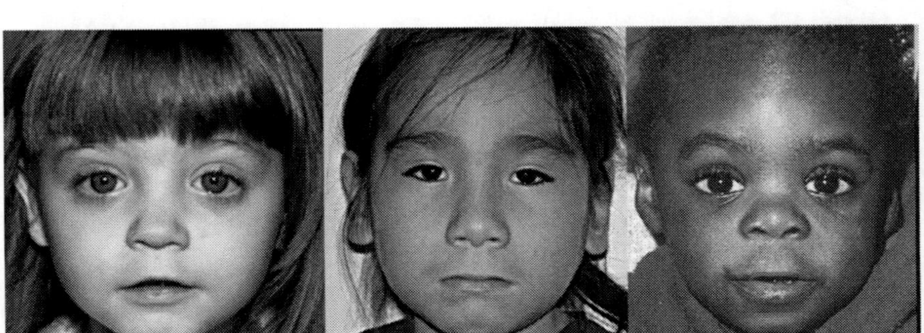

Figure 3. Examples of the FAS facial phenotype (small eyes, smooth philtrum, and thin upper lip) across three races: (A) Caucasian, (B) Native American, (C) African American. Copyright 2014, Susan Astley PhD, University of Washington.

Growth Delay Disorder

This is often seen in the context of Failure to Thrive which has been diagnosed at an early age, including infancy. This is often misunderstood as a product of low birth weight, but it is not. The infants exposed to prenatal alcohol more frequently exhibit a dysmature picture not dissimilar to the diabetic babies. It is the complex neuro-hormonal alcohol induced deficits which relate to the growth delay not a global low birth weight. It is seen in ARND commonly in the context of wt. and ht. below 10th percentile often from birth. It is commonly dismissed as just a reflection of premature birth, but this is not always the case. The Failure to Thrive in ARND is organically based and so 'nurturing treatment' does not necessarily make the infant or young child thrive any faster. Prenatal alcohol affects growth factors in the developing brain including nerve growth factor. Obviously if a birth mother has a history of chronic alcoholism and has poor nutrition with low thiamine, folic acid, iron, glucose and poor liver function then the Failure to Thrive in the infant has two sources needing evaluation and treatment. Transgenerational low folate has been recently identified as one marker for the transgenerational epigenetic effect of alcohol.

The growth and weight delays must take into account factors such as IUGR in pregnancy which may be alcohol related but may also be related to their nutritional or even stress factors. Height and weight should always take into account constitutional factors such as the height and weight of the birth parents. Small parents beget small children. One wonders how much the stereotypic 'Leprechaun' in the Irish mythology and folklore, could be an archetypal representation of transgenerational alcohol in the Irish population.

As well prematurity with subsequent low birth weight less than 5 lbs./2.5 kgs. is a significant factor to incorporate in the diagnostic unraveling of growth height/weight and BMI problems in infants and growing young children. Prenatal alcohol has been shown to increase spontaneous abortions/miscarriages in pregnancy, contribute to blighted ovum's and premature labor and premature birth. (Deirdre Murphy et al., 2011, Coombe).

The criteria include evidence of growth retardation in at least one of the following forms:

a) Low birth weight
b) Decelerating weight over time not due to nutrition
c) Disproportional low weight to height (Ht. and Wt. below tenth percentile) growth retardation, i.e., height and weight below 10th percentile.
d) Growth anomalies

as well as evidence of growth retardations in at least one of the following forms:

a) Low birth weight, not just due to emotional neglect failure to thrive
b) Decelerating weight over time not due to nutrition, or emotional neglect

c) Disproportional low weight to height (Ht. and Wt. below tenth percentile) growth retardation, i.e., height and weight below 10th percentile, not due to neglect.

Intra-uterine growth retardation has been identified in ARND, but far more prevalent is a normal birth weight baby who appears outwardly well, but is not unlike the dysmature babies seen in diabetes where the weight belies the underlying medical and developmental problems.

Here, however, we have the population of infants and young children diagnosed as 'Failure to Thrive' with the spotlight put on parenting and emotional and physical neglect. It is the alcohol effect on the developing fetus that is not seen and has been well documented with effects on nerve growth factor.

Confirmed prenatal or postnatal height or weight, or both, at or below the 10th percentile, documented at any one point in time (adjusted for age, sex, gestational age, and race or ethnicity). Growth problems are integral to the diagnosis of ARND, dysmorphic or FAS, but can be present in varying degrees in patients with ARND. The presence of growth problems can be linked to a diagnosis of Failure to Thrive with organic rather than non-organic/neglect etiology. Therefore prenatal alcohol may effect developing neurotropic growth factor and even growth hormone which underpins this growth development component to the ARND.

The growth features, ht. and wt. below the 10th percentile are core criteria with the facial dysmorphology in the dysmorphic ARND or FAS diagnosis. However frequently the growth delay features are present in ARND without the dysmorphology. Thus the facial dysmorphology does not alone tell you about the brain but it also does not inform you about the growth delay in the ARND.

The Phenotype of ARND, and the resulting Developmental Psychiatric Disorders thus are a mixture of these six Dimensions in varying amounts and varies with the age of the patient.

The only consistent clinical effect that the dysmorphic type of ARND brings to the phenotype is a greater likelihood of earlier recognition. This early recognition does not substantially affect the clinical functional dimensional presentation of the ARND.

Some Phenotypes are Driven by DIMENSION 1.

A 3 year old boy has marked motor and sensory disorder problems, and is quite accident prone. He is sensory seeking and rushes way from his parents in high stimulation areas such as shopping center parking lots, and screams a lot at 3 year old parties with all the party noise. Regulatory disorder, hyper responsive type, diagnosed as early onset ADHD.

A 4 year old boy is seen for assessment of ARND when adopted into a kinship placement home with sister of his birth mother. He had been in one emergency foster home prior from 12 months until 18 months of age prior to his placement with his maternal aunt as his birth mother was still alcohol dependent and could not parent his regulatory problems.

Some are Driven by DIMENSION 2.

Disruptive mood dysregulation with emotional incontinence and unpredictable intermittent explosive episodes (not seizure related|), misdiagnosed as bipolar disorder.

A 6 year old girl with ARND is impossible to manage because of disruptive mood swings with marked emotional incontinence, crying and laughing for no clear reason. She as well has very severe explosive out bursts which seem to have no consistent clear precipitants.

Some are Driven by DIMENSION 3.

Primary language developmental delays with illusion of functioning because of good verbal skills in grammar and syntax, but a fundamental disconnection in the social use of language i.e., the pragmatics of language. Not uncommonly mis-diagnosed as ASD or Asperger's Disorder.

A 10 year old boy with ARND, dysmorphic type (FAS) has been receiving individual play therapy for 3 years at a local UK CAMHS. He has fulfilled the criteria for ASD on the ADOS, but the psychologist remarked on his 'atypical' autism features. One of his unusual features was a pervasive autonomic hyperarousal coupled with physical hyperactivity and significant distractibility.

There have been many clinicians and researchers, who have sought to implicate epigenetic or environmental agents in the etiology of Autism, starting from 1971 child psychiatrist Stella chess and association with Congenital Rubella Syndrome. Alcohol has been associated with a case series of 6 published by Jo Nanson in Saskatoon in 1991. Studies still abound with ever increasing sophistication, MRI findings, serotonin transporter gene correlations, DNA methylation findings. (Fombonne 2002, Dufour-Rainfray et al., 2011.)

Some are Driven by DIMENSION 5.

This is 'the face that launched a thousand dysmorphologists'!

An infant has a clear history of prenatal alcohol exposure and has classic facial features at birth so she is unidentified as at risk for a dysmorphic Alcohol Related Neurodevelopmental Disorder (FAS) by the neonatologist.

Some are Driven by DIMENSION 4. (&6).

Intellectual disability comes in all shapes and sizes. It is not only global intellectual deficits but more frequently significant splits between verbal and performance IQ with core deficits in working memory and processing speed at the heart of the cognitive disorder.

An 18 year old man with ARND, dysmorphic type (FAS) is seen because he has stopped eating. He is gradually losing weight over the last 3 months and keeps changing the foods that he is avoiding. His IQ placed him verbal 1Q 65, Performance IQ 69 (WISC IV). His adult failure to thrive is actually driven by unresolved depressive feelings which he cannot express over the recent suicides of his brother and sister. He responds to liquid fluoxetine, reality based bereavement therapy and vocational support in the community.

A young child who has been taken in to foster care continues to lose wt. and ht. in growth. The initial feeling was it was due to emotional neglect, but the nurturing home environment since 6 months of age invites another hypothesis. The Patient has had a significant history of prenatal alcohol exposure which had been lost in the maternity hospital's records. The boy is assessed and ARND is diagnosed with school problems.

If you combine DIMENSIONS 1 and 4 you can have a girl with dyspraxia and dyslexia in the school system whose history of prenatal alcohol exposure is hidden.

If you combine DIMENSIONS 2 and 3.

You can have a clinical presentation of ADHD with co-occurring Mood Dysregulation Disorder with impulsive suicide risk complicated by alexithymia and the inability to express negative emotions.

If you combine DIMENSIONS 2 and 4 you have disruptive Mood Dysregulation Disorder with cognitive disconnections in coping skills and problem solving in crisis situations, which is compounded by the teenager's emotional dysregulation.

If you combine DIMENSIONS 1, 2 and 4

You can have a 6 year old boy with a history of a Difficult to Settle temperament and Regulatory disorder, Hypersensitive type, who now enters school labeled with severe ADHD, with co-morbid disruptive mood instability and multiple specific learning problems in mathematics, spelling and reading. His IQ is normal, and he has become worse on the Pavlovian methylphenidate prescription, and so the school does not know what to do. He is a Russian adoptive child, well attached to his Irish adoptive parents. They do not have his birth records but they are now going to retrieve them.

The Phenotype of NDPAE. An Update. 2020 (Previously ARND in the Knotted Cord 2014)

The intervening 5 years of continued consultation diagnostic, therapeutic and teaching experience has consolidated my clinical stance to diagnostic approach, as well as broadened its scope to a much greater appreciation of the transgenerational epigenetic, aspect of the condition.

Table 11. The 6 dimensions of NDPAE (previously ARND in the Knotted Cord 2014)

1. Disruption of Motor and Sensory Development

The clinical examination described in 2014 is still valid. Intervening years have produced further evidence of neurological impairment which includes truncal and gait ataxia, co-ordination problems and decreased sensation on one side of the body Prenatal alcohol exposure is reputed to be the commonest cause of acquired Ataxia. (Gill et al., 2018, Rae et al., 2018).
The DSM 5 Diagnostic Classification has a diagnosis which is part of the non –IQ driven, global neurodevelopmental disorder in NDPAE,

Developmental Coordination Disorder, Code 315.4 (F82, ICD 10)

A. The acquisition and execution of coordinated motor skills is substantially below the expected given the individual's chronological age and opportunity for skill learning and use. Difficulties are manifested as clumsiness (e.g., dropping or bumping into objects) as well as slowness and inaccuracy of performance of motor skills (e.g., catching an object, using scissors or cutlery, handwriting, riding a bike, or participating in sports).

B. The motor skills deficit in Criterion A significantly and persistently interferes with activities of daily living appropriate to chronological age (e.g., self-care and self –maintenance) and impacts academic/school productivity, prevocational and vocational activities, leisure and play.

Onset of symptoms is in early developmental period.

The motor skills deficits are not better explained by intellectual disability (intellectual disability disorder) or visual impairment and are not attributable to a neurological condition affecting movement (e.g., cerebral palsy, muscular dystrophy, degenerative disorder).
Witness the amount of children diagnosed with dyspraxia and dyslexia with no etiological criteria.
The other diagnostic category which captures this dimension is in then Zero to Three Classification system,

Regulatory Disorders

- Hypersensitive type,
- Hyposensitive/Under-responsive type
- Sensory-Seeking./Impulsive type

This dimension is also the arena where Seizure Disorder is seen as a neurological sequela of prenatal alcohol not uncommonly kindled by sensory over-reactivity to stimuli.

2. Disruptive Mood Dysregulation Disorder, with impulsive suicidal risk.

The DSM 5 again has a diagnostic code which is often part of the non-IQ global neurodevelopmental disorder, NDPAE.
In this diagnostic category it is important to incorporate the familial loading for Mood Disorder as alcohol dependence/abuse during pregnancy is not uncommonly linked to Mood Disorder or PTSD, with exposure to trauma in the birth mother. Therefore, the child has the epigenetic legacy of alcohol neurotransmitter disruption to the developing brain as well as genetic vulnerability to Mood Disorder.

One of the key factors in making this diagnosis in early childhood is to distinguish from the ubiquitous ADHD or Oppositional Defiant Behavior, which are not uncommonly misdiagnosed in this vulnerable brain- injured group of patients. So this diagnosis has many implications for therapy not the least the potential non- efficacy of stimulants and sequential linear operant conditioning behavioral management which depend on intact memory,
Disruptive Mood Dysregulation Disorder, Code 296.99, DSM 5, (F34.8 ICD 10), criteria include:

A. Severe recurrent temper outbursts manifested verbally (e.g., verbal rages) and/or behaviorally (e.g., physical aggression toward people or property) that are grossly out of proportion in intensity or duration to the situation or provocation.
B. The temper outbursts are inconsistent with developmental level.
C. The temper outbursts occur, on average, three or more times per week.
D. The mood between temper outbursts is persistently irritable or angry most of the day, nearly every day, and is observable by others (e.g., parents, teachers, peers).
E. Criteria A-D have been present for more than 12 months. Through –out that time, the individual has not had a period lasting 3 or more consecutive months without all of the symptoms in criteria A-D.
F. Criteria A and Dare present in at least two or three settings (i.e.at home, at school, with peers) and are severe in at least one of these.
G. The diagnosis should not be made for the first time before age 6 years or after 18 years.
H. By history or observation, the age at onset of Criteria A-E is before 10 years.
I. There has never been a distinct period lasting more than 1 day during which the full symptom criteria, except duration, for a manic or hypomanic episode have been met.

Note: developmentally appropriate mood elevation, such as occurs in the context of a highly positive event or its anticipation should not be considered as a symptom of mania or hypomania.

*This dimension still stands even with the neurological disorder caveat as it is underpinned by the epigenetic effect of alcohol on the developing brain, coupled with familial history of Mood Disorder. My clinical experience over the last 30 years in this area suggests that the diagnosis could be made at 5 years of age in children with NDPAE.

As well the impulsive suicidal risk is a product of this Dimension 2. plus, Language Dimension 3. with alexithymia and Cognitive Dimension 4. with ADHD and cognitive dissonance especially in executive functions such as problem- solving ability.

Table 11. (Continued)

3. Language Disorder, especially alexithymia with impairment in social cognition and social communication
There continues to be much misunderstanding of this Dimension in the diagnosis of NDPAE. as 75% of the total population of those with NDPAE (or FASD) have been shown to have an IQ over 70. Thus it is frequently seen that the patients present with 'the illusion' of good verbal fluidity. The new diagnostic category Social Communication Disorder describes the Language Disorder in NDPAE, and makes the important distinction between this and the overarching Autism which is currently swallowing child psychiatry. Although some researchers and clinicians, myself included, have noted the association but also the critical differences between FASD and Autism or Asperger's Disorder, the truth is the Social Communication Disorder itself which is the clinical source of the communication deficit in NDPAE (Ryan et al., 2006, Mukarjee 2011, O'Malley & Rich., 2013) *Social (Pragmatic) Communication Disorder, Code 315.39, DSM 5, (F80.89, ICD 10), some criteria:* A. Persistent difficulties in the social use of verbal and non-verbal communication as manifested by the following: 1) Deficits in using communication for social purpose, such as greeting or sharing information, in a manner that is appropriate for the social context 2) Impairment of the ability to change communication to match context orb the needs of the listener, such as speaking differently in a classroom than in a playground, talking differently to a child than to an adult, and avoiding use of overly formal language 3) Difficulties following rules for conversation, rephrasing when misunderstood, and knowing how to use verbal and non-verbal signals to regulate interaction. 4) Difficulties understanding what is not explicitly stated (e.g., making inferences) and nonlinear or ambiguous meanings of language (e.g., idioms, humor, metaphors, multiple meanings that depend on the context of the interpretation) B. The deficits result in functional limitations in effective communication, social participation, social relationships, academic achievement, or occupational performance, individually or in combination. C. The onset of the symptoms is in the early developmental period (but deficits may not become fully manifest until social communication demands exceed limited capacities). In the 2014 book The Knotted Cord, the 4 PET scans showed that individuals hear, see, speak and generate words in different pathways of the brain. It is the orchestration of these brain areas working in unison that is essential for normal language development. In NDPAE there is a disconnection between these critical areas, so the spoken, seen and heard word, are severed from their generation. Hence the Social Communication Disorder. Furthermore, the inability to read/understand emotions in others or to generate words for emotions in one self is a specific language deficit in NDPAE, (Alexithymia), as mentioned in the 2014 book. This condition is still not recognized as children are labelled as Oppositional Defiant or adults as Passive Aggressive rather than their language neurodevelopmental deficit being empathetically understood. Finally, the inhibition of the capacity to reflect is often embedded in this social communication and social cognition disorder, but as well the Cognitive Disorder Dimension (Hobson 1993, Monnot et al., 2002, Larsen et al., 2003).

4. Cognitive Disorder especially executive function and working memory deficits.

The basic tenets of understanding the neurocognitive deficits in ARND or NDPAE have not substantially changed in the last 5 years, just become more recognized.

ADHD is the commonest phenotypical presentation of NDPAE and unlike the classical subtypes in DSM 5, NDPAE individuals continue to show an atypical clinical picture of Inattention with Impulsivity. This key dimension includes the non-IQ driven executive function deficits which impair the person's basic functioning throughout life. Problem solving, planning, understanding the gist of a situation, but most destructively the deficits in working memory and processing. In NDPAE the processing is not just of words, letters, numbers but also of emotions and social situations, so the Language Disorder Dimension with the cognitive structural deficits create this core Disconnection Disorder.

5. Growth Development/Delay Disorder

The intervening 5 years since the last book have convinced me that this is a separate Dimension of NDPAE in its own right, and that it is of more clinical importance than the less frequent and also fleeting facial dysmorphology, (which still however have the historical significance).

The concept of "failure to thrive" has been updated to "faltering growth," but the basic clinical tenets remain the same. Height and weight. below the 10th percentile, especially below the 3rd percentile is seen in NDPAE children and adolescents who do not have a history of prematurity and low birth weight.
This growth delay disorder is not just a product of emotional neglect, but a legacy of the epigenetic effect of alcohol on developing systems such as nerve growth factor, brain –derived neurotropic factor, glucose transporter and uptake,
The growth delay/development disorder is not infrequently seen in a patient with NDPAE and no facial dysmorphology. Although it was an essential part of the classic FAS diagnosis with facial features, that condition only occurred in 10 to 15% of those effected by alcohol, and the growth delay problems are much more prevalent and often missed or misunderstood as purely due to poor quality nurturing environment.
This dimension is of critical importance in monitoring response to psychostimulants especially methylphenidate, as poor response to this agent is not uncommon in treatment of the ADHD symptoms and decreased growth hormone is a definite risk in the child the longer the treatment and the higher the dosage used (O'Malley 2008, 2020).

6. Facial Dysmorphology Disorder

In the intervening 5 years the plethora of expensive and cumbersome techniques and also hand held ones to measure, facial configuration has continued to increase exponentially.
However, it is still true that the face, important in the classic FAS, is not an accurate marker for location of brain injury structural, neurophysiological or neurochemical. It also tells the clinician little substantive information about type of management or response to therapy.
Its best value remains that it is a physical marker of the 1st trimester alcohol exposure neurodevelopmental disorder in 10 to 15% of individuals, which is transitory, and needs to be placed in the holistic context of its general importance to the future directions of scientific research in this 'mainly hidden', non-IQ and non –face derived global neurodevelopmental condition.
Unfortunately, the preoccupation with facial pathology harks back to the era of 'FLK', and is currently just as demeaning and stigmatizing to this vulnerable and unappreciated population.
In the de-personalized universe, we now occupy computer-generated facial recognition has become a stamp to validate entry to international corporations or to test or locate potential forensic perpetrators. Both with some dubious conclusions of forensic culpability, and with significant unchartered data protection consequences.

Chapter 8

The Natural History of ARND: A Window into the Future (2014 Book)

The Importance of the Early Nurturing Environment

There is a popular myth that you cannot identify infants with ARND in infancy. This has been driven in the main by the scientific obsession to measure facial dysmorphology as a biological marker for the condition. The common truth is that it is relatively easy to identify 'at risk' infants in infancy. All you need is co-operation from the obstetric, midwifery and neonatal services.

Twenty five years ago I started a FAS assessment clinic in the Child and Family Psychiatric Department of the Glenrose Hospital in Edmonton, Canada, led by Dr Alan Carroll. This hospital was adjacent to a large general hospital The Royal Alexandra Hospital with an obstetric unit that delivered 6,000 to 6, 500 infants a year and also had a large neonatal unit. As chance would have it I had already completed a formal family medicine residency training at that Royal Alexandra Hospital and had been an Attending Staff for 5 years in the Department of Family Medicine. In that capacity I had delivered at least 250 infants. So it was not a problem to approach the Head of Obstetrics, Head of Pediatrics and Head of Neonatal Intensive Care with the news of a new psychiatric assessment clinic which would assess infants and children as young as possible with a clear history of prenatal alcohol exposure. The clinic ran for 5 years, and only closed because the local provincial government cut the funding as too many children under 5 years old were being diagnosed with a chronic neurodevelopmental condition which was too costly to manage. A lesson learned in the 'business' of heath care and the priority infants and children with developmental disability and psychiatric disorder receive in general health care budgeting.

Another twenty five years later working in Ireland as a developmental psychiatrist historically divorced from early pediatric medical liaison it is almost impossible to re-capture that population. But they still exist, and it is the lack of perinatal psychiatry/infant early childhood psychiatry services with no established clinical connections to obstetrics or neonatology that will continue to give credence to the myth that ARND does not appear until you enter school.

All alcohol-exposed infants are subsequently reared in environments that have a modulating effect one way or other on clinical expression of the neurotoxic effects of that exposure.

In particular, a mother who drinks during pregnancy and suffers postpartum depression creates an immediate challenge to parent/infant bonding.

There are multitudinal vulnerabilities and risk factors in the postnatal period and the ensuing Early Childhood developmental time in vulnerabilities impacting on patients with ARND.

1) The pervasive effect of postpartum depression in the birth mother has an immediate and often sustained emotional and neurobiological effect.
2) The specter of multiple early placements in the first 3 years of life has double origins, the difficult to settle temperament of the infant which is an immediate challenge to parenting, and the inability of the birth mother to cope with parenting due to an unresolved addictive disorder, sometimes co-occurring with depressive disorder or even developmental disorder. In the Irish context the entangled influence of transgenerational alcohol dependence roots itself not uncommonly in parents or grandparents who have their own ARND (mostly undiagnosed) which leads to cognitive effect in executive decision making, organization and emotional reactivity. A true recipe for potential chaos when attempting to parent the new generation of ARND. Failure to Thrive became a language to describe the infant with ARND and parental neglect is seen as the culprit, whereas the parent immobilization or cognitive disorganization is missed, and the difficult to settle temperament with sensory reactivity not seen clearly.
3) Reactive Attachment Disorder becomes the 'catch all' for infants from such countries such as Russia or Romania who may be adopted later in life into places such as the UK, Ireland, or USA. These children suffer the effects of early emotional deprivation as well as organic brain damage from their ARND condition. This can lead to challenging, but not untreatable, 'Insecure Attachment' profiles such as Ambivalent Resistant or Avoidant Resistant patterns. Not infrequently, the history of these children's prenatal alcohol exposure is either minimized or not even noted in pre-adoption papers, and only comes to light after placement when behavioral problems emerge. It is important to acknowledge that many children from these environments become very attached to their adoptive or

foster parents. In these situations, especially when the new family environment is protective and nurturing, the challenging behaviors are most likely caused by deficient adaptive, social and executive functioning stemming from the acquired organic brain dysfunction.

4) Unfortunately there are a group of infants and children under 3 years of age who are subjected to direct or indirect violence. These infants are borne into homes with overwhelming alcohol or drug addiction and domestic violence. The infant can incur the rage of a parent or step parent just because of their difficult, reactive nature acquired from the prenatal alcohol exposure.

There is a substantial scientific literature on the effect of traumatic stress on the brain which is more than relevant in diagnosing the full extent of the ARND, and its developmental psychiatric disorders.

Going back over 15 years decreased hippocampal volumes have been described in patients with PTSD compared with matched controls. (Stein et al., 1994, Bremner et al., 1995, Gurvitz et al., 1995, Van der Polk 1995)

Infants born with prenatal exposure to alcohol come from differing social environments that modulates the effects of that exposure.

(i) *Infants born to mothers who are depressed and also drink during pregnancy have vulnerability for psychiatric disorders which begin with an immediate impairment of primary attachment.* This maternal depression may be due to biological/familial inheritability or environmental reasons (such as previous physical or sexual abuse causing PTSD) and should be monitored by a midwives, obstetrician, psychiatric nurse or perinatal psychiatrist (Henshaw et al., 2009).

These infants and young children not only show behavioral and developmental problems related to the organic brain dysfunction from prenatal alcohol, but may enter an emotionally disconnected world due to familial or environmentally caused (i.e., abuse) psychiatric disorder where a parent is emotionally unavailable for active parenting.

Clinical Example 1:

FH was a single Irish/Canadian professional mother who gave birth to her first child AJ, at 34 years of age. Her boyfriend had abandoned her during early pregnancy, and she hid her weekend binge wine drinking from friends and family. Her obstetrician was not aware she was drinking during her pregnancy as assessment of prenatal drinking history was not part of standard clinical inquiry for patients of a certain social class.

Her infant AJ had problems in the neonatal period, and a full neonatal clinical evaluation showed ARND dysmorphic type with classic facial features and growth and developmental delay. AJ had problems feeding and he could not breast feed, due to sucking reflex problems seen in ARND, and had to be bottle feed. FH felt that she was not 'bonded' to AJ. Later, she required hospitalization for acute Postpartum Depression, which included some psychotic features, at 8 weeks post-delivery. AJ went to his maternal grandmother in the same city during the mother's hospitalization. No public health nurse or social worker was involved as the grandmother had taken the acute care of AJ.

FH was managed regularly by an Adult Hospital Psychiatrist after her hospitalization, but had missed a number of appointments in the last 6 months. Also, she did not disclose her return to 'secret' binge drinking at home to her psychiatrist because of the stigma and shame of being called an alcoholic.

As it turned out AJ was taken into emergency care at 2 years of age because the nursery care supervisor complained to social services as the mother had been erratic in picking him up from the nursery and the supervisor suspected that she had smelled of alcohol on some occasions. A few months after the emergency care order an interim care order was obtained and AJ was placed in a foster home because she was deemed to be an unfit mother due to her continuing alcohol abuse. At the time AJ was taken into care FH had been going into work irregularly and was back drinking alone at home. The social service were concerned that her alcohol addiction was placing her child 'at risk'. Her grandmother lived alone and had poor health, and so was unable to help.

The removal of her child precipitated a suicide attempt requiring hospitalization.

Two and a half years later, she was still trying to obtain custody of her child.

The above scenario is more common than one might believe and illustrates the unfortunate disconnect among adult maternity, psychiatric, public health, alcohol counseling and child services in the medical, social service and psychiatric fields. Scales such as the Edinburgh Postpartum Depression Scale are useful, and measures such the Parenting Stress Index may provide a global sense of early parent/infant dyadic problems which are driven by the parent's functioning. (Abidin 2001, Henshaw et al., 2009) Unfortunately, few programs exist that employ advocates who can provide advocacy and supportive services to vulnerable depressed and alcohol abusing pregnant mothers and later to the mother/infant dyad after delivery.

Washington State's Parent Child Assistance Program (PCAP) which was developed in Seattle and replicated in many states in USA and some provinces in Canada is an exception (Grant et al., 2008, 2009). This program uses paraprofessional advocates to form a trusting/nurturing relationship with the substance abusing mother just after she has delivered an alcohol exposed and probably effected infant. The program works for 3 years to help the mother sustain good non- abusive relationships, receive birth control and receive services for her infant/child.

Clinical Example 2:

Another patient, a 29-year-old married UK mother, CD, suffering with a long history of Bipolar Disorder drank heavily throughout all the pregnancy because she had to go off her lithium as it was teratogenic to the fetus and she then became overwhelmed emotionally as the pregnancy progressed. She saw her psychiatric nurse regularly but did not disclose her active drinking.

After her infant girl, ZZ's, birth she was unable to cope with basic parenting. ZZ was diagnosed with ARND and the neonatologist had ordered a cranial ultrasound because of the heavy alcohol exposure to the fetus in pregnancy and the marked difficult to settle temperamental problems at birth. Structural brain anomalies showing decreased cerebellar volume had been identified on neonatal cranial ultrasound. ZZ presented many problems in sensory reactivity. She was hyper responsive to light, sound and especially touch and screamed when upset by these sensory triggers. The mother could not breast feed because of the infant's sensitivity to touch.

However, the neonatologist referred her to a perinatal psychiatrist who explained to her that this was not 'her fault' but rather a recognized neurological consequence of prenatal alcohol exposure and seen in ARND. CD was then actively managed by a combination of the perinatal psychiatrist, neonatologist, public health nurse, and later health visitor. Specialist developmental psychiatric and pediatric consultations were made and ZZ quickly became involved in sensory integration therapy through pediatric OT and the mother CD returned to the psychiatrist and was able to resume her lithium medication which settled her mood swings and gradually she built confidence. Throughout all this traumatic period CD's husband had been consistently supportive and had helped deal with various appointments for mother and infant.

It is in this context that the real risks of postpartum depression within the mother, and its pervasive effect on her immediate nurturing of her infant, were no less of a risk but were lessened by a the combination of services offered which served to form a 'scaffolding' around the mother and infant. Not forgetting an essential component of a supportive spouse.

Clinical Example 3.

JK is a 33 year old Polish married woman who has been suffering from infertility for the last 7 years she has tried to have a child. Her husband's fertility tests were normal. JK had pelvic ultrasound tests which look normal. JK is a steady moderate alcohol, vodka, drinker taking 10 to 14 units a week. She has not disclosed this to her gynecologist and is not aware of a possible the link between alcohol abuse and infertility. JK becomes profoundly depressed but starts a course of IVF.

The 1st treatment is not successful but the 2nd IVF one is. Unfortunately by the time JK has received the good news of her successful pregnancy she has started drinking again because of the stress of the procedure and her returning depression, because she feels she will never be a mother. She does not tell her husband as she drinks at home during the day and she does not tell her obstetrician as she does not think it matters in pregnancy.

She delivers a baby boy LK at 37 weeks gestation. He is under 10th percentile for length and weight at birth although his Apgars are good, 7 at 1 minute and 7 at 5 minutes. A routine pediatric examination reveals Facial features consistent with ARND dysmorphic type, or FAS. The pediatrician chose not to tell the birth mother of his findings because he did not want to upset her.

When LK is 5 years old he is brought to a developmental psychiatrist in referral from a developmental pediatrician because of marked developmental delay and behavioral problems. Unfortunately, LK has core features of ARND, dysmorphic type.

What do you do? What did the parents do?

This is one sad story that is not unique and is told as a warning.

Already a large epidemiological study in Scandinavia of thousands of women receiving IVF treatments has revealed the high prevalence of depression and with it associated self-medication with alcohol.

Sometimes our science and technology removes our ethical sensitivity.

(ii) *There are a group of alcohol-exposed infants who may develop in utero within an intermittently violent, disorganized home setting.* Sometimes this is reflective of the transgenerational socio- cultural legacy of alcohol, which impairs maternal and/or paternal organizational and emotional regulation and attachment abilities.

Clinical Example:

A 7 year old boy JP grows up in a violent home with both parents suffering alcohol addiction.

He was born at 37 weeks gestation and birth weight was below 10th percentile for height and weight as well as head circumference below 2nd percentile at delivery. His mother MP admitted to binge drinking throughout the pregnancy. He was examined by neonatologist in the hospital and was diagnosed Failure to Thrive, with public health to follow up. No mention was made in hospital notes of the prenatal alcohol exposure, and no contact was made with the alcohol counselor then currently involved with the birth mother.

The birth mother, MP herself had been taken into care at 8 years of age as her own birth mother WP was an alcoholic and could not parent her. She was the youngest of 5 children taken into care. The eldest 2 had the same birth father. The youngest 3 had different fathers. At the time MP was taken into care no mention was made of her mother WP's chronic alcohol addiction and probable use during all 5 pregnancies. The reason for placement was one of parental neglect and safety due to mother's inability to meet basic food, clothing and safety needs. WP lived as a single parent with sporadic help from two of her sisters who lived nearby who would take the children over the week- end to let the mother go out drinking. All children, ranging from 11, 10, 9, 8 years to 7 years old (JP) had school failure and the 10 and 11 year olds were already out of school by the time they were taken into care. The 5 were taken into care as a neighbor had called the police because she was aware that all children were left in the house unsupervised over various days. They were all placed in different foster homes.

All the children were eventually examined over the succeeding year and no mention was made of probable exposure to prenatal alcohol. They were all labeled as children of alcoholics (COA) just reflecting the chaos of their home rearing environment. None of the children received any cognitive testing. MP was labeled as Oppositional Defiant Disorder with ADHD and was placed in a school for behavioral problems. She never saw a child psychiatrist. She 'craved alcohol' from an early age and began drinking at 11 years of age. She became pregnant at 16 years of age; the father of her first child was 17 years old. All her 5 children were born in the same inner city maternity hospital, and the midwives in each pregnancy were reluctant to talk to her about her chronic binge drinking as they did not want to upset her. At no stage after delivery was she referred for contraceptive counseling or for postnatal follow up to an alcohol counselor. Her 2 eldest children were documented to have FAS facial features by one pediatric specialist in the hospital, but this information remained in the maternity hospital records, and was not passed on to the public health nurse or local inner city GP.

Now the story returns to JP the 7-year-old boy. At the time of being taken into care MP, his mother, had failed to make her last 3 alcohol counselor sessions and they had removed her from their books for noncompliance. She had recently met a new man who was physically abusive to her and had increased her binge drinking levels. As well her volatile mood changes had increased over the last year. She never had been assessed by an adult psychiatrist.

JP himself had been diagnosed as Failure to Thrive by the local public health nurse at 12 months, but there was no consistent follow–up from the public health or the mother had failed appointments. JP presented as a rather lost child, overcome with sadness and despair. He had major problems in concentration and attention and a WISC IV showed an 18 point split between verbal and performance IQ with verbal 88 and performance 70. He showed many features of social communication disorder with alexithymia and had a marked disruptive mood dysregulation disorder as well. His ht. and wt. were still below 10th percentile and his head circumference at 2nd percentile. At one stage the public health nurse had consulted a doctor and growth hormone was considered but there was no follow up. He is awaiting MRI of the brain and a pediatric endocrinologist consultation. Medication is being considered but only after biochemical tests and MRI results.

This is not a Dickensian story. It is a story of transgenerational alcohol, ARND, current health care complexity in 2013 Ireland. The details change but the story repeats itself. It is told not as unrelenting doom and gloom, but to highlight so many missed transgenerational health, social and alcohol counseling opportunities to attempt to change the natural history course of the transgenerational alcohol devastation.

Some stories are worth re-reading to see wherein the narrative lies an opportunity to intervene and maybe change the transgenerational alcohol trajectory?

This is not about blaming 'present but absent' professionals, but honestly acknowledging how a collective fear of stigma, immobilizes, and can interfere with ethical decision making and communication. It is always easier to blame the victim than the enabler or professional ignorer.

The challenges of a therapeutic connection between adult, addictions, maternity, public health, and social service and child providers is a whole other story!

(Purges 1996, Weitch et al., 2009, Beauchaine et al., 2009, El Sheikh et al., 2009, O'Malley 2011a, 2013)

(iii) *There are other times, however, when it is simply the prevalence of domestic violence*. This is never easy to write about let along acknowledge in the here and now. Trans generational alcohol abuse or drug abuse may be interwoven into this world, but the acquired brain injury due to prenatal alcohol in the infant will be often hidden if the exposure to the domestic violence, either direct or indirect, continues unabated and unrecognized.

Clinical Example:

An infant DS is born to two alcoholic parents. The birth mother AS drinks heavily throughout the pregnancy, and after she comes home with the infant boy the birth father becomes violent to her and physically abuses her on a regular basis when heavily under the influence of alcohol. The maternity hospital has never seen the birth father throughout the pregnancy period. AS does not report the domestic violence to her GP, public health nurse or the police because she is fearful of the consequences. She continues to live in this abusive relationship for the next 4 years with her partner, and the Police are called to her apartment by neighbors on a number of occasions.

In the meantime AS has been unable to cope with her infant son DS, who is very restless, screams daily, is hyper-responsive to noise and light, and becomes very frightened when he sees her partner and especially when he sees Police uniforms. It is only when her partner leaves her apartment and moves to a new city that she is able to have DS assessed. At that time the local CAMHS service is able to elicit acute PTSD features, marked Reactive Attachment Disorder, but as well he has a hidden neurodevelopmental disorder due to alcohol which presented classic facial dysmorphology and delayed height and weight growth and speech development.

(iv) *Prenatal stress coupled with alcohol use in the pregnant mother both have their own emotional and neurochemical sequelae on HPA axis function, which in turn has an impact on fetal brain development, including hippocampal size (Brenmer* et al.*, 1995, Meewise* et al.*, 2009*). The prenatal stress can have varying components, exposure to domestic violence, inability to cope in pregnancy due to chronic addiction, medical complications of pregnancy such as threatened miscarriage, gestational diabetes, anemia, toxaemia.

These are the situations where a referral to a psychiatrist or maybe even the child protection services during pregnancy could be a safety and prophylactic measure for both mother and infant (Henshaw et al., 2009) Additionally, referral to long-term support services for mothers and babies, such as the Parent Child Assistance Program (PCAP), initially started in Seattle, USA (Grant et al., 2008) where a paraprofessional advocate forms a therapeutic alliance with the substance abusing mother has been shown to be effective in safeguarding infants, facilitating appropriate mother/child interactions., and helping the mother to obtain contraception in parallel with alcohol counseling so as to avoid another alcohol effected infant.

A pregnant 18-year-old Caucasian teenager (BD) binge drank during the first and second trimesters of pregnancy. When she entered Adolescent Psychiatric services in mid-pregnancy because she was feeling suicidal and had one serious self-harm cutting episode, she was diagnosed with ARND. BD had a clear history of prenatal alcohol exposure when she was born, with well-documented cognitive testing and school records attesting to a complex learning disability. Her pre-pregnancy personality involved a combination of ADHD and autistic type features that had not responded to individual insight-orientated psychotherapy. She was estranged from the father of her baby, an illegal immigrant who had physically threatened and abused her in early pregnancy. Child protection services were contacted by the consulting Adolescent Psychiatrist, and they obtained a "No Contact Order" and informed the Government Asylum Seeking Agency, which provided information on the father's previous convictions for drug and violence offences in his home country. He was deported, and BD gave birth to an infant with no immediate features of ARND dysmorphic or non-dysmorphic, but with a health care team in support. BD did not know how to measure the milk for infant feeding or how to store it but was trained by the Health Visitor (Public Health Nurse) in these basic mother-baby skills.

Mothers, however, are not the only source of infant, child emotional regulation problems as studies in depressed fathers have shown.

Again Ireland with such a high prevalence of mood disorders has not alone depressed mothers who drink alcohol in, pregnancy, but depressed fathers who drink alcohol as well before, during and after pregnancy.

No wonder the disruptive mood dysregulation seen in ARND is so challenging, as it impinges not alone on maternal parenting skills but as well paternal parenting skills and frustration tolerance (Weitzman et al., 2011).

Further Clarification of the Changing Phenotype of ARND

As the patient ages from infancy through childhood to adolescence and eventually adulthood prenatal alcohol is the primary driving force behind the co-occurring psychiatric diagnoses. However, it is in the infant and early years that the stage of life is set.

Currently in the UK and Ireland infant/child and adolescent psychiatric outpatient (such as CAMHS services) and in patient services manage these patients with the face/mask of a psychiatric disorder but behind this face/mask is the unseen disability of ARND.

The Developmental Psychiatric Disorder phenotype reflects the underlying brain dysfunction which has been well documented, but its expression is obviously modulated by the stress/violence in both the prenatal and postnatal environments.

Several clinical examples illustrate this point:

a) An infant with clear documented prenatal alcohol exposure throughout pregnancy and no exposure to violence in pre or postnatal environment.
THE DIMENSIONAL Presentations of ARND all pertain in varying levels ideally in another time correlated with precise information from the non stigmatized birth mother of the quantity, quality and time of alcohol drinking at each gestational stage in pregnancy.
b) An infant with prenatal alcohol exposure throughout pregnancy but exposed to domestic violence direct and/or indirect in the 1st year of life
Here studies have analyzed the component that the infant's adaptations to various disturbances in early life may actually have a positive/resilience inducing effect rather than the more predictable negative life outcomes. (Giarratano al 2006)
Secondary diagnoses of Reactive Attachment Disorder and early onset PTSD are common. Another disorder is Developmental Trauma Disorder, still looking for a universal voice (Van der Polk et al., 1995).
c) An infant with prenatal alcohol exposure and prenatal exposure to Heroin.
Heroin or methadone in the pregnant mother is becoming a more common issue in urban cityscape of Ireland. It can produce a transitory Neonatal Abstinence Syndrome in the infant due to the withdrawal from the drug exposure. The infant's problems are often put down as this being the only problem and so it is time limited and so needs little post maternity hospital follow-up, the alcohol exposure for some reason is lost in the 'noise' of the heroin, and of course it is more normal.
d) An infant with prenatal alcohol exposure, exposure to domestic violence and removed from birth mother at 6 months of age and placed in a number of foster homes before 4th birthday.
Again the negative impact of the environment cannot be minimized and coupled with the alcohol induced biological vulnerability to stress will increase the likelihood of significant attachment and trauma problems with an inability to form Basic Trust an immediate clinical challenge.

There Are Yet Again Continuing Age Related Shifts in Developmental Psychiatric Disorder Presentations of ARND

Presentation of ARND in childhood is commonly coupled with physical symptoms such as disruptive behavioral problems, chronic headaches, abdominal pain or unspecified pain. These somatic expressions and externalizations are due to the common inability of children with ARND to express their emotional distress in words. For example, in the language disability, alexithymia, patients romanticize their emotional pain and present physical pain as the focus of their distress (Sifneos 1973, Sullivan 2008).

One of the confusing clinical issues in diagnosis and management of ARND is that the developmental psychiatric disorders do not appear at uniform times, but present differently depending on the chronological and mental age of the patient.

According to the Regulatory Disorders guidelines in DC:0-3R (Zero to Three 2005), Sensory Integration problems are identifiable in infancy, while social cognition and communication problems are more easily identified during the toddler years; developmental executive function problems commonly surface in the school setting disguised as multiple psychiatric disorders (e.g., ADHD – commonly the inattention type coupled with impulsivity – disruptive behavior disorder, intermittent explosive disorder, affective instability or ASD, with comorbid complex learning disabilities) that can be quantified on standard cognitive tests such as the Wechsler Preschool and Primary Scale of Intelligence (WPPSI) or WISC (Althoff 2010, Brown 2009, Mukherjee et al., 2008, Nanson 1990, O'Connor 2002, O'Malley 2008, O'Malley and Nanson 2002, Vidal 2012). These developmentally distinct psychiatric disorders form the evolving and shifting behavioral phenotype of infants and children with ARND.

In many ways they reflect changing brain maturation.

Developmental Psychiatric presentations also vary across the age range. This is not unlike the presentation of the dysmorphic ARND (FAS) facial features which are 'fleeting' (i.e., evident in infancy, most obvious from 6 to 12 years of age, but increasingly less identifiable in adolescence or young adulthood).

Thus Regulatory Disorder (hypersensitive type) later becomes diagnosable as ADHD; Regulatory Disorder (hyposensitive type) becomes ASD or mood disorder; and Regulatory Disorder (sensory seeking/impulsive) can become co-occurring ADHD/ASD, (Pervasive Developmental Disorder, PDD).

Recent interest in early onset bipolar disorder (EOBD) in the USA is offering clinical insights into the understanding of the initial psychiatric presentation of dysmorphic or non-dysmorphic ARND (Althoff 2010, Carlson et al., 2009).

In adolescence ADHD can become early alcohol addictive disorder, or mood disorder with impulsive suicide risk (O'Malley 2011a, b, Turk 2007).

As the infant grows older his or her ARND symptoms may be overlooked and misdiagnosed as one or more of these co-occurring disorders:

- For example, in childhood the attention/concentration deficits and physical hyperkinetic activity often associated with ARND is seen and diagnosed by GPs or Pediatricians as Attention-Deficit/Hyperactivity Disorder (ADHD) and treated with standard stimulant medications, (usually methylphenidate) often with only modest or no success.
- Mood Dysregulation Disorder, due to the ARND associated brain dysfunction deficits in self-soothing ability and emotional regulation, may result in a Depressive or Dysthymic Disorder diagnosis that becomes treated with antidepressants and CBT typically with little beneficial result, and sometimes unexplained increased disruptiveness which is explained as deliberate willful defiance.
- A young adult is diagnosed with psychotic disorder but does not respond to anti-psychotics. His developmental history reveals a forgotten diagnosis of ARND in the mid teen years. On closer examination his psychotic features are in fact associated with a deep rooted depressive disorder in which he did not have full words to explain because of long standing alexithymia. He actually has a Major Depressive Disorder with mood incongruent psychotic features and responds quite remarkably to an SSRI alone.

LONGITUDINAL SEQUELAE OF ARND

It was the ground breaking work of Professor Ann Streissguth's group at the University of Washington that really opened the lid and exposed the toxicity of transgenerational ARND, whether dysmorphic or non-dysmorphic. In this study published in 1996, FAE was the term that preceded ARND, and FAS was the same as dysmorphic ARND. The CDC funded study was called a Secondary Disabilities Study, and it followed the natural history of FAS/FAE (or ARND) from childhood to adulthood. The essence of the study was to attempt to capture and quantify the adverse life outcomes that occurred in the lifetime of a patient with ARND. The importance of the early nurturing environment and the importance of early diagnosis, under 6 years became identified quickly as two key protective variables.

There were 415 patients, ranging from young children to young adults, in the study with FAS/FAE (ARND dysmorphic and non-dysmorphic) who were examined with a median IQ = 86, and an IQ range from 29-126. (Streissguth et al., 1996).

The Secondary Disabilities identified and quantified were:

1) Disrupted school experience. which had a lifespan figure of 61%
2) Trouble with the law which had a lifespan figure of 60%
3) Confinement in detention, jail, prison, or a psychiatric or alcohol/drug inpatient setting which had a life time figure of 50%

4) Repeated Inappropriate Sexual Behaviors which had a lifespan figure of 49%
5) Alcohol/drug problems which had a lifespan figure of 35%
6) *Mental health or psychiatric problems which had a lifespan figure of 90% (Attention deficit problems were the most prevalent condition among children and adolescents (60%), while Depression was the most prevalent mental health disorder among adults (52%). (Streissguth et al., 1996, Streissguth & Kanter 1997)

As well and relevant to early nurturing environment was its subsequent disruption with potential toxicity. Streissguth's study showed a marked disruption in the home nurturing environment, and the risk to the biologically vulnerable child in the home environment.

80% were not raised by their biological mothers,

72% were reported to have experienced sexual or physical abuse in their home environments.

Those with dysmorphic ARND or FAS had an average IQ of 78; while their average Composite standard score on the VABS Adaptive Behavior Scale was 61.

A similar discrepancy held for those with non-dysmorphic ARND, or what was previously called FAE:

The average IQ was 90, but average Adaptive Behavior Composite was 67. The Adaptive Behavior Composite score is often a better predictor of life course outcomes than the IQ score. Recent follow-up studies of patients with ARND, dysmorphic or non-dysmorphic, or FASDs in Germany describe adolescents and adults not unlike the USA Seattle sample but they differ in the fact that they show little problems with the Law

This may be due to the stronger social net, and better training programs and living situations that are available for persons with disabilities in Germany than the USA (Nowick Brown et al., 2011).

In one of the first studies of ARND dysmorphic type(FAS) among youth in the criminal justice system, Fast and colleagues 2005, in British Columbia found that 23% could be diagnosed with ARND dysmorphic or non-dysmorphic (or FASD in the Canadian study). Therefore Diane Fast and her colleagues hypothesized that the biological ARND, dysmorphic or non-dysmorphic conditions (i.e., FASD in Canadian terms) should be assessed within the context of the individual's home or community environment.

Streissguth and colleagues also surveyed mothers, parents, or caretakers of the 415 patients with FAS/FAE (i.e., ARND dysmorphic or non- dysmorphic) about a variety of behavioral problems, and by far the most prevalent problems reported (over 90%) were mental health or psychiatric problems. The patients with (ARND dysmorphic or non dysmorphic) had been to a mental health provider, including psychiatrist, for help. The proportion seeking professional help remained the same across the three study age groups: children, adolescents and adults.

This gave the first real glimpse into the world of transgenerational alcohol abuse/addiction as well as transgenerational ARND (Streissguth & Kanter 1997).

It is quite obviously true that if children with ARND are not diagnosed in infancy or early childhood and subsequently provided with positive, structured, and nurturing environments they will invariably suffer. The diagnosis may not be completely certain at the inset due to lack of physical features, but a Neurodevelopmental Disorder, with significant prenatal alcohol exposure, is a good working diagnosis to motivate the medical and social service professionals to serve for an immediate safe placement. This type of structured placement will provide an environment where the child's varied neurodevelopmental deficits will be addressed with a more consistent and coordinated supportive services and appropriate behavior modification strategies.

This grounding in the early nurturing period will have an inevitable positive impact on the predictably that as the children grow and progress in life they will develop one or more co-occurring developmental psychiatric disorders because of the underlying organic brain dysfunction (Nowick Brown et al., 2011).

Therefore in the absence of early recognition in the primary nurturing period of the infant or young child, then by the time this child with an undiagnosed ARND reaches adulthood, he or she has a history of multiple diagnoses, many of which may be inaccurate or incomplete.

Clinical observation and evaluation has shown that not only is the development of co-occurring Developmental Psychiatric Disorders in ARND predictable, it also is sequential. The acquired brain dysfunction, seen from infancy, impairs basic neurodevelopment on global scale, from sensory and motor co-ordination to mood regulation, language ability and cognitive functions. Also, far more studied and recognized are the multitude of neurocognitive abilities which are seen during school years, such as deficits in attention, information processing, cognition, learning, and memory, but the child has already many other features of the ARND before entering school.

Generally, the global impairments in functioning due to the acquired brain dysfunction, and not environmental stressors, inhibit the growing child's ability for an adequate foundation for core resiliency, and the ability to cope adequately with predictable and unpredictable negative life experiences or stressors. Thus it naturally follows that children with ARND who experience traumatic environmental experiences will be less able to deal effectively with those traumas. This would be in comparison to their peers who do not have the biological vulnerability of acquired brain dysfunction.

Much later in development, far removed from the nurturing environment studies, it is documented that adolescents and young adults with undiagnosed ARND and inaccurately or incompletely diagnosed co-occurring disorders, not only have this handicap, but also a twofold stress due to an interaction between their brain dysfunction driven ARND condition and the subsequent adverse childhood or adolescent environments. In this situation a label of antisocial behaviors and antisocial personality disorder is quickly attributed to the patient.

This is not uncommonly in the context of no appropriate treatment being available i.e., psychostimulant or mood stabilizer.

The scientific studies have as well indicated the real risk of early onset alcohol craving and abuse kindled in the womb by the prenatal exposure to alcohol and its effect on the nucleus accumbens. This is very much in keeping with the observations in traditional child psychiatry which has analyzed the benefit of early aggressive management of ADHD and early onset bipolar disorder as a preemptive method of delaying or even preventing subsequent substance abuse, especially alcohol. One can see how countries such as Ireland and the UK, with the highest underage drinking in the world, and panoply of undiagnosed ARND children will continue to fare (O'Malley 2011a, 2013).

The biggest disservice that DSM V has perpetuated is to keep neurodevelopmental disorders in the Intellectual Disability box as they now have created Intellectual Developmental Disorders as a category. This is in the international contact of an recognized acceptance that ARND is not an Intellectual Disability disorder as 70 to 75% of patients with ARND who have normal IQs (Streissguth et al., 1996, Streissguth 1997,) Although the available longitudinal studies suggest that individuals with ARND are at high risk for adverse life course outcomes such as mental health or developmental psychiatric problems and poor social functioning and adjustment, the long-term effects of ARND are not well known. It appears to be the privileged purvey of the relatively small international research community devoted to studying the immediate and long term effects of prenatal alcohol exposure (Streissguth & O'Malley 2000, Novick Brown et al., 2011). The general medical awareness is still really embryonic, and even the psychiatric and psychological professionals have a certain ambivalent resistance, at best, to the ramifications of transgenerational alcohol let alone a specific disorder such as ARND.

The situation is worse in the general population. You only have to think of Ireland where alcohol is the 'uisce beatha' (water of life!). Still many women continue to drink alcohol during pregnancy or when they might become pregnant. This is despite long-standing public health advisory in places such as the USA, Canada, and more recently Australia, New Zealand, exhorting them to abstain. Sadly, a recent national survey data found that 10 percent of pregnant women reported alcohol consumption at some point during their pregnancy, with 2 percent reporting binge drinking or frequent use of alcohol. Each year, more than 40,000 infants continue to be born with ARND in the USA (Ireland a tiny country has at least 700 undiagnosed each year). Which is equivalent to 1 percent of all live births.

There is another hidden static in countries such as Ireland which relates to the lack of public health awareness when it come to the medical risks of early onset and binge drinking patterns, Since returning to UK and Ireland in 2006 I have seen at least a two dozen women die in their mid 30s to early 40s of alcohol related medical problems. All of them were birth mothers to 1 or more children with ARND, and all of them did not have custody of their children at the time of their death. It did not matter if the child or children had dysmorphic ARND or non dysmorphic ARND. Some of the deaths were suspicious accidents in which alcohol was part of the story i.e., a mother died of a fall in a derelict house after sustaining a skull fracture when intoxicated. The deaths due to alcohol related liver or kidney problems are also untold issues in the birth mothers of inter country adopted children i.e., from Russia.

This Needs Formal Study

My anecdotal evidence would point to at least 1 in 30 or 40 birth mothers of children with ARND are at risk for premature death. This obviously has its impact on the birth children at many different and sometimes unexpected levels. One wonders if the alcohol addiction counselors realize that a birth mother of a child with ARND may be at more medical risk, not the least if she has fought to keep her children but is unable to because of continued addiction and potentially violent partners (O'Malley 2011b).

The emotional impact of the removal of an infant or young child from a birth mother is never to be under estimated, irrespective of the birth parent's alcohol addiction or co-occurring psychiatric disorder.

In Ireland this is a continuing balance as the State follows the creed of 'family preservation' at all costs, and so keeps children connected with birth parents even when they are unable to cope. Somewhere in the middle there has to be a way to rise above the overwhelming stigma of a diagnosis of ARND, permanent brain damage in the child, and the so called severe alcoholic label in the mother. Only then can maybe a place can be found to honor and respect the mother, the child and the often essential foster or adoptive paints.

The Prevalence and Nature of Psychiatric Disorders in ARND (2014 Book)

The prevalence of psychiatric or mental health disorders in ARND through the lifespan was initially documented by Ann Streissguth and colleagues at the University of Washington, and still remains the template and in many ways gold standard, to acknowledge these co-occurring disorders within ARND. In this large study of what the research group called Secondary Disabilities 415 persons (6 to 51 years of age) with dysmorphic ARND, (FAS) and Fetal Alcohol Effect (FAE), the older term for non-dysmorphic ARND, were examined for presence of mental health or psychiatric problems (Streisssguth et al., 1996, Streissguth et al., 1997, Streissguth & Kanter 1997).

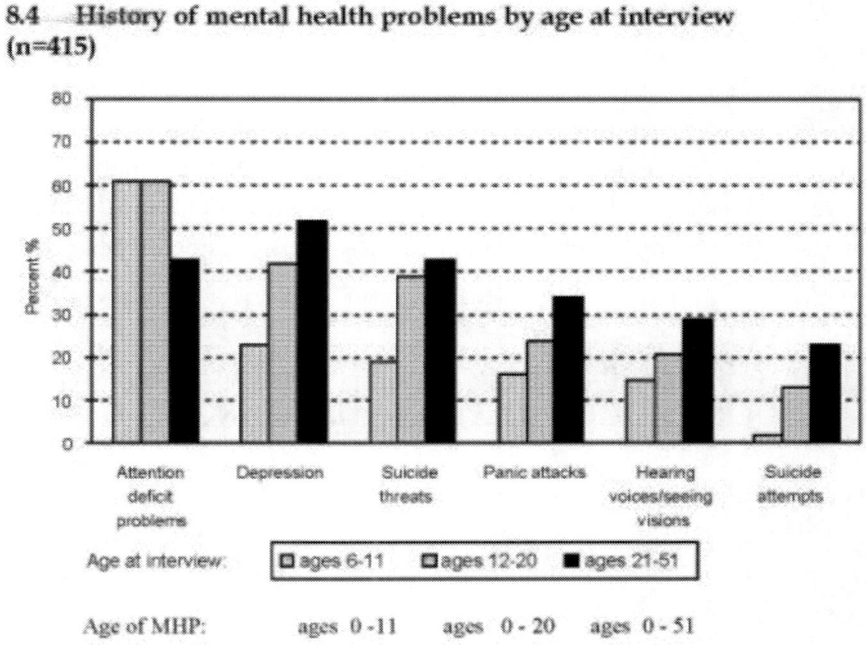

Figure 4. Streissguth et al., 1996.

This figure shows the most prevalent mental health or psychiatric problems for each of the three age groups. The study found a similarly high rate of mental health disorders among 62 adults with FASA/FAE (dysmorphic and non-dysmorphic ARND).

The University of Washington researchers found significantly, a majority (94%) had a positive history of co-occurring mental health or psychiatric problems.

Among both adults and children, attention deficits were the most frequently reported problems (61%) reported whereas in adults alone, depression was most frequently reported (52%) (Streissguth et al., 1996). The lifetime prevalence of mental health or psychiatric disorders in individuals with ARND is as high as 90% (Streissguth et al., 1996, HHS, 2000), highlighting the importance of correct diagnosis and clinical management. Accurate, informed diagnosis is critical in psychiatry to avoid over-medication or inappropriate treatment, leading to worsening of symptoms and poor outcomes.

Table 12. Mental Health or Psychiatric Disorders in patients with dysmorphic (i.e., FAS) or non-dysmorphic ARND across the lifespan

92% had a mental health/psychiatric diagnosis
65% with ADHD,
45% with depression,
21% with panic disorder.

Streissguth et al., 1996.

A preponderance of mental health or psychiatric problems among adult patients with FAS (dysmorphic ARND) was first reported by Lemoine et al., 1992 in their notable 30-year follow-up of Lemoine's original child patients from his 1968 seminal observations on the link between facial dysmorphology, central nervous system dysfunction and maternal alcohol consumption in pregnancy. It is cautionary to note that as adults, these former patients were not located in their familial homes or in institutions for the intellectually disabled but were found most characteristically in psychiatric residential care facilities.

SUMMARY REVIEW OF LONGITUDINAL CLINICAL CORRELATION STUDIES IN ARND

1. A no. of smaller studies have since shown that the proportion of study subjects with a history of psychiatric disorders (74%) was greater than expected from the general population, including alcohol or drug abuse (60%), major depressive disorder (44%), avoidant personality disorder (29%).

Clinical issues such as depression and anxiety are prevalent. (Barr et al., 2006, O'Connor et al., 2002, O'Malley 2011a).

2. Researchers have shown a link between ADHD symptoms and ARND dysmorphic or non-dysmorphic (FASDs) over the past 10 years, indicating an acquired (non-genetic) etiology for a subtype of children with ADHD. (Driscoll et al., 1990, Streissguth et al., 1996, O'Malley & Nanson 2002 O'Malley & Storoz 2003, O'Malley 2008, Coles et al., 2009, Mattson et al., 2011, Kodituwaddu et al., 2011). The link between ADHD and ARND dysmorphic and non-dysmorphic or FASDs, is finding more universal acceptance.

3. Infants and toddlers with ARND have been shown to present with Regulatory Disorder Type I, II, or III (DC Zero to 3, 2005). (O'Malley & Striessguth 2003, 2006, O'Malley 2008).

4. Autistic Spectrum Disorder or Asperger's Disorder type behaviors have been noted in both younger children as well as school age children prenatally exposed to alcohol and the link between Autism and Asperger's disorder and ARND dysmorphic or non-dysmorphic or FASDs will not be far behind. (Nanson 1990, Streissguth et al., 1996, Streissguth & O'Malley 2000, Mukarjee 2008, Mukarkjee et al., 2012, O'Malley & Rich 2013).

5. In Ann Streissguth's groups long-term studies of large numbers of diagnosed patients with dysmorphic ARND(FAS) and non-dysmorphic ARND (called FAE in older studies), it is clear that co-occurring disorders, particularly those involving psychiatric disorders, present the greatest barriers to appropriate treatment. For example, as psychiatric disorders are more readily diagnosed than ARND, the most likely scenario is that the psychiatric diagnosis is observed and diagnosed and thus becomes the primary diagnosis

in determining treatment. As well European studies are finding similar long term trajectories (Lemoine et al., 1992, Steinhausen et al., 1993).

6. However, patients with ARND are likely to have more significant problems in maybe six varied clinical dimensions than the average psychiatric patients without ARND.

Thus, failure to consider their ARND can be a major detriment to effective treatment, throughout the lifespan. Especially in children is the recognition of their ARND is important, as they can become quickly scapegoated at school and the presumptive diagnosis brings more effective multimodal family-based interventions which can be implemented during the early years. (Streissguth et al., 1996, Streissguth & O'Malley 2000, O'Malley 2008, Novick Brown et al., 2011, O'Malley 2013).

The Natural History of NDPAE. A Window into the Future, an Update 2020

The thrust of this chapter combing early nurturing challenges and extrapolating to the natural history of the condition, or Secondary Disabilities (as coined by Streissguth and colleagues in 1996), has not changed in the last 5 years.

However, it is becoming patently apparent that to approach transgenerational alcohol without intervention at the nodal parent/infant or young child dyad level is running the risk of continued scientific research being disconnected from the meat and potatoes of the true public health/psychiatric problem.

The Mortality and Morbidity Risk of Birth Mothers with Children Who Have NDPAE

This new study seeks to re- examine the natural history of NDPAE and specifically the link between a diagnosis of NDPAE in the child, and the death of the biological birth mother The birth mothers of patients with NDPAE are considered to be a high-risk population (Astley, Bailey, Talbot, Clarren, 2000) who may need care in coping with the diagnosis of their child and who may have underlying health issues. The data for this study was gathered over a ten-year period (O'. Malley & Owens 2018).

Sample Demographics

Chosen Through a stratified Random sampling from a clinical population in the island of Ireland past and current patients attending a consultant neuropsychiatrist who were all referred by a medical practioner.

Study Sample

67 NDPAE Patients
44 Male, Age 6 to 26 years,
Ethnic group. 36 Caucasian Irish, 7 Caucasian Non Irish
23 Female Age. 5.5 to 20 years,
Ethnic group. 21 Caucasian Irish, 2Caucasian Non-Irish.

Case Control Sample

33 Patients with conditions unrelated to prenatal alcohol exposure
21 Male. Age 6-27 Years
Ethnic group. 21 Caucasian Irish.
12 Female. Age 6 -21 years.

The Case Control group consisted of patients with depression, bipolar, ASD, ADHD, PTSD/LD The aforementioned ages refer to the age of patients upon last consultation.

Results

NDPAE Patients: The birth mother had deceased in 11.9% of cases,

The birth mothers died before the patient's 12th birthday in 4.48% cases of NDPAE patients.

Non-NDPAE: The birth mother had deceased in 0% of cases.

$X_2\,(1, N = 100) = 0.03, p < .05$, statistically significant.

Discussion

All Barth Mother who died prematurely died as a result of alcohol related medical causes.

There are two main approaches to intervention at this parent/infant or young child, and it is hoped that both of these clinical interventions will have a positive synergistic impact on the natural history of NDPAE in the infant/young child. Thus, decreasing the prevalence of Secondary Disabilities.

1. An Infant/Young Child Centered Approach

The American Academy of Child and Adolescent Psychiatry, AACAP, has a new working 'systems of care' clinical instrument which is for use in planning service provision for children under 5 years with mental health/psychiatric problems.

This instrument is the 'sister' of the older instrument the Child and Adolescent Service Intensity Instrument, CASII which has been used for nearly 15 years with children over 5 years old and adolescents.

This clinical instrument is the Early Childhood Service Intensity Instrument (ECSII).

ECSII has 2 age appropriate parameters (as with the previous CASII).

Domains to Guide Treatment Plans

- Degree of Safety
- Child –Caregiver Relationships
- Caregiving Environment
- Functional and Developmental Status
- Impact of Child's Medical, Developmental or Emotional/Behavioral problems

Service Profiles

- Caregiver/Child involvement
- Services Fit
- Services Effectiveness

This standardized assessment and service intensity model acknowledges the complexity of child's biological status but as well the impact of psychosocial environmental stressors acute and enduring.it is a unique age appropriate child-centered systems of care instrument of diagnostic validity and service needs.

(Rogers et al., 2011, Rutter et al., 2011, AACAP 2019).

Case Example:

A 2/12-year-old Caucasian boy is placed in emergency state care as his birth mother has died in maternity hospital 6 days post-partum of alcohol related medical causes, kidney failure and cirrhosis of the liver.

The boy was placed in permanent state foster care at 1 month of age and is still in the same foster home.

The birth mother had a long history of alcohol dependence and had one previous miscarriage of an alcohol-exposed fetus in the previous year. She had a series of missed appointments to her alcohol counsellor, and attended only one antenatal visit at 2 months' gestation before entering the maternity hospital in early labor.

Emergency caesarian section due to failure to progress in pregnancy with fetal distress and Apgar's 6 and 8.

The infant was born at 36 weeks' gestation, birth wt. 20th percentile and ht. 20th percentile, head circumference 30cms.

The infant had faltering growth with a poor suck reflex and delayed latency to suck, so feeding was a challenge. His ht. and wt. have decreased from 20th to below the 10th percentile at 2½ years old.

Developmental milestones delayed sitting 10 months, walking 21 months,

Language development delayed with 50-word vocabulary, at 2½ years of age

Immunizations were up to date,

Temperament was difficult to settle and a modified Ainsworth/Attachment examination of foster mother and boy showed a secure but disorganized attachment paradigm, driven by the boys Regulatory Disorder.

Clinically he presented clear features of Regulatory Disorder, Hyper-responsive.

Access: Birth father who is alcohol dependent and has history of violence sees the boy once a month in supervised access, but now wants full custody. The boy has soiling episodes usually the night before access visit with father.

2. A Parent-Centered Approach

The transgenerational challenge to management is being approached through work with parents who have mental health disorders are pregnant and delivering next generation of vulnerable children. Birth parents of children with NDPAE have been shown to not infrequently have three clinical challenges, psychiatric disorder, developmental disorder, (often NDPAE itself) and addictive disorder. (Astley et al., 2000, O'Malley 2003). It is, therefore, not good enough to only plan holistic management through the assessment of the child under 5 years old, but a parallel process of parent assessment and management is essential.

a. Parent with Psychiatric Disorder:

Preconception intervention; This involves the active involvement of an adult psychiatrist in the management of the potentially pregnant woman with severer psychiatric disorder such as Bipolar disorder or Schizophrenia. All these psychiatric disorders require medication which can have an impact on the developing fetus.

- Lithium can cause teratogenic effects on the developing thyroid and also can decrease the seizure threshold and cause cardiac irregularities

- SSRIs can cause a neonatal activation syndrome in young infants
- Mood stabilizers such as valproic acid can cause a teratogenic effect on the developing fetus with a dysmorphic neurodevelopmental disorder with ASD features'
- Atypical agents can have an impact on the developing glucose metabolism, cardiac status and prolactin development.

Perinatal depression: This is a complex area needing active psychiatric involvement with the pregnant mother during pregnancy and post-delivery. The clinical impact of the perinatal depression is a holistic problem involving the developing fetus and the subsequent infant. The reactivity of the infant to the immediate postnatal environment can be blunted, and the infant can present with a Slow to Warm temperament or Regulatory Disorder, hypo-responsive. As well, the pervasive effect on primary attachment between the birth mother and infant can be quite profound, and lead to physical effects due to physical and/or emotional neglect. (Winnicott 1984, Stein 2019).

Family support programs have been developed to help parents with new infants in this situation (Carmichael Olson 2006, Henshaw et al., 2018, Walkup AACAP 2019, RSM Parental Mental Health conference 2019)

b. Parent with Addictive Disorder

Preconception Intervention

An intervention, called the Parent Child Assistance Program, PCAP, was started in Seattle by Professor Ann Streissguth and Therese Grant. It involves the use of a paraprofessional advocate who partners with a substance/alcohol abusing woman who has just delivered an alcohol affected infant. One of the primary goals includes management of the substance/alcohol abuse and immediate initiation of birth control to limit the birth of another alcohol-affected infant (Rasmussen et al. 2012).

Antenatal/Perinatal Intervention

This is essential to minimize the teratogenic effect of alcohol on the developing fetus. The hospital team, obstetrician, midwife, social worker are key players in quantifying the amount and nature of the alcohol abuse during pregnancy.

Addiction counsellors are also crucial to monitor antenatal missed visits as well as missed addiction counselling visits during pregnancy and in postnatal period. Continued substance/alcohol, abuse in this period makes the fetus and infant more 'at risk' for neurodevelopmental disorder, i.e., NDPAE.

The transgenerational alcohol effect is displayed in the 'unseen' population of young adult females and males with NDPAE who are becoming parents, whether the abuse alcohol or not in pregnancy. These parents are still at risk for producing infants with complex neurodevelopmental disorders who they cannot parent adequately.

These children then become removed into state care and the parent copes with the of her child loss by drinking alcohol once more, and becoming pregnant with once more.

When Will Society Ever Learn?

c. Parent with Developmental Disorder

Preconception Intervention

This is the most ignored area of medical/social intervention.

The need for trained advocates who understand the impaired of impaired executive function and working memory on decision making and planning is a basic clinical skill. General practice, pediatrics and pregnancy care are still largely disconnected from this special needs population, and so invariably miss opportunities to help the pregnant or new mother in poor decision making about having a baby and bringing up an infant.

In some countries there has been an unfortunate history of forced sterilization for this population of developmental disorder patients (in Canada it remained prevalent in the 1970s).

This is fundamentally against the European Rights for Persons with Learning Disabilities and its practice needs constant monitoring.

Pre/Postnatal Intervention

This is an unexplored area of clinical management .in Native American, First Nations, Irish, UK populations with transgenerational alcohol contributing to the adult developmental disorder population you have a circular never- ending stream of children born to unprepared mothers, and fathers.

Specialist social workers, health visitors, public health nurses trained in learning disability are obviously a much needed basic clinical resource. (Walkup 2019).

This is a critical period for many children vulnerable due to prenatal alcohol exposure, difficult to manage and posing major basic management problems for the birth mother. Unfortunately, this is a period when state Care due to compromised parenting becomes an option. Instead it is the vital time to add developmentally and culturally sensitive support for the mother and parents in general.

Chapter 9

A BROADER APPROACH TO MANAGEMENT (2014 BOOK)

FORMING A DIAGNOSTIC OR WORKING HYPOTHESIS. WHO DIAGNOSES? WHO TREATS?

How Do You Approach Diagnosis in ARND?

The characteristic growth and facial features in classic dysmorphic ARND, i.e., FAS, may sensitize the clinician to explore and quantify the complex learning disabilities, which are a legacy of prenatal alcohol's effects on the developing central nervous system. However, these dysmorphic characteristics of ARND account for only 10 to 15% of the totality of patients affected by prenatal alcohol exposure. While non dysmorphic ARND is far more prevalent, it presents the ultimate challenge to clinicians in terms of diagnosis and management because of its masquerading face/mask.

Management begins with the ability to form a diagnostic or working hypothesis, which is how medical and mental health professionals should begin to approach the clinical presentation of a possible ARND (or any diagnosis, for that matter). As noted earlier in this book, the essential clinical component is the presence of a developmental neuropsychiatric disorder, and the etiology being sought is either genetic or acquired (O'Malley 2011a, 2013).

Pediatricians, General Practitioners and Health Visitors or Public Health Nurses need to be better educated in the immediate and long-term clinical features of ARND. They as well need a greater understanding of the multiple effects of prenatal alcohol not just on the central nervous system development but also organ development such as heart, kidney, eyes, ears, skeletal system., which are collectively called Alcohol Related Birth Defects,

ARBD. Traditionally, clinical medicine still tends to be no better than the old maxim: 'what you look for, you will see,' and so this becomes an enduring clinical diagnostic dilemma for practitioners who examine these infants and children. Even if the dysmorphic ARND, namely FAS, is diagnosed in infancy and early childhood, the diagnosis does not always bring the medical and other services that these children need because conventional wisdom still sees these infants and children as COAs (children of alcoholics) who merely reflect the chaotic alcoholic environments they were born into.

The awareness of the Developmental Psychiatric Disorders related to the prenatal alcohol exposure and the clinical presentation of ARND, (Alcohol Related Neurodevelopmental Disorder) varies greatly throughout the world. Historically the USA, Canada and France have the longest clinical acknowledgement and research related to this problem. However even they are still 'stuck in the moment' so to say, as the diagnostic clinics are dominated by the pursuit of physical dysmorphology and psychiatry is usually a passive observer. Alcohol addiction services when involved seem to be in separate silos with little connection between the alcohol addicted or abusing pregnant woman and the risk to her unborn child. This situation is sometimes compounded by the alcohol addiction or abuse being secondary to a chronic psychiatric disorder such as Depression, Bipolar disorder or Schizophrenia (O'Malley 2003).

Some countries, such as Ireland, still do not 'officially' accept ARND dysmorphic or non-dysmorphic, so NO cases exist. This is in a country with the highest per capita drinking in the world, highest binge drinking in the world, and highest underage drinking in Europe! Furthermore, a recent prevalence study among school-age children in Italy showed 2.5-5% of children in the first grade with ARND, dysmorphic or non-dysmorphic. Unfortunately this did not invite the Italian government to start public health campaigns to warn women to refrain from alcohol use during pregnancy.

Obviously there needs to be international clinical scientific neurological and neuropsychiatric studies to quantify ARND. This needs to be joined with the clinical phenotype descriptions coming from a neurodevelopmental frame of understanding. The plethora of neuropsychological testing seems to be never ending, but unfortunately still continues to not be fully integrated into treatment programmers. It is as if the vast majority of the energy is spent counting the cases, and describing them in detail, but little energy is spent approaching the roots of the disorder coming from transgenerational alcohol, abuse, psychiatric disorder, social disadvantage including domestic violence.

As the understanding of Developmental Psychiatric Disorders continues to grow we are now at a conceptual stage of appreciating that static developmental screening instruments are of questionable utility. The ARND presents differing phenotypes depending on the age of the patient. So the Dimensional mixture in infancy changes in childhood and once more in adolescence through adulthood.

Ironically the change in phenotype is not dissimilar from the change in the presence of dysmorphic facial features, which are well known to be present in infancy and early childhood, but disappear as the summer mists by adolescence and adulthood. Even the so called dysmorphic ARND, i.e., FAS, cannot be 'officially 'diagnosed in adolescence when there are no dysmorphic features seen at the time of assessment.

Does This Negate the ARND?

Yes, and no. As the shifting sands of dysmorphic features are accepted, it has become time to consider and accept the equally shifting sands of the more relevant functional phenotype which offers different clinical developmental psychiatric disorder challenges at different ages of life.

It follows that from infancy through early late childhood and adolescence the developmental psychiatric disorders do not appear at uniform times.

For example, according to the Regulatory Disorders Guidelines in the Zero-to-Three Classification of Mental Health Disorders (DC 0-3, 2005), Sensory Integration problems are identifiable in infancy, while Social Cognition and Social Communication problems are more easily identified during the first few years and early childhood years.

Whereas, developmental executive decision making problems most commonly are identified at 5 to 7 years of age, in the early school setting commonly masquerading as ADHD or Oppositional Defiant Disorder and Complex Learning Disabilities with a normal intellectual functioning.

To complicate matters further, these co-occurring clinical issues, that are in reality the 'functional face/mask' of children with ARND, often become somewhat of a diagnostic Irish stew with;

ADHD and co-morbid ASD,

ADHD with Intermittent Explosive Disorder, or Disruptive Mood Dysregulation Disorder with emotional incontinence. (The latter combination of symptoms is reminiscent of some children with traumatic brain injury). (O'Malley 2013).

Thus, it is also important to be mindful of the developmental trajectory of the shifting diagnostic paradigms in children with prenatal alcohol exposure for the dysmorphic ARND (FAS) and/or non-dysmorphic ARND. This knowledge and diagnostic fine tuning will allow child psychiatrists, pediatricians, and other medical professionals to have a more practical, clearer and more holistic interpretation and understanding of the wide range of neurocognitive, neurobehavioral, and neuropsychiatric disorders affecting the individual rather than simply the degree of facial dysmorphology.

The broader understanding of the developmental psychiatric presentations of ARND will as well clarify in no uncertain terms the lack of association between facial dysmorphology and brain dysfunction. In parallel there is also a clear lack of association between the facial dysmorphology and the psychiatric clinical presentations of ARND.

The Developmental Psychiatric Disorder diagnosis delineating the Dimensional range of the clinical problems is the starting point for setting up management strategies.

Although psychiatrists and mental health professionals treat patients with ARND, there is presently one way within the new DSM-V to code for either the dysmorphic ARND (i.e., Fetal Alcohol Syndrome, FAS) or the non-dysmorphic (Alcohol Related Neurodevelopmental Disorder, ARND). This code is Neurodevelopmental Disorder with prenatal alcohol exposure (ND.PAE, 315.8). Furthermore the intellectual developmental disability is more a hindrance than a help as 75 to 80% of patients with ARND have a normal IQ and it is their complex functional disability not intellectual disability that is the clinical conundrum.

The ICD 10 code has ARND dysmorphic type (FAS) on Axis IV, Physical Disorders, but is much more flexible as it has Axis II and Axis III which address, specific learning disorders, and general level of cognitive functioning.

The in depth diagnostic clinical examination has been dealt with in the previous chapter but suffice to say that the essential 2nd step in management is to establish the Developmental Psychiatric Disorder Diagnostic hypothesis, whether with clear documented alcohol exposure in pregnancy or with 'uncertain etiology' due to conflicting reports and maternal statements regarding alcohol use in pregnancy. (The latter is very common in Ireland because of the stigma and denial of alcohol misuse).

Consequently, Best Practice in terms of diagnosis involves investigating the co-occurrence of both alcohol teratogenic and environmental factors in the patient's developmental, psychiatric presentation whenever there are deficits in basic primary abilities such as attention, learning, cognition, self-soothing, and adaptive and executive functioning. Alternatively, ARND (with its impairments in social communication and cognition, executive functioning and adaptive functioning) may compound and escalate the negative effects that a bad environment has on a patient's behavior, due to alcohol acquired and biologically-created resiliency deficits. For example, with respect to the large numbers of individuals with ARND who have trouble with the law, a number of researchers (Fast et al., 2005) suggest that this problem may stem in large part from an interaction between an adverse environment and the ARND associated primary disabilities in learning, socialization and executive functioning. In other words, the presence of primary brain dysfunction created disabilities beyond the individual's control. These deficits in functioning and understanding undermine his or her ability to withstand negative environmental influences, and so diminish his or her personal culpability for bad/antisocial acts. There must always be an accurate differential diagnosis in such situations requiring careful attention to environmental stressors, as well as the underlying medical condition, and other etiological factors. (Standardized instruments such as the AIMS or SAVRY may be of help).

THE PRACTICAL UTILITY OF A DEVELOPMENTAL PSYCHIATRIC APPROACH TO DIAGNOSTIC FORMULATION

The essential clinical component related to prenatal alcohol exposure is the presence of a Developmental Psychiatric Disorders, and the etiology being sought is either genetic or environmental. Management of psychiatric disorders in ARND begins with pediatricians, child psychiatrists and psychologists 'forming a diagnostic or working hypothesis'.

The challenges in the management of ARND, whether dysmorphic or non-dysmorphic, currently relate to their clinical presentations having an array of apparent developmental psychiatric co-morbidity, but with a general lack of diagnostic clarity. In average clinical practice in both Canada, the USA, Ireland and the UK pediatricians or child psychiatrists who recognize the clinical significance of prenatal alcohol exposure and subsequent ARND, are given either the ICD 10 or DSM V diagnostic classification systems to delineate the developmental psychiatric presentations as they see them.

It is becoming increasingly evident that early onset sensory dysregulation, disruptive mood dysregulation, social communication disorder, ADHD, ASD Features, Intermittent Explosive Disorder, and poorly understood Conduct disorder issues are prominent in the co-occurring presentations of ARND. The interplay with environmental stressors adds to the complexity of the ARND psychiatric presentation introducing a Reactive Attachment Disorder or PTSD component as a legacy of the socio-cultural nurturing environment.

These physicians as well as general mental health professionals will be better served by the developmental psychiatric approach as the initial entry into unraveling the ARND. Too often the attachment issues or the trauma issues are seen as the sine qua non, and when standard psychological techniques do not work the parents are blamed, or that child's noncompliance is blamed. A recent example in Ireland showed a child with ARND, ADHD with co-occurring ASD features and PTSD from exposure to domestic violence became blamed as his deliberate defiance did not respond to play therapy, and his language deficit of alexithymia was unseen. (O'Malley 2003, Rich 2009, Rich & O'Malley 2012, O'Malley & Rich 2012).

a. Embedded in the diagnosis of ARND is the recognition of the possibility of Alcohol Related Birth Defects (ARBD) which is the physical sequelae of prenatal alcohol exposure, i.e., multi system organ involvement cardiac, renal, eye, GI problems and skeletal system.

b. The socio –cultural environmental context that the infant is borne into plays a critical role in modulating the developmental psychiatric disorders due to the organic brain dysfunction.

Therefore:

- childhood direct or indirect exposure to domestic or community violence,
- child physical or sexual abuse or neglect,
- early institutionalization with social isolation,
- multiple caregivers,
- multiple home moves,
- multiple school placements,
- death of birth mother in her mid late 30s before patient is out of teen years,
- death of special pet
- loss of special friend due to moving to new city,
- divorce or separation of birth, foster or adoptive parents

All may contribute to development of well documented childhood psychiatric disorders such as:

1) Reactive Attachment Disorder (RAD),
2) Post Traumatic Stress Disorder (PTSD),
3) Developmental Trauma Disorder, especially if exposure to stressful situations are in the early years of life before the child has the language to describe the experience.

The interaction of the childhood experience on the developmental psychiatric presentation of the ARND phenotype cannot be overlooked. Thus, the developmental biological vulnerability profile of ARND during infancy, toddlerhood, childhood, and adolescence predisposes the individual to adverse psychological outcomes resulting from these psychosocial stressors. (Cummings et al., 2000, Elias et al., 2012).

Any one of these psychosocial stressors can impact the clinical presentation related to the acquired organic brain dysfunction and of themselves add more co-occurring psychiatric disorders to be dealt with. There is not necessarily a hierarchy of impact of these stressors, although Besel Van der Polk was the first to distinguish between the isolated stressor and the chronic enduring stressors. Within the socio-cultural familial environment of alcohol addiction the enduring stressors are the norm rather than the exception, and must be taken into account when formulating a management plan. This, for example, could include removal from a toxic home environment to a more structured emotionally calmer foster or adoptive home placement. The diagnostic assessment of the patient prenatally exposed to alcohol must take into account the impact of the postnatal and early childhood environment as a significant protective or potential risk factor for the continuing development of the child (Besel van der Polk et al., 1995, O'Malley 2003, Rich 2009, O'Malley 2008, Rich & O'Malley 2012, O'Malley & Rich 2012).

An early diagnosis or developmental psychiatric working hypothesis is crucial as it avoids the common impasse of a Reactive Attachment Disorder or PTSD diagnosis. These former diagnoses place the infant or young child's difficulties with the parents, instead of attributing them to complex brain damage acquired through prenatal alcohol exposure. So in making such a diagnosis, the professionals often invalidate the valuable objective observations of foster or adoptive parents and immobilize many of them. Thus, through misdiagnosis, denying the child's effective parenting.

However, in some birth families where parents continue to abuse alcohol and provide an adverse rearing environment, these diagnoses, although painful, may offer an opportunity to break a cycle of transgenerational addiction and subsequent transgenerational prenatally created brain damage.

The one area where the coupling of acquired brain dysfunction due to prenatal alcohol with PTSD is quite problematic is in the field of inter country adoptions. In these private adoptions the theory is that the infant has attachment problems solely due to the foreign adoption process, but the reality is that the infant has brain dysfunction from undeclared alcohol exposure in pregnancy, and has been exposed to some inappropriate caring i.e., left in wet nappy for days, not fed properly.

Constructing a Scaffolding Containment System

The first principle in effective clinical case management of ARND is the construction of a 'scaffolding containment system' around the patient and his/her family (Stressguth & Kanter 1997, Page 2008).

The quality and stability of the childhood home environment is a crucial factor in the ultimate outcome of those with ARND whether dysmorphic or non-dysmorphic. It has been recognized and scientifically studied for many years that children, especially in early childhood, who are provided with positive, structured, and nurturing environments, will be more likely to cope with their developmental or psychiatric disabilities. This is in no small part because their developmental challenges are met with consistent parenting Therefore, it is essential to contain the vulnerable infant or child early in development in a suitable safe, structured, and predictable nurturing environment.

The Social Services have an critical role in assessing the safety of the home environment, and, if necessary, facilitating placement into safer environments.

The impact of transgenerational alcohol addiction in home environments is multi-factorial: it affects physical, emotional and cognitive development at many levels, as well as possibly exposing the vulnerable infant or child to risk of abuse and exposure to domestic violence due to lack of safe boundaries. (Abudabo and Cohen 2011, Dumaret et al., 2009, Streissguth et al., 1996, 2004).

The current standard of care or 'treatment as usual' for individuals with ARND is inadequate due to lack of diagnostic clarity, and lack of accepted developmental psychiatric treatment protocols.

As with Autistic Spectrum Disorders, the diagnosis of ARND and the treatment involves early intervention with a multimodal team approach (genetics, developmental pediatrics, psychologists, psychiatrists, PT/OT, speech, special education) (O'Malley 2008, 2011a, c, Kodituwakku et al., 2011).

Clinical presentations of patients with dysmorphic ARND or non-dysmorphic ARND show a combination of developmental disorder and co-occurring psychiatric disorder, or more correctly Developmental Psychiatric Disorder. The psychiatric disorder(s) may arise and be a combination of the acquired brain dysfunction and the environmental impact of the rearing home. All alcohol-exposed infants are subsequently reared in environments that have a modulating effect one way or other on clinical expression of the neurotoxic effects of that exposure. Clinicians need to adopt a family-based systemic approach that identifies key environmental supports and stressors in the patient's environment (Grant et al., 2009, Nowick Brown et al., 2011, O'Malley 2008, 2011a, Page 2008).

In particular, a mother who drinks during pregnancy and suffers postpartum depression creates an immediate challenge to parent/infant bonding. The rearing environment must therefore be assessed, especially if there is evidence that direct or indirect violence (i.e., abuse or witnessing domestic violence) has occurred beyond the typical impact of a chaotic home environment and/or insecure attachment disorders often seen in the children of alcoholics (COA).

When the family environment is protective and nurturing, challenging behaviors are most likely to be caused by deficient adaptive, social and executive functioning stemming from the neurotoxin central nervous system dysfunction (Streissguth & Kanter 1997, Novick Brown et al., 2011, O'Malley 2011a). However, as well as organic brain damage from their ARND condition, children (including many of those adopted from Romanian and Russian orphanages) may suffer the effects of early emotional deprivation.

Prenatal stress impact on the fetus (e.g., due to developing in utero within a violent, disorganized home setting) or post-traumatic stress disorder (PTSD) in a pregnant mother also have certain neurochemical sequelae on the hypothalamic pituitary adrenal axis (HPA) function resulting in a synergistic effect on fetal brain development from combined cortisol and prenatal alcohol (Meewise et al., 2007). Emotional deprivation may also be due to familial mental illness where a parent is emotionally unavailable for active parenting.

Sometimes this is reflective of the transgenerational cognitive legacy of alcohol, which impairs maternal and paternal organizational and emotional regulation abilities.

This can lead to challenging (but not untreatable) insecure ambivalent resistant, or ambivalent avoidant attachment patterns. As a result, among the postnatal and early childhood vulnerabilities in ARND is a tendency for infants and young children to experience multiple placements before the fifth birthday due to their difficult and unpredictable behaviors. This needs to be acknowledged. So the child has Reactive Attachment Disorder features, but as well co-occurring Developmental Psychiatric Disorders as a result of their ARND due to the multi Dimensional Disorders which are interwoven with the environmental stressors. So, it might be expected that their Phenotype profile would be different than those without ARND.

For example, in a study of children with ADHD, those who also had ARND demonstrated significantly poorer social cognition and emotion-processing ability than those without ARND. These researchers reported a distinct behavioral profile for children with ARND and concluded that problems in social cognition and emotion processing may contribute to the higher incidence of social behavioral problems in children with both ADHD and ARND.

Ensuring Multi-System and Then Multi-Modal Treatment Approach

The involvement of different health, education and social service systems in the diagnosis and management of ARND is essential, and, when you are acknowledging the transgenerational alcohol component, should include Addiction services. Although the USA, Canada and France are regarded as many years ahead of the rest of Europe in the integrated understanding of these issues, they have still not developed consistent diagnostic or management strategies which incorporate a developmental psychiatric understanding.

This Multisystem involvement begins and ends with the transgenerational approach to alcohol.

The idea that alcohol craving and subsequent abuse or dependence in pre-pubertal children, adolescents and young adults with ARND may have their origins in prenatal alcohol exposure has been demonstrated by animal and human researchers for many years (Baer at al 2001, Barr and Streissguth 2001, Barr et al., 2006, Reyes et al., 1985). Thus effective management of transgenerational drinking has to involve general acceptance that maternal drinking may reflect a prenatally kindled biochemical craving for alcohol, or what is called fetal programming, due to the effect of prenatal alcohol exposure on the developing brain, especially the nucleus accumbens (Abate et al., 2008, Haycock 2009, O'Malley 2003, 2011a,c), When children or adolescents with ARND live with birth parents who have ARND themselves, this can cause diverse clinical management problems at many levels. This disorganized family functioning dynamic is compounded by the historical pervasive disconnection between addiction services for adolescents and adults and psychiatry and/or learning disability (O'Malley 2003, 2011a, 2013).

The multiple impacts of parental ARND associated difficulties include the chronic crisis and chaos arising from problems in dependent living and employment, and also those associated with problem solving (e.g., poor judgment, poor organizational skills, coupled with impulsivity, difficulty in making decisions and inadequate interpersonal relationships (Fast et al., 2001, Streissguth et al., 1996). These are not only due to alcohol addiction, but can be seen in binge drinking, seeming functioning, alcohol abusers. The important variable is the transgenerational legacy of ARND is a brain based biological vulnerability often not recognized through the fog and noise of alcohol use and abuse. These adult parents began life with this ARND vulnerability and now find themselves attempting to cope with their own child with ARND similarly disorganized, impulsive and with impulsive disruptive mood dysregulation.

Example: a 19 year old UK young adult with ARND which presents ADHD and Disruptive Mood Dysregulation becomes father to an infant at 18 years of age. The mother is 17 years old, also has ARND. She lives with her maternal grandmother as her birth mother died 2 years ago of alcohol related medical problems at 36 years of age. She was dropped out of school at 15 years because of academic problems and started binge drinking at that time, and continued throughout pregnancy. She now has a child with global developmental problems from birth. She has a love/hate relationship with the father and so changes the rules about access visits on a weekly basis. He cannot cope as he wants dearly to be a father and become acutely suicidal when access visits are stopped or changed for no reason. The maternity unit and midwives did not see this pregnancy as a 'at risk' one and there was no follow up arranged with child psychiatry, pediatrics or public health. The maternity hospital did not recognize the father's rights, and he was prevented from any contact with his girlfriend throughout the pregnancy hospital visits. The birth father still lived with his UK foster parents who are both professionals and very committed to support their son in his fatherhood. The maternity hospital was not aware of their existence as a support network for the birth father. After delivery the 17-year-old mother was told to go back to her GP.

At this juncture there is little formal connection between and child or adolescent psychiatric (CAMHS), social services or child learning disability services and adult psychiatric or adult learning disability services and so there is no natural case management forum to discuss the family or parenting challenges. Transgenerational alcohol abuse and dependence management requires Health and Social Service systems collaborating across traditional age-divides (i.e., child/adolescent/adult). Obstetricians and midwives need to become sensitive to implicit risks in the developing fetus from alcohol use in any trimester of pregnancy.

An effective model for this type of situation is the Parent Child Assistance Program (PCAP), an advocacy program in Seattle, which began working with substance abusing pregnant mothers in the mid-2000s. They acknowledge the complexity of working with a parent/infant dyad if the parent has ARND (Grant et al., 2009, Werner et al., 1985).

In the UK, hospital based services are beginning to address the critical area of perinatal psychiatry which seeks to identify mentally or developmentally vulnerable pregnant mothers and their potentially vulnerable newborn infants. The vulnerable pregnant woman may have a mixture of psychiatric disorder, addictive disorder and even developmental disorder (Henshaw et al., 2009).

Early Multi-modal treatment can improve the developmental, social, academic, and mental health trajectory of these children (O'Malley 2008, Novick Brown et al., 2011). Brain organization and function is affected in many individuals with ARND whether dysmorphic or non-dysmorphic, and can be enhanced by appropriate multi-modal treatment strategies.

There Are Many Barriers Existing to Effective Multisytem Management in ARND

a. There may be multiple providers who have different conceptualizations of the child's problems, resulting in lack of coherence in the service plan and conflicting treatment approaches.

Example: The infant in care has a well-documented history of significant alcohol exposure in pregnancy but the social worker does not 'believe' in the medical model so the foster parents are blamed as poor parents as the behavioral problems in the child are seen as attachment disorder.

Example: The adoptive parents of a Russian child do not believe in the medical model and so see their child's problems solely due to attachment issues and not related to neurotoxic exposure to alcohol during pregnancy. The OT feels that the problem is solely sensory integration and so the pt. must has sensory integration therapy. The dietician feels that it is just a nutritional problem and so is supplementing the child's diet with heath food products. The pediatrician wants to seek a specialist psychiatrist opinion related to developmental psychiatric problems.

b. The providers may not be targeting the problems that the child or family is most concerned about.

Example: the psychologist is providing insight orientated psychotherapy but the birth parents want an understanding of the impulsive suicidal risk and academic problems in school.

c. The child or family may not accept services because their concerns and apprehensions are not being understood or respected. This is especially relevant to minority children or families.

Example: the foster parents do not believe in medication and so cannot accept the role of medication in the management of acquired brain damage due to prenatal alcohol exposure.

d. The child or family may not engage in services because their social or concrete needs (i.e., for housing, vocation or recreation) are not being met.

Example: the family does not link with services as their child is still out of school because of severe behavioral and academic problems and no agency is taking responsibility for this dilemma.

e. Adequate consultation is not available to assist in diagnostic clarification or formulation of the problem, development of an appropriate treatment plan, and problem solving difficulties in team functioning.

Example: A child is failing in school and has had a number of failed drug treatments. The foster parents are concerned that there may be a problem related to the birth mother's pregnancy and delivery which included prenatal exposure to alcohol. There are no developmental psychiatrists or neuropsychiatrists available in the local area. The local CAMHS team does not deal with children with developmental disability, so the child and family are referred back to the local GP to have him access services. The pt. is diagnosed with ASD but the ASD services say he does not fit their remit as he is too disruptive.

f. The services needed (such as specialized services or culturally competent clinicians) may not be available within the service continuum. It has been well documented that minority youth have poorer access than non-minority youth to any mental health services, as well as inadequate access to culturally competent service providers. (Pumariega 2003, US Department of Health and Human Services 1999, 2001, Winters & Terrell, 2003).

Example: There are no joined- up services in the area. Thus the tertiary care dysmorphic FAS diagnostic clinic is disconnected from primary care and pediatrics and psychiatry. The patients that are seen in the tertiary care dysmorphic FAS clinic are referred back to social service or the primary care physician (GP) with no holistic management plan and no specialist follow –up.

No suggestions are given to the parents about practical management, including medication, of the immediate significant behavioral problems.

No specialist wants to take responsibility for follow up management as the tertiary care dysmorphic FAS clinic model is separated from active management and subsequent clinical follow-up.

There is no connection to child psychiatry and so the child receives mental health care only after another crisis in school or at home.

There is no connection between the tertiary care dysmorphic FAS clinic to culturally competent service providers and thus the foster or adoptive parents are left to their own devices. For instance when I worked in Western Canada it was not uncommon to see children who had been diagnosed 2 or 3 years earlier at the local dysmorphology clinic in the tertiary center. The foster and adoptive parents had sought a referral from a GP after being overwhelmed with complex learning and psychiatric issues which were not addressed in the dysmorphology clinic at initial diagnosis.

g. Another situation which causes problems is a child moving between three different placements as he/she can be acutely traumatized by this experience.

Example: The child as well has ARND, dysmorphic type (FAS) with marked features of Regulatory Disorder, Hyper responsive type and is pervasively hyperactive, disorganized and impulsive. The primary placement with the single adult mother figure is challenging but slowly becoming more settle with social service support to the foster mother.

Unfortunately the child has mandated access visits to birth mother weekly which are chaotic mainly due to birth mother still being alcohol addicted. There are also mandated 2 weekly visits to grandmother with 3 half sibs all with different fathers but all alcohol effected in pregnancy themselves (none diagnosed with possible ARND). These visits are even more chaotic as the grandmother cannot cope and may have undiagnosed cognitive problems herself which impairs her own judgment and management.

h. Kinship placements are expedient but create their own barriers to multi-system management.

Example: A kinship placement with maternal aunt of a 4 year old boy with ARND is opposed by birth father who is still alcohol and drug dependent. He has mandated access visits to his son which are unpredictable due to his addiction. The birth father refuses blood alcohol testing and refuses to go to alcohol or drug counselor, preferring to go to the GP who gives him the sedatives and methadone he desires. He, as well, has hepatitis C and other unspecified infectious diseases but is not being followed by infectious disease specialist.

This has been a problem in Ireland, but also in Native American and First Nations communities. It invites minimization of the alcohol problem and can enable the birth mother or birth father to continue drinking and parenting more alcohol effected children. Obviously this situation creates a barrier for multi-system involvement in management.

Although this clinical approach to management is less well integrated in other health care systems in UK, Canada, Australia it is really the most holistic, logical and respectful manner of management.

Specific Systems

1. The Social Service System

There are situations when a referral to child protection services during pregnancy would be a safety and prophylactic measure for both mother and infant. There is a need for more parent/family support services for alcohol-abusing pregnant women who are often exposed to domestic violence.

Social services in Ireland are caught between a rock and a hard place, as they often have to intervene in a child protection role to take a child into emergency care because of neglect etc., including alcohol addiction/abuse in mother. However, when the child is in care they are mandated/obliged to maintain the State's principle of 'Family Preservation'. So you not uncommonly have a situation where a child is apprehended on one day and the next day the birth family, still abusing alcohol, are asked by the social worker which day they would like access to their, probably brain damaged, child. (A situation unheard of in the initial management of potential ARND in the USA or Canada).

All is not lost in Ireland, as the court appoints a Guardian ad litem if the child is being placed for a Permanent Care Order to the State Care. This Guardian has a role as a potential voice for the child in further diagnostic and treatment issues, which includes an assessment for possible ARND. There are complex ethical issues in this stage of care in Ireland as there is still no true functioning Charter of Rights for Children. Thus the child's rights are pitted against the birth parents rights and re-unification is always mooted, irrespective of the state of alcohol sobriety and violence in the birth family. It becomes not unlike the messy custody battle between two warring parents. In this case you have a biologically vulnerable child with some, but effectively, little voice.

The plight of foster and adoptive parents is quite shocking at times in Ireland, especially if kinship or/family, placement. (This is not much different than the kinship placement problems with the Native Americans or the First Nations).

So foster parents and adoptive parents have to fight for their rights. In a country where the diagnosis of ARND does not exist, but is of course present abundantly they a have a hard road to hoe.

The adoptive parents of children from other countries have a particular problem accessing professional specialized medical support to clarify their fears and worries about their adopted child in contrast both the USA and Canada recognize ARND as a special needs disorder so adoptive and foster parents can avail of specialized parent training and also extra financial support for their child's complex medical and psychiatric needs. As well there is a post adoption agreement which has details of financial and medical need support.

But, there are green shoots appearing. It's Ireland! It is quite apparently obvious, in the last few years, that the social service, guardian ad litem, probation and indeed the school service recognize that ARND is real, and yes it does exist in the Island.

2. The Educational System

School failure was first identified as a major problem by Streissguth and colleagues in the mid 1990s, and continues to present significant management challenges. These children are often 'hidden' under diagnoses such as ADHD, ASD, ODD or bipolar disorder and the organic roots to their learning, behavioral, psychiatric and language problems are not recognized (Streissguth et al., 1996, Carpenter et al., 2013).

School-based assessment typically focuses not only on the child's learning disabilities, but also any classroom behaviors that may be affecting a child's learning progress. This may include history of suspension or even expulsion from school.

However, standard school testing is often limited and can miss the multiple developmental psychiatric, academic, social and language impairments associated with ARND which impede the child's ability to learn in a standard classroom environment. Most frequently it is when the child displays attention, concentration or distractibility problems and/or disruptive behaviors in the classroom, ADHD is usually considered if the child displays attention problems and disruptive behaviors in the classroom, an attention deficit disorder is often the presumed etiology, and a recommendation may be made for a medication assessment. A referral is then made to a physician which commonly results in a prescription of methylphenidate (or Ritalin). However, as noted in medication review section, this type of medication has sometimes little impact on dysfunctional behaviors arising from CNS impairment (as is the case in ARND).

Traditionally in countries such as Ireland, if Attention Deficit Hyperactivity Disorder or some other psychiatric disorder, such as Oppositional Defiant Disorder, is considered to be the cause of the learning and/or behavioral problems, then this closes off initial further inquiry. However, for ARND patients, often methylphenidate is not effective and so the school based problems continue. It is at this juncture, or in the context of a suspension or expulsion, that a comprehensive child psychiatric assessment of a possible undiagnosed developmental psychiatric disorder should be carried out, preferably by a pediatrician.

The early recognition of ARND is critical to school success and the avoidance of disrupted school experiences identified by Streissguth and colleagues (Streissguth et al., 1996), and a Developmental Psychiatric assessment is the kernel of understanding the ARND clinical presentation.

Embedded in the Streissguth and colleagues Secondary Disability study (Streissguth et al., 1996, Streissguth & Kanter 1997) was the demonstration that over 60 per cent of children with ARND, dysmorphic (FAS) or non-dysmorphic, (then called FAE) had a disrupted school experience which progressively increased during the adolescent years. Obviously school systems were not meeting the patients' needs. There was therefore a critical need to understand the complexity of the developmental and/or psychiatric ARND in terms of broader based functional assessments including six Dimensions described in previous chapter.

This type of approach to diagnosis was mooted by:

(O'Malley 2003, 2008, Rich 2009, Rich & O'Malley 2012, O'Malley & Rich 2012, Carpenter et al., 2013).

Summarizing again these Clinical Dimensions:

1) Motor and Sensory Disorder.
2) Disruptive Mood Dysregulation Disorder.
3) Language Disorder.
4) Cognitive Disorder
5) Facial Dysmorphology Disorder.
6) Growth Delay Disorder.

Within the school setting an assessment of functional ability compared with IQ (e.g., using the Vineland Adaptive Behavior Scales (VABS) or ABAS (Streissguth et al., 1996, Elias et al., 2013)) is really a critical part of the evaluation.

So often the school systems, in countries such as Ireland or formerly the UK, have been caught in the old thinking of mental retardation or Intellectual Disability (based solely on IQ under 70) as the criteria to assess the need for special needs support and this standardized assessment of functional ability brings a new language to the table.

Already the introduction of a formal functional assessment within a school's evaluation of a child or adolescent has resulted in many new insights in knowledge and understanding of ARND, dysmorphic, but especially non dysmorphic, in the USA and Canada. It has, for example, informed school curriculum planning in places such as British Columbia and Alberta in Western Canada.

Early school recognition of ARND could become one lynchpin of multi-system intervention, including a more holistic approach to essential Vocational Training, (Sadly lacking in Ireland) which could incorporate the many strengths of learners with ARND, such as art, music, drama, sport, beauty care, mechanics, woodwork, home cooking, to name but a few.

School-based assessment typically focuses on learning disabilities plus any classroom behaviors that may be affecting a child's learning progress. However, standard school testing is often limited and misses the multiple varied ranges of Dimensional disorders associated in ARND with chronic, enduring failure to learn.

IQ level is typically the accepted benchmark.

So if a child underperforms on achievement tests compared to the IQ-based normal expectation, 'learning disability' is the conclusion, which triggers a search for the 'cause', as well as mobilizing resource room and SNA (special needs attendant) educational supports.

As children enter their Secondary (or in USA/Canada middle and high school years) the persistent academic failure and ultimately increasing disconnection and disinterest are assumed to be volitional or deliberate in nature. Now comes a new period for looking for the 'cause'. Usually this time the pre-pubertal child or adolescent parents are informed the problem is one of lack of motivation.

At this juncture, and especially in Ireland, so few children with ARND have been recognized or diagnosed, this crucial underlying developmental psychiatric disorder is missed. As a result the pre-pubertal child or adolescent is excluded from special education support or at least some change in school curriculum to offer vocational activities.

Cognitive testing can have hidden information such as a significant difference (15 points or more) between verbal and performance IQ, which can point to organic brain dysfunction, and the need for a more comprehensive holistic testing. In Ireland neuropsychological testing is generally not available so best ancillary help comes from a formal assessment of adaptive functional ability as assessment using VABS or ABAS which is readily available.

It is more common sense in the later grades or years in school to guide the student towards a vocational training certificate rather than a diploma/A level, Leaving Certificate track, or to master the basic life skills to be productive, employed in a semi-skilled trade (e.g., construction worker, brick mason, landscape worker, plumber's assistant, etc.).

Nevertheless, for many individuals with a higher degree of functioning and with appropriate academic/examination support it may not be unreasonable to expect completion of secondary/high school and even the entering of a two or four year college or university programmer. This is especially true for ARND non dysmorphic or, patients with an ASD profile and average or above average intellectual functioning (O'Malley 2011a, 2013).

3. Multimodal Management Strategies

Ideally for children and adolescents with ARND, multidisciplinary management teams should include other developmental specialties as well (e.g., speech and language, social work, occupational and physical therapy, family and psychological therapy, education). The principle of multimodal therapy is well known in the fields of developmental disability or intellectual disability.

Unfortunately the local CAMHS teams in many parts if Ireland and the UK do not see themselves as having the professional expertise to manage children and adolescents with ARND as they are not seemingly sufficiently trained in Developmental Psychiatry, and still only see patients with ARND as presenting the problems of intellectual disability or mental retardation. An outdated view. This reluctance to become involved is a major stress for many parents, birth, foster or adoptive, as they are often in dire need of a professional, measured opinion on the calming role of medication, but unable to find a suitable expert.

This is not the situation in the USA or Canada, but there they have the not uncommon disconnection between the Fetal Alcohol dysmorphology clinics and follow up clinical care. So the child psychiatrists or pediatricians are often asked to see patients with ARND in crisis quite removed in time from their dysmorphology diagnostic process. Also with no guiding Developmental Psychiatric Disorder hypothesis to inform their medication management strategy.

There are a number of standard modalities of therapy which are used in ARND and each one has different age periods that they are best suited to. (O'Malley 2008)

They are:

1) Occupational Therapy.
2) Physical therapy
3) Speech and Language Therapy
4) Special Education
5) Psychological therapy
6) Family therapy
7) Group therapy
8) Case management through the lifespan
9) Therapist Support
10) Legal System
11) Medication therapy

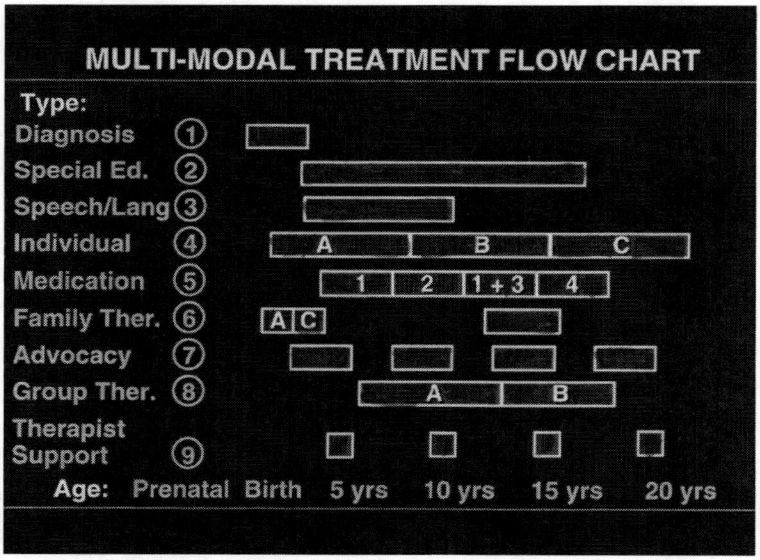

Figure 5. KD O'Malley 2003, use ruler from top to bottom, i.e., 5 yrs. or 15 yrs.

1) Occupational therapy is most useful in the first 5 years of life, specifically for Motor and Sensory Disorders embedded in the ARND. The well-respected sensory integration techniques are especially useful. The children at this stage commonly have Regulatory Disorders and the OT intervention is essential as initial management. The Dunn assessment or the University of Washington sensory assessment are both useful measures.

2) Physical therapy is useful at early ages as well, and helps with Developmental Coordination Disorder and dyspraxia.
   The brain of a developing infant or young g child is still quite 'plastic' in the 1st 3 years of life and so this under stated therapy can have a significant regeneration, healing effect on the ARND damaged brain. This has been shown in animal studies where part of the cerebellum has been oblated, and then somewhat regenerated with motor training.
3) Language therapy is one of the key intervention from early childhood to adolescence.
   It clarifies not just expressive language early onset problems, but with standard assessments such as the CELP 4 the pragmatics deficits in language discourse are identified and form a template for individual therapy. They also educate the parents, teachers and physicians in this commonly hidden disability which is *not* Asperger's Disorder or ASD, but a true Social Communication Disorder (Adnams et al., 2007).
4) Special education is an ever changing challenge and as the diagnosis of ARND is not made in Ireland there are no specialized designated services in school, but the functional ability and Dimensional Disorders within the ARND can often build a case for SNA and resource support on an individual basis.
   This Is a Societal and Ethical Issue
   It is not just about Ireland, but in all countries UK, USA, Canada, and Australia. It is about the 'value' of the special needs child, the 'value 'of the child with a developmental psychiatric disorder, whatever the cause.
   It is not about the plight of marginalized populations, which some politicians still perpetuate to aid an avoidance of an inconvenient truth to borrow from Al Gore.
   Money creates services, services create a better quality of life, and you never know may improve treatment strategies by funding outcome research not just case finding, and mapping.
   I remember, in another lifetime, when I was working in Oil rich Alberta, Canada, the local provincial/city government in Calgary decided to save money by cutting the number of school psychologists in the Public System from 40 to 8 in one year! Needless to say the special needs services died a death.
5) Psychological management
   Although few evidence-based psychological treatments have been shown to work consistently in FAS or ARND populations, and few have scientific validity (Kodituwakku and Kodituwakku 2011), some psychological management approaches have proven value (Streissguth & Connor 2001, O'Malley 2008, Coles 2009, Olson et al., 2009, Novick Brown et al., 2011, Mattson et al., 2011, O'Malley 2013).

Unfortunately, as mentioned earlier in this book, standard outpatient Child and Adolescent Mental Health Service (CAMHS) practice in UK and Ireland generally does not incorporate developmental psychiatric patients. When this is the case, children or adolescents with ARND become further disadvantaged by being effectively excluded from mainstream psychological or even psychiatric systems.

A psychological management approach may include any of the following:

a) Individual play therapy, especially if child has also experienced abuse or domestic violence. (Music, art, pet, water all has roles). Music and art therapy are particularly good for dealing with mood dysregulation and language problems such as alexithymia. They also offer an opportunity for the child to show his or her talent in different areas than school work, and so contribute to self-esteem. One 13-year-old girl with ARND was able to teach herself the guitar and compose a song called 'Paralyzed' which captured her life struggles at the time.
   Pet therapy has a role as well and helps with children who have motor and sensory dysregulation. In the Dublin clinic a Tibetan spaniel who is quite docile is involved in regular Saturday follow up clinics and is well received.
   Dance and Drama therapy both have roles in this patient population. In Native American communities dance and music are very much part of the culture and help include children with ARND in to the general community.
   As well drama therapy has been shown to have a role in helping with social communication skills, and a successful programme exists in Trinity College Dublin dealing with ASD/Asperger's Disorder children and teenagers which has clear connection to the ARND population.
b) Reality based therapy to help child or adolescent navigate life stages, such as relationships, losses, school setbacks, and family or home transitions.
   This is helpful approach to teach the parents and also communicate to the school teachers.
   NB There is a Strategies Document at the end of the book which offers a range of clear strategies for use with children with ARND.
c) Trauma based therapy for severely vulnerable child with features of developmental trauma disorder as well as dysmorphic ARND (FAS) or non-dysmorphic ARND. This is essential in patients with a clear documented trauma exposure history and the nonverbal modality using art, music, water, sandtray are most helpful in calming and helping the patient process the trauma experiences.
d) Dyadic therapy for child and parent (usually the mother) at different stages (i.e., early childhood, later in adolescence, etc.); this may include work on identity, conflict and antipathy towards birth parent.

This type of therapy is useful at many times in the developmental life of the child and later adolescent. It helps to clarify misunderstandings due to social communication problems and as well approaches the insipient attachment issues which may or may not be present. The complicated dance of attachment between the birth parent and the foster or adoptive parent is a key issue, and often made all the more stressful with the premature death of the birth parent due to alcohol related medical factors. (O'Malley & Streissguth 2006, O'Malley 2008).

e) Parallel therapy between adult psychiatric and addiction providers and child psychiatric/psychological providers to address the transgenerational issues (O'Malley 2003, Novick Brown et al., 2011, and Turk 2007).
This is in an ideal world. In Seattle, with a long history of knowledge of FAS, this type of collaboration was more common and of obvious benefit to all concerned. In this context the successful PCAP program evolved from Seattle (Grant et al., 2008).

f) Intergenerational psychotherapy and support is needed, especially in countries with transgenerational ARND such as Ireland and the UK.
This would be on a wish list as well, but has been instituted mainly in the psychoanalytic world in addressing the transgenerational trauma of Holocaust survivors. It is not a major leap of imagination to see its role in communities such as the North of Ireland. When I worked there I did attempt some inter-generational work but the pervasive denial, minimization, and resistance due to stigma was an impossible impasse. One only has to see the intransigence related to the recent Haas talks over flags, parades and dealing with the traumatic past to see the problems in the path ahead.

g) There needs to be integration of services between adult psychiatric and addiction providers and child psychiatric and psychological providers (O'Malley 2003, Turk 2007).
This does not happen in Ireland or the UK to great extent and until it does transgenerational ARND will continue to grow, despite any latest science showing the epigenetics of alcohol.

h) Addiction counseling is an important approach for birth mothers, but this type of therapy may not be suitable for birth parents who have ARND themselves and therefore have differing levels of cognitive processing impairment.
Animal research is now involved in exploring models of experience based interventions to decrease or manage the behavioral deficits caused by prenatal alcohol exposure (Hannigan et al., 2007). A recent review by Bertrand et al. in 2009 delineated a number of interventions that had positive results.

6) Family therapy related to:

- Family education, regarding the immediate and long term consequences of prenatal alcohol exposure. This is a critical part of therapy in countries such as

Ireland where the condition ARND officially does not exist and there is so much disinformation about the effects of alcohol in pregnancy.

Web sites:

- FASD.IE
- NOFAS.co. org
- FASDTrust. co.uk
- NOFAS. org (USA)
- BMA FASD 2007
- EUFASD.org

- Family instrumental work on daily living organization, this is a more sensible approach to help the family and a child with ARND, than the more 'wordy/sophisticated' Narrative and strategic systemic family therapy which miss the mark due to language and memory, processing issues.(Also they are likely to 'blame' the birth, foster or adoptive mother as they are not properly attached to their infant or young child).
- Family stress resulting from the burden of caring for someone with chronic neurodevelopmental disorder

Parent support with respite care and utilizing the concept of the parent becoming an 'auxiliary brain' for the patient with ARND to help them navigate life's tasks and stages (Bertrand 2009, Densmore 2011, Kulp 2004, Malbin 2011, Novick Brown et al., 2011, Olson et al., 2009, O'Malley 2008, 2011, 2013).

7) Group therapy has been used sporadically but has real potential in the realm of socialization, communication and problem solving skills training in adolescents and young adults.

Groups have been run in Canada for young adult males and young adult females and the issue of delayed processing of information in a group setting was an interesting part of the group process, as patients processed emotional information at different paces. (O'Malley 2008).

This is the area for the incorporation of drama therapy techniques.

8) Case management through the lifespan.

This is the sine qua non in the management of ARND. It is really true that the foundation of effective service provision is lifelong case management and regular multidisciplinary team monitoring.

A key to building this foundation is the acquisition of developmental pediatric and/or disability services as soon in life as possible, which typically requires a diagnosis of ARND with the varying Dimension disorders delineated.(in Ireland developmental pediatricians are a rarer bird and usually in the hospital rather than the community). Disability service is elusive at best. This is not a given in other countries, but there is a general recognition that early intervention is the essence of better outcomes in ARND.

Most important in this service delivery process is long term case management to assure consistent overview and monitoring of treatment needs and effectiveness. This begins with the social service team and guardian ad litem in early placement, continues in nursery and early school placement. It continues in secondary, middle, high school, and of course is vital in the no man's land of young adulthood when there are traditionally little if any specialized services for any youth with psychiatric disorders, let alone ARND, on both sides of the Atlantic.

Because Cognitive psychological disorders in ARND tend to be lifelong, it is clear that as youth with ARND mature into adulthood, case management needs to continue indefinitely.

At this current juncture most adults with ARND are unable to live independently and support themselves. Thus, the vast majority need residential assistance (ideally, a structured living environment) and assistance with adaptive tasks (e.g., nutrition, shopping, transportation, money management, time management, leisure activities and socialization, job coaching, acquisition of medical and dental care).

The introduction of a legal guardian or trustee/protective payee in USA is crucial to protect the adult with ARND from exploitation. When they also have an alcohol addiction programmed from fetal time, then they need to be involved with medical alcohol counselors, and may need appropriate medication to cut down the alcohol craving.

Since many adults with ARND who are not living in structured, supervised living environments may inadvertently and or willfully have trouble with the law, structured living situations that involve some form of supervision and staff assistance will enhance their chances of success.

9) Therapist support is essential for psychiatrists and mental health workers, social workers, school teachers, and especially foster, adoptive and birth parents involved in the area of ARND management. It is essential to prevent compassion fatigue. In psychiatry the use of peer groups as mandatory part of continuing professional development is very useful, in keeping one ' honest and sane'! Parent support groups can and do serve a similar function.

10) The Legal System.

This is another area in ARND where the USA and Canada are at the forefront. Lead by such pioneers and spark plugs, as Ann Streissguth, Kay Kelly, Billy Edwards, Hon. Anthony Wartnik in the USA., and Diane Fast, Julie Conroy, David Boulding in Canada.

Already the American Bar Association has set out criteria for dealing with potential FASDs patients (i.e., ARND dysmorphic and non-dysmorphic) in August 2012, and the Canadian Bar Association set out their own criteria for dealing with potential patients with FASD (dysmorphic and non-dysmorphic ARND) in August 2013.

There are many legal protections for patients with ARND through the lifespan in place.

a. The unborn fetus has rights if the mother continues drinking alcohol during the pregnancy and social service can make plans for a safe placement after birth which is portable between Provinces (States) as happened when I was consulting the over 15 years ago.
b. Miranda rights protect the adolescent or young adult with ARND who has a legal problem if they had not given a statement with a third party present.(A major problem in Ireland, especially in the North, where the police have long experience in obtaining guilty statements, and sensitivity to developmental psychiatric disorders such as ARND varies).
c. Capacity laws are well honed in the USA and Canada, so it is easier with the Adult Dependent Act legislation to obtain guardianship and trusteeship (Protective Payee, USA) to help the young adult with ARND navigate life, especially daily living and budgets.

   In Ireland the old Ward of Court is going and the new Capacity Laws are soon coming into place. They are not IQ driven, as far as I can gather, and include items such as decision making assistant, co–decision maker, and decision–making representative. All relevant to the ARND population. (They are based on the long standing UK legislation). (Leonard, Kelly et al., 2013).
d. In the USA there are a number of people, usually male, with serious violent charges which include admitting to crimes where no body, money etc. was found,

   There is so a Seattle-based legal team, with Natalie Nowick Brown, Paul Connor, Billy Edwards (LA), Rich Adler, and Fred Bookstein whose advocacy job is to 'bring the brain to the table', using patient history of alcohol exposure in pregnancy, neuropsychology, psychiatry and brain imaging.
e. In the USA there are actually Mental Health Courts which have trained Judges and advocates to spot the mentally ill, including ARND patients.(There is a new initiative in the UK to incorporate mental health nurses in selected police stations, and hopefully this will identify patients with psychiatric disorders including undiagnosed patients with ARND).
f. Again in the USA there has been a long history of collaboration between Juvenile Justice and the American Academy of Child and Adolescent Psychiatry, run by AACAP (Bill Heffron from Kentucky was an early leading light).
g. The Guardian ad Litem role is very helpful for children who are taken into Care by the State, and may be the sole reason that the child has an n assessment for ARND. (Many are previous social workers who understand the ins and outs of the legal system,) In Ireland experienced Guardians include, Maura Lagan, Brain Lavery, and Harry Law.

(Kelly 2009, Edwards 2011, Leonard et al., 2013).

BRIEF SUMMARY STATEMENT (2014 BOOK)

Few evidence-based mental health interventions have been shown to work in ARND populations. According to a review by Bertrand, several interventions show promise. Important elements in these interventions include parent education or training and teaching children specific social and executive function skills that children typically learn through observation or abstraction. Another promising aspect of these interventions was their integration into existing mental health treatment systems (Nowick Brown et al., 2011).

NB. There is 'A Strategies for Management of children or adolescents with ARND, dysmorphic (FAS) or non-dysmorphic' at the back of the 2014s book. It has been piloted in Ireland, and is undergoing further field research in Kamloops, British Columbia. It has become 'Standard of Practice' in Ireland the last year for all new patients diagnosed with ARND, dysmorphic, or non-dysmorphic, and is given to parents, birth, foster or adoptive as well as social worker involved.

It has also proved useful for the school teachers involved with the patient.

The instrument is available for use; all you have to do is inform the primary author, (Dr Kieran D. O'Malley,).

The Broad Parameters Described in the 2014 Book in This Chapter Update Have Not Fundamentally Changed in the Last 5 Years, Except That ARND Is Now NDPAE a Diagnosis in the DSM 5, Code 315. 8

I will briefly expand on then basic tenets described in the first book.

Constructing a Scaffolding System in NDPAE

Oftentimes the clinician does not know where, or how, to begin this process critical first stage process. The intervening clinical practice over the last 5 years have helped me in formulating a more logical approach to where and how to begin the scaffolding process. It naturally is driven by the ecological environment in which the child or adolescent with NDPAE dwells.

a. Birth family in which an infant/child is at risk or diagnosed with NDPAE.

As seen in the previous chapter update the scaffolding must take on a simultaneous double strand approach, which collides with the traditional medical silos of adult and pediatric medicine.

Not unreasonably, it is the obstetrics specialty which bridges adult/parent and infant/young child care which is the key ingredient in this scaffolding. It is during pregnancy that the' at risk parent' and 'at risk infant' has to be identified. The midwife has a central role in this identification and as well earning the trust of the birth mother who is alcohol dependent or abusing alcohol, in the pregnancy. This requires a level of co-operation with the pregnancy mother not just about alcohol, but also exposure to partner stress in pregnancy, attendance at ante natal visits and involvement with addiction counsellor. It is not fair to a birth mother to minimize her alcohol usage and missed antenatal and addiction counselling appointments, and then present her with the diagnosis of alcohol –acquired brain injury, NDPAE, in her recently born infant.

This is the first level of the scaffolding.

The birth father has a role in this obstetrics driven scaffolding, and it can be positive or negative. Either way it contributes to the stability of the fist level of scaffolding.

The hospital social worker is another key component in developing the scaffolding for the birth mother who is a functional alcoholic or alcohol dependent and has an infant/young child with NDPAE. He/She needs to be an integral part of the obstetric team and be appraised of the potential 'At risk' mothers and 'at risk' infants.

This is the 2nd level of scaffolding.

The hospital social worker can then liaise with the community social worker to set up a family support team after the birth of the infant.

In parallel the midwife can liaise with the health worker and/or public health nurse regarding the 'at risk' mother/infant dyad regarding basic feeding and nurturing needs.

This is the 3rd level of scaffolding.

b. Foster family with infant/child at risk or diagnosed with NDPAE.

The community social worker needs to inform the prospective foster parents that the child they are taking into care is a special needs child, and is at risk or probably has NDPAE because of exposure to alcohol in pregnancy. The foster parents need to be honestly appraised of the potential complexity in care needs for this child. This means family support is built into the initial care plan, the placement is, if possible, of a more stable permanent basis, and the community social worker is sensitive to the probability that the child's untoward behaviors and reactivity are not just due to an attachment disorder, but a product of the alcohol- acquired brain injury in the child.

This is level 1 of scaffolding.

The Community Social Worker who places the child in State Care needs to liaise with the Hospital Social Worker to obtain the maternity record, especially as it pertains to alcohol in pregnancy. (in some countries this may involve obtaining a Judge's Court Order as the Maternity hospital sometimes refuses to release data on the birth mother for data protection reasons)

This is level 2 of scaffolding

The foster parents need to connect with care provider/family physician with access to specialist consultation i.e., pediatric and/or child psychiatrist

This is level 3 of scaffolding.

The community social worker and the foster parents need to have a diagnostic assessment for NDPAE done ASAP by a treating physician (there are problems with tertiary care hospital dysmorphology clinics and private multi- disciplinary clinics who generally do not follow up the child. Thus the diagnosis of NDPAE or FASD is given in a potential therapeutic vacuum.

This is level 4 of scaffolding.

The community social worker has to balance the access to the birth parents who may still be alcohol dependent and the child with NDPAE, as this can potentially undermine the attachment to the foster parents. However, if managed respectfully it can be of lasting benefit to all involved, the child with NDPAE, the birth parents and the foster parents

This is level 5 of scaffolding.

c. An adoptive family with a child at risk or diagnosed with NDPAE.

The adoption social worker needs to inform the prospective adoptive parents that the child they are probably receiving a special needs child.

This is level I of scaffolding

The adoptive social worker should have all the medical information on the child's birth and early history, especially alcohol in pregnancy. This can be obtained from private agencies such as Bernardo's adoption agency, Catholic adoption agencies, Russian or Romanian orphanages and Inter- country adoption agencies.

This is level 2 of scaffolding.

The adoption social worker and adoptive parents need to organize a medical assessment of the child ASAP, to establish the potential diagnosis of a neurodevelopmental disorder and anticipate service needs.

This is level 3 of scaffolding.

NOTE: The adoptive parents of a child with NDPAE are the most likely to have little if any scaffolding protection.

This is especially so for those inter- country adoptive parents from countries such as Russia or Romania (Rutter et al., 2011). Although the emotional problems related to institutions, orphanages in these countries have been well documented it is still less universally recognized that these children also have frequently significant prenatal alcohol exposure (which is commonly to 40% alcohol/vodka, rather than 5% beer in Ireland or

UK). Unfortunately, the 30,000 to 40,000 Euro fee does not guarantee an unblemished Caucasian child or medical professional diagnostic or management follow up. Many of these new adoptive parents have no assigned adoptive social worker to help them navigate service needs, and no entry into the health system for specialist special needs services.

In my recent 14 years' practice in the UK and Ireland I was only was involved with 2 international adoption social workers who maintained contact and support with the adoptive parents. Both were marvelous, but are sadly rare.

Cultural Competence and Cultural Sensitivity

This is a major problem in inter-country adoptions in certain countries such as Ireland, less so the UK. The children are privately adopted from countries such as Russia, Romanian, or China but there is no organized system of 'inclusion' in the new society. So, no groups of parents with children from similar countries, no Russian, Romanian, Chinese professional support networks to help the new adoptive parents and their children.

This is in contrast to countries such as Canada or the USA which have a long history of cultural connectedness for these inter- country adopted children with special needs such as FASD or NDPAE.

Ensuring Multi-System and Then Multi-Modal Treatment Approach in NDPAE

This is not taken from Henngler multi- systemic therapy, but a practical approach to involvement with different health, education, social service, and legal systems due to the nature of the non- IQ, non- face driven global neurodevelopmental disorder, NDPAE.

> It is also worth reviewing the current situation of these specific health care systems in follow up to my 2014 book observations.

As well, I would like to add that in my years of psychiatric consultation work in his clinical area I have participated in 100's of case management meetings in multiple settings, and it has been the most consistently rewarding part of my professional work.

The Social Service System

a. A formal case management meeting at the beginning of the diagnostic formulation review is essential. This meeting will clarify the diagnosis of NDPAE and review the different dimensions which are impaired in the child which will require longer term remedial support or even active treatment. (At this stage many of the specialist evaluations will be incorporated in the diagnostic formulation i.e., psychological testing, occupational therapy (OT) testing, speech and language testing and so on). It is better to have these professionals present their findings at the initial case management meeting so as to facilitate constructive multi-disciplinary planning.

It is also essential that the foster parents are present at this meeting

Finally, it is important to hold this initial case management meeting in offices of the social service department where the child is being managed, and to have it lead by the senior social work supervisor or team leader.

b. The psychiatric or psychological consultant involved with the child with NDPAE in care should formally meet with the Social Services agency at least once a year as part of the yearly review.

It is always a good idea to have scheduled a recent clinical follow up session with the child and parents, just before the yearly social service case management meeting.

The meeting should be held in the social service offices and lead by social service management as in the initial meeting. Individual professionals i.e., education, special needs teacher, speech and language therapist, occupational therapist, individual therapist, family support worker should be present in person to present and discuss collaboratively their ongoing work with the client with NDPAE.

Again, it is essential that the foster parents are at this yearly follow up meeting. Sometimes one or both birth parents may be invited to this meeting depending on the therapeutic success of the access visits.

The One Key Professional Very Uncommonly Seen Is a Learning Disability Specialist

Key Points

a. It is better for a child with NDPAE to enter care for a longer period of time to afford a secure predictable attachment to the foster parents. (2 to 3years placement is not in the best interest of the child and undermines the structured home of the foster parents).

b. The issue of access to the birth parents is a major factor and often continues to emotionally disturb the child and undermine the authority and parenting of the foster parents.

- The child can be subject to chronic PTSD as he/she experiences missed access appointments due to birth parent absences.
- access visits which are anxiety - provoking due to continued alcohol dependence of birth parents and child continues to be triangulated between foster parents and birth parents but has ‘no voice’.

- access visits are planned with no communication between social services and the alcohol counsellor treating the birth mother, or father, so no professional communication of the suitability of the visit relationship to the birth parents' level of treatment compliance.

c. Kinship placements are the ones commonly most undermined by both social services and birth families. It is as if the aunt/uncle or brother/sister is wanted, but is also not wanted so is in a state of constant negative' double bind'. Stigma and denial are critical factors in this situation.

d. Children who are adopted from other countries not infrequently suffer from issues of cultural identity disconnection in pre-teen and teenage years. This is more likely a problem for later adopted children after 5 years of age, and can be compounded by speaking 2 languages i.e., Russian and English in Ireland or UK.

The Educational System

Case management meetings are an essential part of the holistic treatment plan for children with NDPAE.

There ae generally 3 opportune times for these meetings which, of course should only be held in the pupil's school, and lead by the principal or special needs coordinator.

a. An initial school meeting as soon after diagnosis of NDPAE has been made. This involves sharing the psychiatric consultation report with social services or/and parent permission (and permission of adolescent or older pupil if being discussed). The availability of specialist reports, or better the professional themselves, such as psychologist for cognitive testing results: WPPSSI and WISC IV, OT for developmental coordination assessment or speech and language for language results, such as CELP-4.

This meeting forms the template for understanding the rubric of NDPAE, which is a non-IQ, non-face global neurodevelopmental disorder which effects functioning in many area, but does not subscribe to the older learning disability model of IQ under 70.

As well it brings the concept of alcohol acquired brain injury to the table which has psychiatric presentations which are not just ADHD or ASD, but a separate global neurodevelopmental disorder which need a different management paradigm. Functional assessment through Vineland Adaptive Behavior Scales (3rd edition) or Adaptive Behavior Scale (ABS) is essential information for school understanding.

The foster, birth or adoptive parents should be present.at the meeting.

b. It is a good idea to have a case management meeting, in the school led again by school professionals, at the beginning of the school year, usually September as this affords the time to do a measured approach to resource time or SNA needs for the coming year.

The foster, birth or adoptive parents should be present.at the meeting.

c. The third time for a meeting in the school, led by school professionals, is at the end of the school year. This affords the time to review school academic and social progress as well as maybe response to therapy, individual or medication.

This also is a time to plan appropriate school academic setting and support for the following year, which may even include a change of school to Junior High, Middle or High School all critical environments which have different impacts on learning ability.

The foster, birth or adoptive parents should be present.at the meeting.

Unfortunately, as with the social service meetings the elephant in the room is invariably the absence of a special needs learning disability administrative official.

This is a major 'bone of contention; in the main stream schooling environment as in truth there are never enough special/learning needs schools or places so the reality continues to be that complex children with conditions such as NDPAE are managed as best as possible in the regular school environment.

It is only fair to acknowledge that countries such as Canada and USA have an over 20-years history of recognizing the unique learning needs of children with NDPAE (previously FASD), and even have sensory sensitive classes and learning environments for these pupils. A true luxury for many other parts of the world.

Key Points:

a. The transition from Primary/Grammar school to Secondary or Junior High is a major problem for a child with NDPAE, as they go from one classroom and one teacher to many classrooms and many teachers.

b. Mathematics is a core learning disability in NDPAE, and is at the center of executive functioning i.e., deductive reasoning, decision making, organization, problem solving and planning, dyscalculia. A specific mathematics learning strategy and resource support is an important remedial education tool.

c. A specific individualized educational plan (IEP) is necessary for a child with NDPAE, remembering it is not driven by IQ under 70. Resource hours in key subjects, and SNA when needed, especially during unstructured 'play periods' due to impulsive/hyperactive behaviors.

d. Sometimes it may be useful to have a time of blended home tuition and in-house school teaching coordinator, so as to settle an impulsive, intermittently aggressive and disruptively moody child with NDPAE.

e. Examinations bring many challenges including processing of information, working memory anticipatory and performance anxiety, and the introduction of a scribe or reader, individual or together have proven of great benefit through the years.

f. Lastly there are school programs, such as DARE and others, which allow student to achieve a lower level of points or mark to qualify for second level education. This is not just the vocational system but is built into regular university/technical

g. college entrance application (Carpenter et al., 2014).

The Medical System

a. A case management meeting should be held in the hospital children's or general if the child is diagnosed with NDPAE. under 5 years of age, especially if there are issues with faltering growth, seizure disorder or motor or sensory problems.

These meetings are best if held and chaired by the hospital social worker in liaison with the community social worker, perinatal psychiatrist, neonatologists, pediatric, physical therapy, maybe neurology are useful participants and the foster or birth parents are important as well. The busyness of hospitals makes these types of meetings less common, but if they do happen they form a good scaffolding for the child with NDPAE and can create a link between the hospital specialists and the community child psychiatrist or community child psychologist (the traditional CAMHS services do not deal with patients under 5 years old with NDPAE so generally would not be part of this type of meeting).

They can also form a gentle reminder of the real legacy of prenatal alcohol exposure and inform cared of subsequent pregnancies.

b. Case management meetings in children's hospital or adolescent hospital centers should be able to incorporate a pre-admission/early admission and pre-discharge meeting but this rarely happens for many reasons, and invariably leads to communication about management and response to treatment issues.

c. It is a central issue in the systems of care management of children or adolescents with NDPAE as the hospitalizations are usually only short chapters in their lives but can often, unintentionally, de-rail holistic community management.

It speaks volumes about the dearth of community/hospital linked learning disability services which are able to manage dual diagnosis patients i.e., developmental disability and psychiatric disorder (see USA National Association of Dually Diagnosed, NADD).

The Legal System

The Court system becomes part of the life of a child or adolescent with NDPAE and his/her family due to various serious clinical antisocial issues:

a) Sexually inappropriate behavior
b) Stealing and compulsive lying
c) Fire setting
d) Violence to people or animals
e) Drug or alcohol involvement.

There are a number of basic principles to be addressed when the legal system is involved:

I. The NDPAE has an effect on functional capacity of the client, which is directly related to the level of global neurodevelopmental disorder which has been diagnosed using the 6 Dimensional criteria. described in previous chapter. and 2014 book and expanded and clarified in this update.
II. The general principles of assessing the client with NDPAE as suitable for court:

- Assess the reliability of the general comments and replies to questions in the initial police interview (assess the need for an inclusion of an adult advocate to be present).
- Assess the possible presence of suggestibility to leading and open-ended questions (the presence of an advocate is important).
- Assess whether the client/defendant understands the nature and seriousness of the charge.
- Assess if the client/defendant understands the workings of the court and is ‘fit to plea’.
- Assess whether the neurodevelopmental disorder, with co-occurring psychiatric problem or addiction problems, have influenced the client’s responsibility for the offence.

(iii) The NDPAE in the client may have an impact on his/her court appearance/demeanor.

The person may have limited understanding of court proceedings; this includes the client saying that they understand the questions or questions when in fact they do not.

The person may agree too much with Attorney/Barrister or be easily lead by the Attorney/Barrister.

They may blurt out things inappropriately unrelated to the court questions.

They may become suddenly very agitated or emotional in court with no clear precipitant from the court proceedings.

This can include a tendency to confabulate when anxious about question meanings.

(Burd 2012, Church et al., 2007, Brown et al., 2015, Kelly, 2018,)

It is also important to be aware of:

(i) Sexually inappropriate behavior in clients with NDPAE must be seen in the light of their neurodevelopmental challenges but also possible environmental challenges such as abuse. In working with a number of specialized sexual abuse agencies the professionals within these organizations have recognized that sexually aberrant behavior is not solely 'binary' in clients with NDPAE, but often the patients are both victims and perpetrators at the same time.

The vulnerability from early exposure to physical or sexual abuse coupled with social communication deficits lead to misunderstandings. about culpability and motivation.

Clinical Example:

A 9year old with NDPAE is placed with 2 younger sibs all with NDPAE. He begins to start physically and sexually abusing his 7year old brother every time he returns from an access visit to his birth father who is still alcohol dependent. The birth father has a history of violence and probable abuser of his children especially the eldest son. The social worker is unsure of the veracity of 9-year-old boy's story.

(Nowick Brown 2008).

(ii) Violent behaviors

The violent behaviors maybe impulsive, unplanned and reactive, or part of a general aggressive, angry provocative demeanor. In either case the careful developmental history of the age of onset of violent behaviors and possible precipitants is key.

It is important to have a developmental history with attention to developmental disorders, ADHD, mood disorder or seizure disorder.

Cognitive or neuropsychological testing is the first level of functional assessment.

Standardized psychological instruments, such as Structured Assessment of Violent Risk in Youth (SAVRY) and AIM3 assessment for adolescents who display harmful sexual behavior, are helpful in specifying and quantifying risk.

Sleep Deprived EEG or MRI of brain may be useful tests to quantify the acquired alcohol brain injury underpinning the violence. These are both useful clinical tools

(Rich 2016)

(iii) Fire-setting can be a serious risk-taking behavior.

An 8-year-old child sets his mother's mattress on fire because he is very angry with her. They both could have died of smoke inhalation, but were saved by the local fire service.

A teenager sets a fire in his hospital unit as he is angry with the locked-door policy.

A young adult is admitted to prison and is allowed to smoke and have a lighter, even though his psychiatric record showed a history of repeated childhood fire setting.

The history of fire-setting with troubled aggressive angry children is well established from a psychoanalytic perspective, but the neuro biological roots of this focused impulsive behavior, seen in NDPAE are being more recognized (Stafford Clark 1969). Kolko, (2002) provides a practical handbook on fire-setting in children and youth which includes a number of assessment measures, such as the Federal Emergency Management Agency (FEMA) interview tool and guidance on how to take a fire-setting history.

(iv) Cruelty to animals may be an indicator of severe anti-social behavior.

One child breaks the leg of a young dog, another child puts a kitten in a microwave oven, and lastly a child squashes a hamster to death.

Conversely a number of children have petted their animals to death. One over- petted a rabbit, another a gerbil, and another 2 pet snakes. All these children had sensory-seeking temperaments, and were in many ways over-attached to their pets. They did not understand that over-petting could harm their pets.

(v) Drug and alcohol abuse or dependence are interwoven with violent or sexually inappropriate behaviors and must be assessed in the light of the possible epigenetic kindling of early onset alcohol craving due to prenatal alcohol exposure (O'Malley 2003).
(vi) Stealing and compulsive lying also need to be assessed within a developmental frame with attention to early onset, exposure to neglect or abuse, cognitive functioning and working memory and social communication problems.

The Multi-Modal Treatment in NDPAE Continues to Be Expanded and Revised

Occupational Therapy

This is very much part of a young child's therapy under 5 as Developmental Co-ordination Disorder is a problem in NDPAE.

Motor training continues to be an integral part of work to remediate the neurological disconnections, often related to disturbance in developing cerebellum.

The sensory issues underpin the regulatory disorders and lead to significant disconnections due to visual, auditory, tactile over sensitivity.

In older school-aged children problems, such as dyspraxia and dyslexia, benefit from Interventions including graphic writing, penmanship, use of computer. visual training (sometimes needing special blue tinted glasses).

The sensory issues need many individualized interventions, including sensory room in class or residential center.

Physical Therapy

This is very much part of neonatal care with more medically vulnerable children and progresses in concert with occupational therapy as the child ages. Problems with feeding are a particular area of concern as prenatal alcohol can have neurological effect on the sucking reflex delaying sucking and also causing a long latency to suck.

As well poor habituation is a feature of NDPAE which ushers a difficult to settle temperament.

Speech and Language Therapy

Delayed language development is a key dimension in NDPAE.

The language disorder is in the area of pragmatic use of language or social discourse/communication. Often the standard language tests do not shed a light on this disability and secondary tests such as CELP-4 or Pre-school CELP are necessary (for example WPPSS or WISC IV show verbal IQ over 70 or even 80 with significant split with performance IQ, but the verbal cognitive test score hides the disability in social communication and social cognition which is most troublesome and often misunderstood as deliberate defiance).

Special Education

Specific learning disorders in mathematics and visual processing of information are key neurocognitive disabilities embedded in the core of NDPAE.

The specific learning problems of dyscalculia, dyslexia are often coupled together needing specific remedial education approaches. They are sometimes associated with ADHD symptomatology and so general educational approaches for ADHD, especially inattention/impulsivity subtype are warranted.

Psychological/Individual Therapy

This is abroad, ever-expanding area.

a. Music therapy has proven benefits having been shown to enhance mathematics learning in the 1960s Philadelphia child guidance clinics. It has also been used in schizophrenia/psychosis, mood disorders, with explosive episodes, and PTSD. All potential clinical parts of the phenotype of NDPAE.

The music therapy can be done in the context of a music therapist treatment center or individualized in the family home.

Clinical Example:

A Russian adoptive boy learned to play the tin whistle but could only play tunes under 2 minutes long due to his working memory problems.

A Romanian adopted teenage girl taught herself the guitar and was able to express her emotion s about break up of a relationship with a boy through the medium of music and lyrics. (her birth parents were musical Romany gypsies.

A very explosive angry teenage foster boy was able to express his emotions in a more nuanced fashion through the medium of music, rain sticks.

b. Animal therapy Equine or Dog (especially). Equine therapy has been used and studied in autism, for example in USA (Belmont Stables, NY), Thailand, UK, Canada and Ireland.

Clinical Example:

A number of foster and birth teenage girls have responded instantly to horse therapy, and were able to understand the horse's feelings which became a bridge in therapy to understanding their own emotions (one girl joined a national circus group and became the 'carer' of the horses).

Many younger children, especially, have responded to the calmness of our Tibetan spaniel, Mollyo in therapeutic situations and their hyperactive, impulsive, aggressive behaviors have visibly diminished (a number of parents have used the therapeutic experience to buy a dog as a pet for their child in the home with consistent success).

c. Art therapy. Has long usage in psychiatry and neurodevelopmental disorders and is central in enhancing communication when the individual has problems in language communication with alexithymia.

Clinical Example:

A number of children and adolescents with NDPAE have been able to express their emotional state through drawings and are particularly graphic with use of bold colors. (very useful if child has experienced the trauma of death of birth parent, or has been physically or sexually abused in early placements or residential centers/schools). Standard 'house/tree/person' still valid, as well as 'draw a person, 'outer and inner self'.

d. Dance Therapy has a particular value with dyspraxia and coupled with music brings much joy to clients and increased self-esteem. Long utilized in Downs Syndrome patients.

Clinical Example:

First Nations and Native American children have benefited from Pow Wow dancing in their local tribes and have gained much self-esteem in the process. (however, one boy who was very good at this dancing become quite disturbed and out of focus when the drummer changed from an elder one with steady rhythm to a younger drummer with a faster rhythm. He could not cope with the change in the beat cadence).

e. Body awareness/dance therapy also has been used with violent offenders in such countries as Holland to aid with body sensitivity/awareness, physical boundaries and help with aggressive impulses.
f. Drama therapy is more useful in older adolescents as it affords them a script and role with clear boundaries and objectives. Open-ended stories driven by trauma or violence are dramatic and cathartic and often shocking show and tell when portrayed in a collaborative play. They can also be a self- destructive, as I have seen a number of adolescents with NDPAE/FASD who have acted out their life story in a play to raise funds from Corporate sponsors, but the following week have felt' violated, used and abused' by this show and tell experience.
g. Last but never least there are a host of Psychological therapies which have been utilized in people with intellectual disabilities. Many are not a good fit for patients with NDPAE, because of the pervasive problems in working memory and social communication.

However, a number of chapters in the book are quite relevant to NDPAE population:

Chapter 1: Identifying and meeting the emotional and mental health needs of people who have intellectual disabilities through psychological therapies.

Chapter 7: Solution - focused brief therapy

Chapter 9: Group interventions.

Chapter 10: A systematic review of the outcome measures used in psychological therapies in adults with ID.

(British Psychological Society, 2016)

Family Therapy

This has been described in 2014 book, but needs continued emphasis as it is an essential part of the 'emotional scaffolding' holding the patient with NDPAE and his/her family together no matter which context, birth, foster or adoption. The most useful approach remains instrumental or structural family therapy which places concrete roles and goals/expectations on all family members in the general family functioning.

Narrative therapy is the most destructive with NDPAE as patients, and sometimes birth parents, have cognitive disconnections and memory problems. Therefore, they are unable to consistently incorporate this process.

Group Therapy

This is a woefully underused form of therapy.

I have had personal involvement in both pre-teen and adolescent groups and both are most rewarding modalities of management package.

There is a specific area, not recognized in addiction circles, and this is the children of parents with NDPAE or alcohol dependence, or the adolescents of patents with NDPAE or alcohol dependence.

Now, as populations age and struggle with many medical illnesses there is a new era of adult patients with NDPAE who are able to discuss the transgenerational medical sequelae of their condition. They are the present, but as well, the potential 'change – makers' or 'influencers' of the future. Warning us of the coming generations of prenatal alcohol exposed infants and children.

For example; 15 to 20 years ago when I referred adolescents with FASD (or now NDPAE) with neurodevelopmental, psychiatric and addiction problems to a major hospital. Addiction center in Calgary the patients were rejected as this addiction center did not deal with addiction disorder in adolescents with 'organic brain dysfunction'. New science shows us the organic roots of addiction (Tomkins 2001, Volkow 2015).

Therapist/Parent Support

a. This is still an unheralded area of the multi modal management strategies.

Anthem first strategy is to give Strategies for Management Document (SEE END OF 2014 Book) to parents after the diagnosis of NDPAE is made. This offers a 'script' for management which differs from the traditional operant conditioning/behavioral modification instruments which generally do not work with this global neurodevelopmental disorder.

This empowers the therapist in the initial approach to management and the implications of the diagnosis. (The strategies document is most useful if given to the social worker in charge and the current school, so that all three areas of wrap around care are in sync.)

b. Support meetings on a regular basis are very helpful as long as they do not only dwell on the negative aspects to diagnosis and management.

c. A yearly FASD/NDPAE summer camp for children with NDPAE or FASD and their families is a welcome supportive environment, and has been successful in Canada, USA, UK and most recently N. Ireland. The inclusion of professional staff support for children and parents is important to the camp process.

(Catterick et al., 2014)

Social Care

This is the area often most neglected in the management of children and adolescents with NDPAE, diagnosed or undiagnosed. (Chasnoff et al., 2015).

International research has documented the prevalence of medical, psychiatric and developmental disorders in children in care. Not uncommonly in children with NDPAE there is he further added risk of epigenetically- kindled addictive disorder (O'Malley 2003).

Already in the UK Professor Anne Lingford-Hughes is posing the question in her psychiatry in dialogue with society distinguished lecture:

Can neuroscience influence national policy on addictions and should it do so? RSM Lecture, London, March 19th 2020.

The complexity of patients in State Social Care continues to be an under sourced clinical area of diagnosis and management. These children present many hidden disabilities, the most prevalent is probably NDPAE.

This acquired brain injury has a synergistic effect on psychiatric, developmental presentation and in adolescence addictive disorder risk.

Chapter 10

MULTIMODAL MANAGEMENT: (2014 BOOK) MEDICAL MEDICATION MANAGEMENT

INTRODUCTION

Although medication is used quite extensively (especially poly drug therapy in the USA and Canada) with children, adolescents, or adults with ARND, there are still no US Food and Drug Administration (FDA), National Institute of Mental Health (NIMH) or UK National Institute for Health and Clinical Excellence (NICE) approved medications for these conditions. Thus, the use of medication in ARND non dysmorphic or dysmorphic ARND (FAS) has not been properly evaluated, and as O'Malley and Hagerman (1998) have commented, the brain of a prenatally brain damaged infant, young child, or adolescent is especially vulnerable to an atypical medication response or side effects.

There is literature on the pharmacological management of many Developmental Psychiatric Disorders such as ADHD, Autistic Spectrum Disorder, Fragile X syndrome. There is also a wealth of literature in the treatment of aggressive disorders, and alcohol and other addictive disorders (Hagerman 1999, Lee et al., 2001, Glancy et al., 2002 a, b, Vocci et al., 2005, Turk 2012), which is often inappropriately extrapolated to apply to individuals with ARND. It appears the lack of a code/billing diagnosis in the DSM system has hampered any interest in the USA or Canada for large scale clinical trials in Developmental Psychiatric Disorders which are co-occurring in ARND. These types of randomized controlled clinical studies are needed to begin to determine 'Best Practice' as it pertains to medication management in ARND from childhood to adulthood. There are not even smaller studies with reasonable study numbers to determine safety and efficacy, or to try to gain FDA or NICE guideline approval for use of the medications in this unique Developmental Psychiatric Disorder population (Turk 2009).

Currently, there currently are no FDA, AACAP, APA, Royal College of Psychiatrists, UK, guidelines for medication usage in children, adolescents or young adults with ARND who present with these developmental psychiatric disorders through their lifespan.

Therefore, as of 2013, all medications that are used in ARND are 'off label' or 'off license."

> A sorry situation to be in with a chronic debilitating condition originally described in the Lancet 40 years ago...

What makes this clinical situation even worse is the fact that there are no medium or large scale scientific drug industry or government-sponsored randomized clinical studies in any age group of this patient population in any part of the world.

Why are doctors so shy to treat this complicated population of patients with totally preventable so called, permanent, incurable, acquired brain dysfunction?

Why did the doctors not shy away in the mid-20th century from jointly tackling another so called incurable disease, AIDS ?(and low and behold they jointly developed triple therapy regime which changed the course and prognosis of this ravaging illness forever).

So with ARND we have a context in which co-occurring readily identifiable Developmental Psychiatric Disorders such as ADHD, Disruptive Mood Dysregulation Disorder or Chronic Anxiety present in some shape or form in almost all children and later adults with ARND. Amazingly there are no medium or large scale scientific drug industries or government-sponsored randomized clinical studies in any age group with single or poly drug combinations in this patient population (Kodituwakku and Kodituwakku 2011, Novick Brown et al., 2011, O'Malley 2011a).

> Is this an under-appreciated ethical issue of ignoring an 'orphan', dependent disability population who are unable to advocate for themselves due to the very nature of their Developmental Psychiatric Disorder?

The Role of Medication Is One of Symptom Control in Order to Facilitate Other Modalities of Treatment

There is extensive literature on the psychopharmacotherapy of patients with mental retardation and also with brain injury, both of which are relevant to this patient population. Only a small number of studies have been performed on children or adolescents with mental retardation and co-morbid psychiatric disorder. They have been reviewed by, (King et al., 1998, O'Malley 1997, O'Malley and Hagerman 1998, Hagerman 1999, Byrne 2008, and O'Malley 2008, 2010, O'Malley & Rich 2013).

Moreover, medication may improve the participation of ARND patients in other important treatment modalities such as nonverbal play therapy, speech and language therapy or sensory integration therapy. As well, family therapy, especially structural type, and family support to reduce the compassion fatigue in the foster, adoptive or birth parents is essential.

Therefore it is no harm to re-iterate that if medication management is selected for patients with ARND, it needs to be embedded in an array of services for both the child and his/her family. This is a challenge for harried child psychiatrists working in a time limited (15 to 30 minutes) consultation role in HMO system of care. Unfortunately it has become a similar challenge for child psychiatrists working in the Child Adolescent Mental Health Service systems in Ireland and the UK.

As is standard in general psychiatric practice if medication is being considered, it is essential to have a recent complete medical examination by a family physician or pediatrician to rule out any Alcohol Related Birth Defects (ARBD) such as kidney, cardiac problems or liver metabolism problems, for example (Stratton et al., 1996). Thus FBC, LFT, B. Sugar, T4, TSH, S. Creatinine, Folate, S. magnesium and ECG should be routine pre medication work-up.

The clinical presentation in childhood is frequently coupled with physical symptoms such as, chronic headaches, abdominal pain or unspecified pain, self-harm or angry explosive behaviors. These differing somatic expressions and varied externalizations are due to the common language inability of children with ARND to express their emotional distress in words. This phenomenon has been well described, mostly by speech and language specialists, in ARND as an often primary language disability called Alexithymia. So patients with ARND who cannot verbalize their emotional distress in words begin to romanticize their emotional pain and thus can present physical pain as the focus of their distress.

The risks of combined psycho pharmacotherapy in children and adolescents have been highlighted in the USA and Canada recently, and patients with ARND have amazingly very few studies of single medications and naturally none with combinations of medications (Coles et al., 1997, Oesterheld et al., 1998, O'Malley et al., 2000).

Inevitably combined pharmacotherapy involves more risks in this unpredictable brain damaged population due to potential ARBD associated cardiac, renal or even liver dysfunction. There have been few studies of single medications in ARND, let alone combinations of medications (Wilens 2009). Although medication, and especially polydrug therapy, is used extensively in co-occurring psychiatric disorders associated with ARND, this is also done without approval from the Food and Drug Administration (FDA) of the United States) or from the National Institute of Clinical Excellence (NICE) in the United Kingdom. In fact, despite co-occurring mood disorders presenting in almost all children and adults with ARND.

There is some sporadic continuing research on new medications, such as choline, that may modulate or decrease the neurotoxic alcohol damage (Savage et al., 2010). It is medication that truly has the opportunity to improve the participation of ARND patients in other important treatment modalities such as OT, physiotherapy, art and play therapy, speech and language therapy or sensory integration therapy (O'Malley 2008). It therefore stands to sense that medication management should always be part of a multimodal array of services for both the child with ARND and his/her family (O'Malley 2008, 2013).

There Are Cautions in the Use of Medication in ARND

While research is scarce in patients with ARND, this population may be even more vulnerable than those with brain injury sustained in the postnatal period, childhood, adolescence, or adulthood. Individuals with ARND whether dysmorphic (FAS) or non-dysmorphic, have had whole body alcohol exposure to the fetus during prenatal development, leading to the potential for unrecognized Alcohol Related Birth Defects (ARBD) in a number of organ systems (kidney, heart, liver/G.I. system, eye, immune system, neurological) (Stratton et al., 1996, O'Malley 1997, 2010).

These underlying problems with physical organs and structures may lead to unanticipated side effects to even low doses of medication.

For example:

i. cardiac problems such as conduction anomalies, structural defects, and pathologic murmurs may be linked with adverse events with stimulant medications.
ii. Overt seizure disorders and irritability of the brain (associated with random and triggered electrical discharges) may be present due to neuro-anatomical changes in the ARND brain. Therefore, safety issues related to decreased seizure threshold for certain medications should be considered prior to treatment of this population. (O'Malley & Barr 1998, Hagerman 1999, Bonthius et al., 2001).
iii. Other medical complications associated with alcohol-related birth defects (ARBD) need to be considered prior to beginning medication.
iv. Therefore, caution in use of medications should be given due to the unique vulnerability of these ARND patients for severe and catastrophic side effects of certain medications due to:

There are a number of medications that should be used with caution in children and adolescents with ARND

- Lithium carbonate causes cardiac, renal, and thyroid problems.

- Tricyclic antidepressants (amitriptyline, imipramine, desipramine, clomipramine) cause cardiac toxicity, sudden death, and lower seizure threshold and are lethal in overdose.
- New antidepressants affecting serotonergic and noradrenergic systems. (Effexor) may cause cardio toxicity due to noradrenergic activity.
- First generation antipsychotics (chlorpromazine,*stelazine, nozinan, and haldol) cause excess sedation, increased risk of EPS and possible liver toxicity, and sun sensitivity*.
- Second generation atypical antipsychotics can affect weight and glucose metabolism.
- Paroxetine (SORI) has now been recommended by FDA not to be used in under 18 year old patients. It causes increased interaction with other psychotropic medication because of its inhibition of cytochrome P450 2D6 isoenzyme liver pathway.

(O'Malley 1997, 2010, 2013)

(v) More general medical clinical risk factors include:

It has been recognized for quite a long time that the use of multiple psychotropic medications is a risk for toxicity and acute confusional state, even in absence of underlying neurocognitive problems. The mechanism of multidrug interaction leading to toxicity relates to individual drugs competing for absorption through the liver cytochrome P450 2D6 enzyme system. In turn, certain medication blood levels increase (i.e., paroxetine is well known to increase blood levels of other psychotropic medications).

Rather frustratingly, in a recent lecture at the First European Conference on FASD in Rolduc, Holland (Nov 3rd to 5th 2010), Ken Warren, Acting Director of NIAAA, mentioned concern in the USA about medication interactions in patients with ARND dysmorphic (FAS) and non dysmorphic, but no data was given or studies forthcoming.

- differential or paradoxical medication response; SSRIs can unmask or precipitate a manic switch in patients with ARND who have an underlying brain dysfunction. Also SSRIs may bring on extra pyramidal side effects in adolescents or young adults with ARND an effect which is not dose or length of usage related,
- prenatal alcohol induced neurochemical or structural CNS changes (i.e., acquired brain injury),
- complications related to multisystem organ involvement (absorption, metabolic or elimination problems related to kidney, gastro-intestinal or liver problems related to ARBD); an increased incidence of seizure disorders in this population (i.e.,

lower seizure thresh hold); lithium carbonate or tricylic antidepressants pose this special risk,

- overall greater risk of side effects from: multiple drug combinations,
  - higher doses of medications,
  - and sensitivity to psycho pharmaceuticals.

(O'Malley 1997, O'Malley & Hagerman 1998, O'Malley 2013a, O'Malley & Rich 2013).

The Pathophysiology of ARND as It Relates to Psychopharmacological Agents

Over the last 30 to 35 or so years there have been a number of scientific animal and human study reviews demonstrating that heavy doses of alcohol administered to a wide range of laboratory animals produced a spectrum of Central Nervous System (CNS) effects beginning with the cell death seen in the nerve cells (neurons). (Behnke et al., (2013), Kodituwakku and Kodituwakku 2011, Streissguth and Connor 2001).

As well, numerous animal studies have demonstrated that prenatal alcohol exposure interferes with the embryological development of most of the neurotransmitters. (Manteueffel 1996, Hannigan 1996, Stratton et al., 1996; O'Malley and Hagerman 1998, O'Malley 2008). Deficits have been found in the dopaminergic, noradrenergic, serotoninergic, GABAergic, cholinergic, glutaminergic, and histaminergic systems. Human studies are progressing replicating the animal study findings. The deficits in dopaminergic and noradrenergic systems most likely are connected with the Attentional Deficit Hyperactivity Disorder (ADHD presentation of patients with ARND non dysmorphic or dysmorphic. For example, previous animal research on rats has demonstrated that the D1 receptors of the mesolimbic dopamine system are affected by prenatal alcohol more than the nigrostriatal or tegmental dopamine D1 receptor system.

There is also current neurobiological/pharmacological research analyzing the clinical effect of the prenatal alcohol in the disruption of the balance between GABA, the inhibitory, and Glutamate, the excitatory, neurotransmitter in the brain. Scientists in the USA have shown the kindling of seizures due to the effect of prenatal alcohol on the GABAergic cells in the hippocampus which leads to a lower seizure threshold.

Separate brain imaging studies utilizing such radiological techniques as MRI, fMRI, SPECT, PET scans or even Diffusion Tensor analysis studies have been used for almost 20 years and are constantly becoming more focused in their brain area delineation. They have and continue to map more specific areas of brain dysfunction related to prenatal alcohol exposure married to the Developmental Psychiatric presentation. Unfortunately they are mostly done in tertiary center academic centers removed from the cut and thrust of real psychiatric diagnosis and practice. As well they have not entered into any coherent treatment plan of management linked to the morbidity of the ARND in the child, adolescent or adult as clinically assessed on the Dimensional overview described earlier. (Riley, et al., 2005, Kodituwakku et al., 2011, Mattson et al., 2011, Coles et al., 2011).

The medical history of scientific knowledge of damaged or diseased brain structure was associated with infections such as syphilis, more recently AIDS or lesions associated with cerebrovascular accidents, less common genetic intellectual disability disorders such as Fragile X syndrome, Downs syndrome, Velo Cardio Facial syndrome. In the past and even currently, in these developmental psychiatric disorders or illnesses with neuropsychiatric problems the brain imaging has informed/guided medical diagnostic accuracy and informed treatment progress.

Therefore it should not be unrealistic to expect that correlations between the structural and functional deficits in individuals with ARND, with documented alcohol exposure at certain points during pregnancy, could dramatically improve our understanding of brain function.

All we need is the will and the institutional structures to do this collaborative clinical psychiatric and neurological research.

General Principles of Medication Usage in Addressing the Developmental Psychiatric Disorder(s) in ARND

1) It is well known in psychiatry and neurology that patients with an acquired brain injury respond differently to medications than individuals with no brain injury.
2) International clinical experience with this population indicates that individuals with alcohol acquired brain dysfunction (dysmorphic ARND or non-dysmorphic ARND) can often respond to medications similarly to those with other types of acquired or traumatic brain injury.
3) A solid therapeutic approach in this specific group of patients is to immunize or streamline the numbers of medications the person is taking in order to reduce drug-drug interactions and prevent complications from over-medication (Stratton et al., 1996; O'Malley & Storoz 2003; Byrne 2008; O'Malley 2008).
4) Medications need to be started at low doses and increased slowly. The ultimate therapeutic gold being to maximize efficacy and minimize side effects to the sensitive and/or vulnerable central nervous system in these ARND patients, especially children.
5) Psychotropic agents do improve brain organization and/or brain function, and the psychiatrist or pediatrician can facilitate the child's cognitive processes by using

judicious medication to dampen down the spontaneous or random firing of the misshapen and distorted neural pathways in the ARND brain.

6) Also it should not be forgotten that psychotropic medications may improve mood, behavior, and academic performance in individuals with ARND by altering the physiology of the acquired injured brain structure and function. It is not unreasonable to believe that correctly chosen, appropriately managed medications can have a positive effect on cognitive functioning and decision making.
7) There is a pressing need for scientific testing and evaluation of new clinical instruments which combine cognitive, language, and behavioral or emotional response as the 'gold standard' for assessing medication efficacy and safety in patients with ARND. Currently there are no validated clinical instruments to evaluate the Developmental Psychiatric Disorder Dimensions present in ARND, and so no baseline quantifiable psychiatric clinical evaluation with which to measure the medication response in this specific patient population.

There is a non-specific neuropsychiatric rating scale, but most drug rating scales (with the exception of those used in Alzheimer's disorder) evaluate clinical symptoms related to psychiatric disorder (i.e., Connor's Questionnaire, Beck Depression Inventory, Hamilton Rating Scale, CBCL).

(FAS Diagnosis, 2005; Byrne 2008, Coles 2009; Novick Brown, et al., 2011, Hosenbus et al., 2012, O'Malley 2010, Turk 2012, Rich & O'Malley 2012, O'Malley & Rich 2013, O'Malley 2013a)

Medication Management of Specific Developmental Psychiatric Disorders

(i) ADHD Symptoms

ADHD Symptomatology (usually predated by Regulatory Disorder, Hyperresponsive type, or Sensory Seeking/Impulsive type in less than 5 years of age). This symptomatology comes from the alcohol effects on the Motor and Sensory Dimension, the Cognitive Disability Dimension and the Disruptive Mood Dysregulation Disorder Dimension.

Attention, Distractibility, and concentration deficits, more frequently inattention combined with impulsivity, are the most common developmental psychiatric presentation of both children and adults with ARND (Hagerman 1999, O'Malley & Nanson 2003, O'Malley & Storoz 2003). Medications such as psychostimulants do have an ameliorating role in the management of ARND, and some early clinical studies have shown that Dextroamphetamine seems more efficacious than Methylphenidate (Synder et al., 1996, Cole et al., 1999, O'Malley et al., 1998, Oesteheld et al., 1999). The animal research, coupled with the evidence from Hannigan (1996, 1997) and reviewed in Hagerman (1999), and O'Malley (2008), has indicated that prenatal alcohol affects the developing Dopamine

D1 receptors in the mesolimbic and not the fronto-nigral dopamine neurotransmitter system (which is the site of action of methylphenidate).

Long-acting biphasic or bimodal (in USA) agents such as Concerta (USA), Equasym, and Medikinet (UK) may be helpful and can increase medication compliance. However, proper double-blind placebo studies are yet to be performed in patients with ARND. Compared to other co-occurring developmental psychiatric disorders, there is a greater recognition of the prevalence of ADHD in ARND.

Long-acting guanfacine (which are not available in the UK) may be useful in such cases, as is the short-acting version, but this needs to be studied in this patient population. There is a study of this medication versus atomoxetine in ADHD being carried out in Ireland (McNicholas 2012, O'Malley 2013a).

In mental retardation or intellectual disability studies on children, Methylphenidate relieves ADHD symptoms, but is less effective if the IQ is under 50. The previous research on animals and humans, as reviewed by O'Malley and Hagerman 1998, Byrne 2008, and O'Malley 2008, 2010, 2011c, has indicated that dextroamphetamine (short or long acting), including lisdexamfetamine dimesylate, may be better first-line psycho stimulant choice than methylphenidate (short or long acting) for ARND non-dysmorphic or dysmorphic patients with ADHD symptoms, as it modulates the mesolimbic dopamine system, whereas methylphenidate modulates the fronto-nigral dopamine system. A dose of 1 mg/kg/day is a good maintenance dosage. The short acting product should be started initially in case of individual sensitivity or even allergic reaction. As mentioned above it is important to do baseline biological screening before medication, FBC, LFT, B. Sugar, T4, TSH, S. Creatinine, Folate, and ECG. Sleep disturbance, decreased appetite, nausea or vomiting and irritability, labile personality change are key side effects to monitor. In pubertal children some affective instability may be seen.

Methylphenidate still remains a reliable medication and is probably a good second-line choice, but side effects can be more common especially aggressive behavior, tics, sleep or appetite disturbance, schizoid demeanour.

The biphasic newer preparations such as Concerta XL (Methylphenidate HCL) and Equasym (Melthphenidate HCL) appear to be useful after initial stimulant response is established. They seem to be particularly efficacious in pubertal and older teenagers. The long acting psycho-stimulant products are a good fit for children in pubertal age or adolescence because they are more compliant to take because of a once a day dosage, and they also have a lower risk of abuse potential.

A clinically significant but often unrecognized negative side effect of psychostimulants in ARND is their ability to increase arousal and help the patient focus, but at the same time contribute to an increased level of perseveration especially in patients with co-existing ASD or obsessive features. (Stanley 2007)

- Atomoxetine (Strattera) seems to be more helpful in older children or teenagers with ADHD symptoms.

It also seems to have a particular efficacy if there is a co-morbid Disruptive Mood Dysregulation Disorder with the ADHD.

Lastly it has less risk of dependency.

Patients can show hypersensitivity with increased grumpiness and irritability.

Liver function, FBC, T4, B sugar, electrolytes and ECG need to be tested if atomoxetine is given.

Studies need to be done to clarify the pharmacokinetics and pharmacodynamics in these preparations, as patients with ARND often metabolize psychotropic drugs at a faster rate than patients without this developmental neuropsychiatric disorder. This has implications for the efficacy of the longer acting preparations as they may have a clinically shorter duration of pharmacological action than anticipated.

It is worth remembering the *Alcohol Related Birth defects (ARBD)* because prenatal alcohol exposure can affect the developing heart, kidney, and even liver, so side effects are more unpredictable. Blood pressure, ECG, blood sugar, and thyroid function should be tested.

ARND, dysmorphic type (FAS) is a growth retardation condition, and long-term stimulants run the risk of lowering the growth hormone. A number of patients have shown decreased bone age or decreased linear growth due to long-term high dose psycho-stimulants (usually, methylphenidate). Finally, the lower the IQ, i.e., under 60 more likely an unfavorable favorable response to any of the psychostimulants.

The BMI is a good measurement to follow these patients on longer term basis, remembering that the psycho-stimulant products can decrease the trajectory of linear height growth.

- The complexity of ADHD co-morbidities has been long recognized (Brown 2009). The co-occurrence of ADHD appears to be the commonest psychiatric condition in ARND, most often presenting inattention and impulsivity, without physical hyperactivity, in both children and adults (O'Malley 2010, O'Malley and Nanson 2002, O'Malley and Storoz 2003, Streissguth et al., 1996). Medications such as psychostimulants do have an ameliorating role, and some initial small clinical studies have shown that dextroamphetamine seems more efficacious than methylphenidate (O'Malley 2008).As well as mentioned, long-acting biphasic or bimodal (in USA) agents such as Concerta (USA), Equasym, and Medikinet (UK) may be helpful and can increase medication compliance. However, proper double-blind placebo studies have yet to be performed in patients with ARND.
- In addition, prenatal nicotine also has been identified as a synergistic biochemical agent that kindles ADHD (Altink et al., 2009, Mick et al., 2002, Milberger et al.,

1996) The long-acting guanfacine (available in the USA) can be useful in such cases, as has been shown with the short-acting version, but this needs to be studied in this patient population (Salee et al., 2009).

- ADHD can occur with comorbid Disruptive Mood Dsyregulation Disorder or Intermittent Explosive Disorder in both cases the combination of a psychostimulant with a mood stabilizer such as carbamazepine or valproic acid shows good efficacy.
- As well if the appears to be a sensory overload or Generalized Anxiety component to the ADHD and the co-morbid Disruptive Mood Dsyregulation ADHD with co-morbid Anxiety (seen in young children as Regulatory Disorder, Hypersensitive (cautious/vigilant), Sensory Seeking/Impulsive, Underresponsive in under 5 years old)

  This is the clinically most difficult area to assess as the child may have been subjected multiple placements in early years or subjected to direct or indirect violence. In these cases, co-occurring Post Traumatic Stress Disorder (PTSD), early onset and/or Reactive Attachment Disorder (RAD) compound the ARND presentation.
- The GABA ergic agents can play a role with the psychostimulants, i.e., Neurontin, Lyrica, Frisium.
- Also Guanfacine, clonidine, frisium (Clobazam), lyrica (pregabalin) are all useful by themselves or they can be added to a psychostimulant.

It is important to check BP and pulse while lying and sitting and do a pre-treatment ECG, blood tests as before. As well liquid fluoxetine or tablets alone may be of help, or sertraline in older patients.

(ii) Mood Disorders

Mood disorders in ARND vary significantly in their range and quality. It often appears at an early age and has a Disruptive Mood Dysregulation quality which sets it apart from the general mood disorders.

In ARND, the disruptive mood dysregulation has been attributed to emotional dysregulations caused by the effects of prenatal exposure on developing neurotransmitters. These can range from deep rooted depressive feelings to uncontrollable mood instability which mimics a rapid cycling bipolar disorder. Early childhood Regulatory Disorders are often a combination of a disturbance of autonomic arousal, attention, behavior, and mood. Recent interest in early onset bipolar disorder (EOBD) in the USA is beginning to offer clinical insights into the understanding of the initial psychiatric presentation of ARND (Carlson et al., 2009, 2010). Patients with co-occurring mood disorders may present with what is called 'emotional incontinence', or unprovoked cascades of crying or laughing.

As well, these patients with the emotional incontinence, and/or unprovoked cascades of crying or laughing are not true Bipolar Disorder. (This type of emotional incontinence has been described for years in children and adolescents with traumatic brain injury).

This appreciation that early childhood Regulation Disorders are often a disturbance of attention, behavior, and mood, recent interest in early onset bipolar disorder (EOBD) in the USA and this scientific work is beginning to offer clinical insights into the understanding of the initial developmental psychiatric presentations of ARND.

Carbamazepine, valproic acid or even GABA agents such as gabapentin or progablin can be effective in treating these symptoms (Wozniak and Biederman 1996). If these agents are used, there must be awareness of potential teratogenic problems if the Bipolar patient becomes pregnant. Fetal valproate syndrome, as an example, has many of the physical and some of the CNS hallmarks seen in dysmorphic ARND.

Medications that are useful for mood disorders include fluoxetine in liquid or tablet form, sertraline, and citalopram. Therefore, it is best to start with low dosage fluoxetine liquid or tablet depending on child's age and weight, and build slowly. It is important to be especially aware of an activation effect in the first week which may bring forth increased agitation or even increased suicidality. Also a problem if SSRIs are used during pregnancy.

If the antidepressants, serotonin-specific reuptake inhibitors (SSRIs) are used, and the patient becomes pregnant, dosage needs to be carefully monitored as neonatal neurobehavioral effects have been described as a result of prenatal exposure (Oberlander et al., 2009). Nevertheless, Oberlander and his Canadian research group did also note that the clinical challenge is to unravel the effects of the prenatal Selective Serotonin Reuptake inhibitors (SSRI) exposure on the infant from the impact of the mother's depressive disorder.

The more commonly accepted efficacy of SSRI does not necessarily hold true for ARND children or adolescents which and can lead to unmasking a Bipolar diathesis, or in young adults or older patients contributing to extra pyramidal symptoms. This is especially a problem in Ireland which has a high prevalence of Affective Disorder which is quite common in the mothers who drink alcohol during pregnancy, and so this genetic vulnerability can be brought forth by too aggressive use of SSRI.

As well for example, Selective Serotonin Reuptake Inhibitors (SSRI's) such as fluoxetine, paroxetine, or citalopram, may be more likely to precipitate agitation, activation, or suicidality in these brain damaged adolescents due to augmentation of a pre-existing, organically-driven impulsivity.

At the same time, given that individuals with ARND may have deficiencies and/or differences in neurotransmitter systems such as serotonin and dopamine, low doses of sertraline and fluoxetine have proven anecdotally beneficial for some patients.

As a warning, the tricyclic antidepressants increase the risk of cardio-toxicity in a patient population related to unpredictable liver metabolism and potential cardiac problems from their prenatal alcohol exposure (O'Malley & Hagerman 1998, Hagerman 1999). If tricyclic antidepressants have to be used, and the patient becomes pregnant, dosage needs to be monitored carefully as neonatal neurobehavioral effects have been described in infants.

The tricyclic antidepressants are generally contraindicated in ARND because of this risk of cardio-toxicity which is compounded by the potential developmental cardiac problems (ARBD effect) from prenatal alcohol exposure (Byrne 2008, Hagerman 1999, O'Malley 2008). Therefore, a pre-treatment ECG, BP are essential before prescribing any psychotropic medication for mood disorder in ARND.

Mood disorders in ARND of whatever variety, must always be assessed in the context of the family, as environmental factors (e.g., abuse, recent losses or separations, change in family constellation such as arrival of a new sibling, or illness in a parent) may have a profound kindling, or synergistic effect, on the appearance or severity of the mood disorder (O'Malley 2008, 2010, 2013a).

- Carbamazepine, valproic acid, lyrica, frisium have also been anecdotally helpful in patients with generalised anxiety, aggressively, impulsivity, and mood dysregulation.
- Lamotrigine is also useful but safer in adults because of risk of Steven Johnson Syndrome

(iii) Conduct Disorders

Significant Conduct problems are seen in children who come from family environments where there is a transgenerational history of disorganized or even absent parenting. The unrecognized nature of ARND is its transgenerational nature, and the fact that it tends to run through multiple generations in a family.

Recent clinical work in the UK and Ireland is beginning to understand and consider the risk of Conduct disorders when ARND affects several generations within a family. It remains to be seen if the prevalence of transgenerational violent community and personal trauma, in countries such as Ireland, coupled with acquired biological vulnerability due to prenatal alcohol exposure will be scientifically approached?

Conduct Disorders do include aggressive or explosive episodes in ARND and may progress to fire setting or even cruelty to animals.

A Sleep Deprived EEG may rule out a Complex Partial Seizure Disorder, and a supplementary clinical examination may uncover sexual or physical abuse.

Medications such as carbamazepine and valproic acid are useful, especially if Disruptive Mood Dysregulation Disorder or Intermittent Explosive Disorder is present with the Conduct Disorder.

Also, fluoxetine in liquid form for young children and tablet form for adolescents 10 mgs or 20 mg tablets may help if there has been a traumatic history, because of its antidepressant quality.

In this clinical situation the role of individual interpersonal therapy, verbal trauma centered or nonverbal art, music, is essential in forming a bond with the child or teenager who may have hidden trauma in their past.

- Carbamazepine or valproic acid added to a psychostimulant may be useful dual medication therapy (where ADHD, Explosive Disorder and Conduct disorder co-exist).
- In situations where the explosive episodes are escalating and no seizure disorder is present then atypical antipsychotic agents are useful, but need careful monitoring i.e., risperidone and olanzapine, quetiapine are helpful with aggressive/disruptive behaviors the newer atypical antipsychotics (i.e., aripipisal or clozaril) may have a use here (only after failed treatments with the other antipsychotics, or in very ill hospitalized patients). Recent work on the atypical antipsychotics has shown that they can double the risk of abnormal glucose metabolism including diabetes, hyperprolactinaemia, and pancreatitis. The population of patients with ARND is also more likely to need benztropine as they develop extrapyramidal symptoms (EPS) easier. As has been recognized for many years in psychotropic treatment of Intellectual Disability, rarer serious side effects do occur such as neuroleptic malignant syndrome needing hospitalization. This is a particular risk with some atypicals especially olanazepine if the IQ is under 50, or if there is the presence of identifiable structural brain damage on MRI or CAT Scan.

Parenteral medication such as fluanxol has proven effective in once a month regime, useful in noncompliant older patients with schizoaffective symptomatology. (O'Malley & Rich 2013, O'Malley 2013a)

(iv) Chronic Anxiety

Chronic anxiety often co-occurs in children and adults with ARND, partly due to a chronic inability to self-soothe, but as well an over sensitivity and reactivity to visual cues, especially faces.

This may have its origins in the effect of prenatal alcohol on the developing amygdaloid nucleus which primes facial recognition.

- Anxiety agents such as buspirone have a role and have less a risk of dependency.
- lorazepam (be careful of potential dependency if used for too long a period)
- frisium (clobam) can also address the pervasive anxiety.
- clonidine or guanfacine are also helpful (ECG and BP check essential)
- propranolol can help if the anxiety spills into more of a social panic variety (ECG and BP check essential)

- A combination of psychostimulant and guanfacine or clonidine has been effective in the treatment of such symptoms, if there is a co-occurring ADHD with the anxiety disorder.

It is important to check blood pressure and pulse and do an ECG prior to prescribing these particular medications due to their possible cardio toxicity when used in combination.

Remember However - If the anxiety disorder is the primary developmental psychiatric presentation, it also is essential to unravel the environmental stressors in the history and techniques such as individual non-verbal play therapy may be better than medication as the first option in young children.

(v) Panic Attacks and Generalized Anxiety Disorder

- respond to lorazepam (short acting),
- buspirone (longer onset of action and less risk of drug dependency),
- propranolol, (check ECG)
- bupropion if mood symptoms are present.
- GABAergic agents such as gabapentin or frisium (clobazam) could be used if there is disruptive mood instability present.

(vi) Sleep Disorders

This is commonly a critical disturbing feature of young children and has been shown in animal and human research going back 25 years to be a primary neurological effect of alcohol on the developing arousal system (Havichek 1977). The sleep problems often underpin the ADHD behaviors and the Disruptive Mood Dysregulation Disorder components to the ARND.

- do show good response to melatonin (liquid or tablet form),
- phenergan,
- trazodone,
- l-tryptophan (safe if the patient is pregnant).

(vii) Psychotic Symptoms

Psychotic symptoms may be quite difficult to diagnose and unravel in patients with ARND and working memory deficits in brighter children have an innate capacity to tell fantastical stories that are not delusional (i.e., confabulate), and have a rather a creative a way to 'fill in the blanks' because of their memory and recall problems which is part of the Cognitive Disability Dimension.

As well problems in social cognition or social communication which lie in the Language Impairment Dimension influence and derail narrative story telling.

- Newer atypical agents are used in such cases but are still unpredictable.

For example, atypical agents such as risperidone with its differential effect on 5HT receptor can also prove problematic in management of psychosis with a prenatal alcohol exposure history. In this case the longer and prolonged use of the medicine can make the clinical situation worse by unmasking an affective instability. Also it is important to carefully monitor weight, cardiac status, blood sugar and serum prolactin, as for all the atypical agents, (O'Malley 2010, Rich & O'Malley 2012, O'Malley 2013 a)

- Clinically, olanzapine seems to be most effective if the patient is displaying features of acute mania, but here the weight gain can be a significant problem.
- seroquel (quetiapine) seems to have a good sedating effect for night time sedation and settling evening restlessness
- abilify (aripiprazole) is usually well tolerated, and can be used concurrently with carbamazepine if intermittent explosive disorder, or severe mood disruption dysregulation is a problem.
- ziprasidone, is used in the USA. (Rich & O'Malley 2012).

(viii) Symptoms of ASD or Asperger's Syndrome

1. Historical and Evolving Clinical Perspective. The potential epigenetic or environmental link between prenatal alcohol exposure, ARND, and Autism Spectrum Disorder or Asperger's Disorder has a long history. Environmental agents, diseases and postnatal interventions have had a rather varied and controversial past, as pointed out by Cathy Lord, So Hyun Kim and Adriana Dimartino in an International book on Autism (Fitzgerald 2013).

As long ago as 1971 the American child psychiatrist in New York, Stella Chess reviewed cases of Rubella and Thalidomide and implicated these prenatal infectious and medication exposures as etiological factor in Autism Spectrum Disorder (however a small number in the case series).

Scandinavian researchers Gilberg and Gilberg in 1983 later identified a cluster of adverse prenatal complications which may contribute to a clinical presentation of Autism Spectrum disorder in early childhood.

In 1990, Canadian child neuropsychologist Jo Nanson in Saskatoon, described 6 cases of FAS (dysmorphic ARND) with autism. Also there has been a developing interest in prenatal risk factors contributing to Autism, pursued by a number of authors and this potential etiological link which was published in 1991 by International Autistic Spectrum

Disorder researcher neuropsychologist Cathy Lord and colleagues. (O'Malley & Rich 2013).

Since 2009-2010, adult psychiatrist in London, Raja Mukarjee, has clinically analyzed the clinical presentation of Autistic Spectrum Disorder in patients with ARND dysmorphic (FAS) or non-dysmorphic FASD. Furthermore the complexity of diagnostic issues within ARND, dysmorphic and non-dysmorphic were recently illustrated in a 2011 on line book chapter by Natalie Novick Brown, Kieran O'Malley and Ann Streissguth in which the developmental psychiatric presentations of FASD were shown to include sometimes unrecognized Autistic Spectrum Disorder or Asperger's Disorder.

In the international pediatric and child psychiatric field the last 5 years have brought a wealth of clinical case descriptions and case studies indicating the presence of ADHD co-morbidly with PDD or Autistic Spectrum Disorder. Clinicians and researchers such as Professor Jeremy Turk in the UK have commented on as much as a 25-30% co-morbid link between ADHD and PDD/ASD (O'Malley & Rich 2013).

2. Basic Scientific Research in the Autistic Spectrum Disorder and the prenatal alcohol exposure link has formed one strand of study in alcohol teratogenesis. Here, researchers have been identifying brain areas that are more sensitive to alcohol damage. Areas such as the corpus callosum, hippocampus, prefrontal cortex, temporal lobe collectively and individually contribute to a clinical presentation of social disconnectedness, lack of social cognition and awareness, impulsivity, and inability to understand another person's cognitions or feelings (alexithymia). (Bookstein et al., 2001, 2005, Sullivan 2008).

The underlying organic brain dysfunction at a cellular, neurotransmitter and structural level related to prenatal alcohol exposure sometimes shares significant congruence with ongoing neuroscience research in Autism Spectrum Disorder and Asperger's Disorder, and awaits collaborative work between the two academic fields.

There is also accumulating research which highlights the biological roots of fundamental functional problems in ARND which relate to sustained impact on working memory (Congdon et al., 2012, O'Malley 2011a).

3. Neuropsychological Research framework of understanding ASD and Asperger's and its relationship to patients with ARND (reviewed by Pennington 2009).

1) The psychological deficit in the child must be present before the onset of the disorder and so very early in development.
2) It must be pervasive among individuals/patients with the disorder.
3) It must be specific to autism, or ASD.
4) There have been a number of different psychological theories in autism orASD;
   a. theory of mind theory
   b. the executive theory
   c. the praxis/imitation theory
   d. the emotion theory

e. the empathizing-systematizing or ' extreme male brain' theory

(Hobson 1989, Russell 1997, Baren Cohen et al., 2000, O'Malley & Rich 2013).

4. The ARND Dimensional Perspective: Some symptoms on the autistic spectrum disorder are invariably coupled with ARND, with its Dimensional Impairments in Cognitive Function, Language Function and Motor and Sensory Function.

It appears that the language impairments in social cognition and communication bring the most secondary developmental psychiatric problems such as anxiety disorders and possible psychotic disorders.

As well patients with ARND who have ASD features are more likely to have co-occurring ADHD features. Thus they have this unique blend of compulsivity and impulsivity which is clinically very challenging to understand, let alone treat. (O'Malley & Rich 2013).

- Psychostimulants might be used with caution as they can precipitate a schizoid personality change, sometimes described as 'zombie' type states in the USA, or increase perseveration due to enhancing focus. Atomoxetine seems to be a good fit in some patients. This type of medication can have a positive effect on visual or auditory focus. This increases the child's social awareness and connection.
  The psychostimulant must be used advisedly, as it can bring on a 'hyper'-focus' which increase perseveration in the vulnerable ARND patient with ASD symptomatology. (Stanley 2007).
- Atomoxetine seems to be a good fit in older teenage patients, but may show a hypersensitivity response of increase in moodiness or irritability. (ECG, BP essential).
- Fluoxetine in low dose seems to help if the anxiety and obsessive thinking are an issue with the ASD presentation of the ARND.
- Seizure disorders can be related to prenatal alcohol exposure and the effect of alcohol on the GABA ergic system is one hypothesis. Unexplained explosive episodes, rage attacks in ARND children and adolescents with Autism Spectrum Disorder or Asperger's Disorder may have origins in seizure disorders which are not related to the lower level of cognitive functioning or IQ as is the accepted rule. (Bonthius et al., 1992, O'Malley and Barr 1998).

(vii) Alcohol Dependency

Alcohol dependence is still a poorly understood phenomenon in adolescents and young adults with ARND.

Epigenetic fetal programming for early alcohol craving and later dependence has been recognized from animal research some 40 years ago. These animal studies, and more lately human studies have shown that prenatal alcohol exposure increases the risk for alcohol craving probably via its effects on the developing brain, specifically the nucleus accumbens.

Ireland and the UK have the highest under-age and binge drinking patterns in the world. Animal researchers for over 40 years have established links between teratogenic prenatal alcohol exposure and alcohol craving. This concept and its potential impact for the developmentally delayed, alcohol craving children of the Irish and UK binge drinking generation has still not been fully realized in the adult mental health or adult addiction field (Baer et al., 2003, Abate et al., 2008, O'Malley 2011a, Orakwue et al., 2010, Reyes et al., 1985).

Lack of understanding of children's difficulties by the school authorities, can precipitate disconnection from school leading to school expulsion, leading in turn to aimless behavior, excessive alcohol consumption, impulsive early sexual intercourse and pregnancy, giving rise to the next generation of children with ARND.

Where addiction counseling is ineffective, the use of psychopharmacology (borrowing from work in cocaine addiction) has been used successfully in blocking the central nervous system craving (Sinha and O'Malley 1999).

- Agents such as Naltrexone or Acamprasate have been used successfully in patients with ARND but still require rigorous scientific testing, especially if considered as a strategy in pregnancy with the alcohol addicted patient (O'Malley 2008, Handley and Chassin 2009). Treatment strategies can be borrowed from studies on narcotic dependent mothers and the mother/infant dyad (Velez and Jansson 2008).

Naltrexone has been shown to have a dual role in preventing alcohol craving and reducing impulsivity, both very useful treatment strategies in the ARND adolescent or young adult with ADHD and co-occurring early onset alcohol addiction. (Prof. Lingford Hughes, 2013).

The interest in developing more scientific methods of managing addiction and the role of neurotransmission in the cause and eventual treatment of the addictive disorder continues to be an area of ever changing research, and ARND offers a unique clinical model. (Tomkins et al., 2001).

This is a critical area for future psychopharmacological research as the trans-generational effect of alcohol abuse and dependence in ARND appear to have their roots in the epigenetic effect of prenatal alcohol on the developing fetus, which kindles the fetal programming of early alcohol craving in each succeeding generation.

Neurological Co-occurring Disorders in ARND

Seizure Disorders

Children, adolescents and young adults with ARND can present with unrecognized co-occurring seizure disorders which underpin the complex clinical presentation of their Developmental Psychiatric Disorders. They are not necessarily a product of lower IQ as measured in the Cognitive Disorder Dimension, but can be anticipated by the level of Disorder in the Motor and Sensory Dimension.

The seizures are the result of a prenatally alcohol kindled organic brain dysfunction and its neurological impact on the developing brain, not just in structures (the corpus callosum, cerebellum or hippocampus), but in neurophysiology and neurotransmitter balance as alcohol is a false inhibitory neurotransmitter. The prenatal effects of alcohol can also result in a change in the balance of the developing neurotransmitters. Animal research has shown that prenatal alcohol can induce decrease in inhibitory neurotransmitter GABA in the hippocampus, and this neurochemical imbalance can underpin development of seizures (Hannigan et al., 1996, Riley et al., 2006).

- There is still only anecdotal clinical evidence (from Ireland, UK and the USA) that anticonvulsants (i.e., carbamazepine, valproic acid, neurontin, and to a lesser extent lamotrigine,) can be effective in preventing or modulating this kindling effect. The effects of antiepileptics should be weighed carefully since some medications for seizures may also increase anxiety, affective or mood liability, and reduce learning and cognition.
- Anticonvulsants such as carbamazepine or valproic acid if the patient with ARND has an epileptic focus in the temporal lobe and clinical presentation of auditory hallucinations as part of complex partial seizures. (O'Malley 2013).

New Directions for Medications and Interventions for Patients with ARND

1) The holistic concept of prenatal and postnatal nutrition including dietary supplementation such as Omega 3 fatty acids, iron, tryptophan, crinoline continue to be studied in patients with ADHD clinical profiles. (Lucas 1991, Royaguru et al., 2013)
2) Glutaminegic agents are gathering interest internationally and borrowing from seminal work in Alzheimers disorder, (Paponastasion et al., 2013).
3) Neuroprotective agents have already been used to counterbalance the effect of prenatal alcohol on the developing fetus. They include folate, vitamin B12, thiamine, Vitamin B6, and choline (Kodituwakku et al., 2011).

Some current work is being done with choline in the European setting and the USA is now considering entering into this pharmacological preventative arena. This research needs to recognize the risk that the alcohol dependent pregnant woman may inadvertently feel the alcohol risk to the developing fetus is now much less, and so she can continue drinking. (Thomas et al., 2000)

4) N- Acetylaspartate (NAA) has attracted attention as it is found primarily in neurons and axons. It has also been identified as a potential biological marker for neuronal integrity, and specifically neuronal degeneration, especially in the prefrontal and frontal areas of the brain.
5) Stress/Trauma management.
   Increasingly, researchers, medical, psychiatric and mental health professionals show that patients exposed to prenatal alcohol are frequently exposed to stress at many different levels i.e., domestic violence, abandonment by partner, and physical or sexual abuse which predates pregnancy.
   Postnatal stress includes multiple placements due to in ability of birth or foster carers to cope with unpredictable disruptive behaviors, or continuing tension between birth and foster parents due to shared parenting (especially if birth parents are still alcohol dependent).
   The role of the hypothalamic-pituitary axis is being reconsidered in the population of patients with ARND who have been born into environments of high stress (Meewisse et al., 2007). Excess cortisol has been shown to stop many metabolic, neuronal, and immune systems, including potential nerve growth factor.
   It remains to be seen if psychopharmacological agents affecting the balance of the HPA axis have an ameliorating or neuroprotective role in ARND. (O'Malley 2010, 2013a).
6) Multimodal behavioral, family and school support and medication especially psychostimulant interventions, although more complicated to orchestrate, still have a utility and have been shown to have a positive effect in decreasing later adolescence substance abuse when given to disruptive 6 year olds which also have a role in the ARND population (O'Malley 2008, Castellanos et al., 2013).
   These are again a general, list of relevant references regarding medication use in ARND. A subject sadly receiving little if any scientific quantification.

(Stratton et al., 1996, Hagerman 1999, Streissguth and O'Malley 2000, Chudney et al., 2005, BMA 2007, O'Malley 2008, Novick Brown et al., 2011, O'Malley & Mukarjee 2010, O'Malley 2010, 2013 a, Densmore 2011, CDC 2011, HHS).

Medical Medication Management. An Update. 2020

The intervening 5 years have had a few initiatives in this area of management.

1) British Medical Association, BMA, consensus NICE Guidelines on the management of ADHD with FASD were developed and published (Young et al., 2016).

These guidelines validate the presence of ADHD symptomatology resulting from prenatal alcohol exposure and postulate a differential positive effect of dextro-amphetamine psychostimulant over the standard methylphenidate in primary medication management. (a clinical proposition mooted over 20 years ago, but not validated, in the USA.).

The basic medical triage investigations and algorithm is no different than described in the 2013 book The Knotted Cord, and elaborated in O'Malley 2016, 2020.

2) There is a proposed follow –up in 2020 to the to the initial BMA Consensus NICE guidelines.
3) Risks, Cardiac and Addiction -related, to GABAergic agents are now well documented and so should not be used in NDPAE patients, without a 2nd opinion. Pregabulin has rapidly entered the illegal drug market as a secondary or synergistic drug used in conjunction with more stimulating agents such as cocaine or opiates.
4) Some research has continued on neuroprotective agents, notably choline.

(Bearer et al., 2015) but with mixed results.

No systematic approach has been implemented on the use of folate, vitamin B12, thiamine, magnesium, zinc in pregnant alcohol abusing pregnant mothers. Nevertheless, ongoing transgenerational animal research on prenatal alcohol exposure shows low folate passes through generations, and has an impact on the developing cardiac system. Animal studies have shown this is ameliorated by folate supplementation in pregnancy. (Linask KK 2015).

It would be good to develop agents which are linked to the teratogenic effects of alcohol. So, antioxidants, alkalizing agents or glutamate antagonists would be a start. Already work on purifying water has developed this potential curative quality, related to its antioxidant and alkalizing properties.

5) Nevertheless, researchers in British Columbia have doggedly pursued Iron supplementation studies to quantify its positive impact on the abnormal sleep-wake

behaviors of infants and young children exposed tom prenatal alcohol (Jan et al., 2010, Ipsiroglu et al., 2016).

6) The newer field of pharmacogenomics has played a helpful role in decision making about safety in prescribing psychotropic agents in patients with NDPAE.
   - For the last number of years, I have used HLA typing before prescribing Carbamazepine for mood dysregulation or intermittent explosive disorder.
     HLA A 3101 is used to screen European patients at risk for Steven Johnson Syndrome (useful in both Irish and UK patients).
     HLA B 1502 is used to screen Asian patients at risk for Steven Johnson syndrome. (Helpful in Russian adopted patients from with NDPAE from Chinese side of Russia).
   - Cytochrome P450 liver enzyme system is well known in other medical specialties but is proving of specific clinical use in psychiatry. The cytochromes are membrane –associated proteins located in the inner membrane of mitochondria or endoplasmic reticulum. They metabolize thousands of endogenous and exogenous chemicals Their use in guiding psychiatric management in the early stages, but poses much promise for a more person –centered approach to medication management (Mc Donnell et al., 2013)

     Clinical example:

     A patient who has developed side effects, increased prolactin, gynecomastia, to atypical agent such as Risperidone which is metabolized through the 2 D6 system can be changed to another agent which uses a different system, 3A457, i.e., Aripiprazole. (This is a real example which showed a positive result, with disappearance of adverse side effects and better clinical effect).

     This type of clinical informed decision making or personal medicine is already present in other medical specialties and child neuropsychiatry and NDPAE in particular awaits its entry.

7) The basic problem with medication use in NDPAE is that the condition remains uncharted territory in management. within the Medical world., No medical specialty, whether pediatrics, child psychiatry, child neurology, public health seems to wants to take ownership of this transgenerational alcohol problem. Therefore, no sustained active medication interventions have been performed or studied on this complex acquired brain injury.

Until such time as medical professionals begin to take ownership of this non-face, non-IQ driven global neurodevelopmental disorder nothing will happen.

(It makes Goldin's 1999 paper on the demedicalisation of FAS all the more prescient)

Conclusion

1) The intervening 5 years have not changed the fundamental problem in management as the Diagnosis of NDPAE or FASD is still divorced from Treatment.
   So the model of care used in still frozen in a late 20th Century dyspmorphology/genetic paradigm where the diagnosis is disconnected from medical care so no RCT trials on medication have been done to any extent, except choline which is still exploratory and few trials on psychostimulants.
2) The Treatment model of many Child and Adolescent Mental Health Services CAMHS, in countries such as the UK and Ireland are still also outdated, as they do not see patients deemed as not displaying an' acute mental health disorder', thereby excluding any children or adolescents with acquired brain injury due to alcohol or other cause and showing neuropsychiatric/brain -driven disorders. Although Neuro-CAMHS departments exist in the UK they are few and far between and serve Traumatic Brain Injury patients rather the epigenetic acquired brain injury patients such as NDPAE.
3) The systematic use of narcotic antagonists or agents decreasing alcohol craving are still not fully integrated into the management of transgenerational alcohol craving and dependency in NDPAE. The brain-driven epigenetic origins of this alcohol craving have been long established but need to be integrated into pediatric, psychiatric and addiction medicine. There needs to be a more static use of agents such as naltrexone, acamprasate and selencro in transgenerational alcohol abuse/dependence with attention to age, gender and ethnic class differences in efficacy.

Chapter 11

The Systems of Care Approach to Management (2014 Book)

Introduction

Historical overview of the diagnostic dilemmas described in previous chapters in this book serve a salutary function by demonstrating that health care professionals in the main have failed to appreciate appropriately the broad implications of transgenerational ARND.

As long as diagnostic treatises fail to acknowledge dysmorphic ARND (FAS) non dysmorphic ARND as developmental psychiatric disorders, then it will nigh impossible to conduct scientific research on management or outcome.

Despite these significant constraints, it is becoming increasingly obvious that a transgenerational management perspective with alcohol abuse at the core of understanding is the only effective way to approach ARND.

The family-centered, transgenerational approach spans all age groups and is, by its nature, multi-systemic and multi-modal as it encompasses all the professional disciplines, medical and non-medical, disciplines involved in ARND assessment and management: i.e., medicine, psychiatry, alcohol services, education, social welfare, psychology, occupational and language therapy, and legal advocacy.

Although this type of new perspective may seem rather daunting in its scope, ultimately the goal is to produce a scaffolding containment system for the affected child with ARND and his or her family that achieves a balance between over-ambitious parenting and 'good enough' parenting, as well as locating a suitable level of health care delivery which marries the patient's needs. This includes identifying key environmental supports and stressors in the patient's environment.

The core concept for this type of delivery of services comes from the basic tenets of Wraparound Services (Goldman 1999). This was seen as a way of delivering services to children and families with multiple problems, which commonly were being served by multiple agencies.

There are a few key elements mentioned in Goldman that are equally critical for services to patients with ARND and their families.

Therefore:

1) The services are based in the community.
2) The services and supports must be individualized, build on strengths, and meet the needs of the children and families across the life's domains in order to promote success, safety and permanency in home, school and the community.
3) Families must be full and active partners in every level of the wraparound process.
4) The wraparound process must be a team –driven process involving the family, child, natural supports, agencies, and community services working together to develop, implement, and evaluate the individualized culturally competent service plan.

(From Goldman p 12- 13)

To extrapolate from the general wraparound principles the management approach to the zero 5 year old age group begins by entering a particular age appropriate systems of care paradigm.

The systems of care approach in this age group begins with early identification of potential ARND.

1) It is essential that the addiction counselors or adult psychiatrists communicate to the maternity units the risk of alcohol to the unborn child when they are aware of their patient's pregnancy and continued drinking. This is the first area to break down traditional stigma.
2) The GPs, midwives and/or obstetricians need to communicate with the pregnant mother and each other about the risks of alcohol in pregnancy to the unborn child. This is the next challenge to the pervasive stigma.
3) When an infant is identified as 'at risk' due to alcohol exposure then the hospital social worker should be informed.
4) There should be an in hospital case management meeting at least once, or better twice, in the pregnancy to look at suitable specialist for post-natal diagnosis and planning for suitable placement, so it is not done ad hoc or in an emergency.
5) The Public Health nurse should be involved as soon as the infant is born, and have a post-delivery meeting with the allocated physician for the infant, parents and social worker.

This is the time that parenting issues will be highlighted.

6) If the infant needs to be placed out of home it is essential to have a diagnostic assessment for ARND as soon as possible, as the diagnosis of a potential developmental psychiatric disorder has implications for complexity in home management
   This will inform the social service as to the better type of foster parent if needed. (i.e., one with more experience, training, no children in the home).
7) The parallel issues of the mental health and stress in the substance abusing mother need to be addressed, and her addiction therapist, GP or, psychiatrist need to be formally involved in liaison meeting/communication at this point.

Otherwise the child will be taken into care by default and the mother stigmatized and blamed with her psychiatric/addiction issues placed on the so called 'back burner'.

(There is a standardized instrument for the under 5 population (developed by the Committee of Systems of Care at the American Academy of Child and Adolescent Psychiatry), the ECSIII (Early Childhood System Intensity Instrument), which is still in early use.

It is probably currently less compatible for the UK or Irish health system, mainly due to the dearth in perinatal psychiatric, early childhood/infant service professionals available in the basic health systems. However, it is the author's hope that the earlier, and more consistent, recognition of conditions such as ARND will encourage field testing in other countries besides the USA).

For children and Adolescents there is a standardized systems of care instrument which has been tested, validated and used for at least 10 years in the USA.

The development of a standardized instrument of psychiatric clinical assessment, called the CASII (Child and Adolescent Service Intensity Instrument) by the American Academy of Child and Adolescent Psychiatry was a method of combining clinical assessment of mental health complexity, made through Dimensional assessments, with a Level of Care determination being made depending on the complexity of Dimensional assessments., which were mathematically calculated by a simple ordinal point score equating to service intensity need. (The child and adolescent instrument had been developed from an Adult instrument used in level of service care called the LOCUS developed initially by the American Association of Community Psychiatrists, AACP).

As stated in the CASII manual;

> "The CASII employs multi-disciplinary, multi-informant perspectives on children and adolescents and is designed to be used by a variety of mental health professionals. Although it may be used for initial level of care placement decisions, it can be used at all stages of

> treatment to assess the level of intensity of services needed." (CASII user's manual, March 2005, p. 15).

Time has given the space to acknowledge hidden mentors of creative thought, cultural sensitivity and simple humanity, Mark Chenven, Andy Pumariega, Bob Klaehn, Tommy Vaughan, Al Zachik, Nancy Winters, Larry Marx, Bill Heffron, Graeme Hanson, Ted Fallon, Peter Metz, Gordon Hodas, Kay Mc Ginty, Debbie Carter, and the omni present Kristin Kroeger, and the effervescent Charley Huffine! This grounding in 'systems of care theory' is the well respected and much appreciated fruits of the author's long involvement (1997-2006) with this Systems of Care Work Group, now Committee, in the American Academy of Child and Adolescent Psychiatry (AACAP).

The Dimensions are:

I will only describe the essence of the instrument because of copyright issues.

Risk of Harm

This is the first clinical Dimension and in many ways the most immediately of clinical importance for triaging services.

> "It is a measure of the child or adolescent's risk of harm to self or others by various means, and an assessment of his/her potential for being a victim of physical or sexual abuse, neglect or violence"

(CASII user manual, March 2005, p. 16)

It is divided into five levels which the rater scores depending on clinical basement or clinical information available. (Each level has a score 1 to 5).

They are:

- Low risk of harm
- Some risk of harm
- Significant risk of harm
- Serious risk of harm
- Extreme risk of harm, this current suicidal or homicidal intent

Functional Status Is Equally Described in Detail, at Each Level Using the Same Scoring System

So you have:

Minimal functional impairment, Mild functional impairment,

Moderate functional impairment, Serious functional impairment, and Severe functional impairment.

Co-Morbidity

This is where the instrument has the most utility for children and adolescents with ARND as it is the only current psychiatric clinical assessment tool that fully acknowledges the unique complexity of co-morbidity in assessing this type of patient morbidity and need for service.

> "... for the purpose of this dimension only sources of impairment directly related to developmental, psychiatric, and/or substance use problems should be considered" (CASII user manual, p. 25).

Therefore, you have:

No co-morbidity, Minor co-morbidity, Significant co-morbidity, Major co-morbidity and then, Severe co-morbidity.

Recovery Environment

This is very interesting as it captures both the environmental stressors, but also acknowledges the environmental supports in the child or adolescent's life, personal, family and community and is at the heart of the ecological model underpinning the instrument. Naturally it has a significant role in trying to quantify the current lives of children and adolescents with ARND.

Environmental stress with a 5 point scoring scheme, from minimally stressful environment to severely stressful environment.

Environmental supports, with a 5 point scoring scheme, from highly supportive to no support.

Resiliency and Treatment History

This dimension is informed by the long history of research on resiliency in child psychiatry. As well it offers a practical analysis of the success or failure of previous treatment, more than a little relevant in the case of ARND children and adolescents.

The 5 point scoring scheme goes from Full Resiliency and/or Response to Treatment to Legible Resiliency and/or Response to Treatment.

Treatment, Acceptance and Engagement

This Dimension in the instrument shows the influence of the psychiatrists in the production of the instrument and its testing , especially those who had training in psychoanalysis and family therapy.

It differs from other Dimensions in that it is the first Dimension to assess both the opinion of the carer and also the child or adolescent (still a rather foreign concept in the more conservative climate of child psychiatry in the UK and Ireland).

a) Child or Adolescent acceptance and engagement
   This goes from Optimal, to Constructive, Obstructive, Adversarial and finally Inaccessible
b) Parent and/or primary caretaker acceptance and engagement
   Similarly, this goes from Optimal, to Constructive, Obstructive, and Adversarial to Inaccessible

The Level of Care Services were:

> "These levels of care described in the CASII represent a graded continuum of treatment responses designed for use with the CASII dimensional assessments and composite score." (CASII user manual, March 2005, p. 40). So it is not a generic triage model to be patched into disparate communities.

There are 7 levels of care delineated which go from: (CASII User's Manual, March 2005, p 40-52)

Unfortunately, when you think about it the children and adolescents with ARND, currently undiagnosed and untreated, are all at the higher levels of care.

There is another problem that the continuum of care does not really exist in the post Celtic tiger finance poor Ireland, not dissimilar to many Native American or First Nations communities. The UK, however, with its National Health System (NHS), has a much better chance of benefiting from the CASII in the management of children and adolescents with ARND.

LEVEL 0: Basic Services. Each level of care has identified a specific range of services available as indicated;

Clinical services i.e., "It is imperative that Basic services in all settings provide screening for mental health and developmental disorders. Comprehensive, multidisciplinary assessments for children and adolescents who, after initial screening, emerge with multi-faceted problems should be readily available"...

Support services i.e., Basic services should be available to children, adolescents and families through collaboration with religious and culturally distinct community groups and in a variety of community settings, including schools and adult education centers, day care and recreational facilities, vocational and social service agencies and medical facilities."

Crisis stabilization and prevention services i.e., "24–hour crisis services should be publicized, accessible, and fully integrated into Basic services in all community settings."

Care environment i.e., Prevention and community support activities may occur in many settings, from a child or adolescent's home, in schools, churches, medical and recreational facilities, or mental health settings."

As can be appreciated in many parts of the UK and Ireland there are not even Basic Services available for child mental health, let alone a range to Level 6, however this does not negate the need to establish some baseline for basic duty of care.

To *Level* 5 Non Secure, 24 hour Services with psychiatric monitoring.

It is important to note that this is a community psychiatry based instrument, so the 24 hour services are not necessarily hospital based.

Clinical services, Support services, Crisis intervention and prevention services, Care environment

and

Level 6. Secure, 24 hours Services with psychiatric management.

Clinical services, Support services, Crisis intervention and prevention services, Care environment.

The intermediate Levels of Care are:

1) Recovery Maintenance and Health Management
2) Out Patient Services
3) Intensive Out Patient Services
4) Intensive integrated Service without 24-hour psychiatric monitoring

There is a grid scoring system which needs training to use, but is not too complicated, and which allocates the child or adolescent needs profile to an appropriate level of care determination.

A Needs Assessment is a common concept in the social service system dealing with children, but, although I am a wee bit biased, this brings some science to the equation.

The rest of this chapter is devoted to clinical vignettes and stories which maybe could be used if the professionals choose to contact the American Academy of Child and Adolescent Psychiatry, (AACAP), Committee on Community Systems of Care, for an official training in the CASII instrument, which is still very much part of the working health care scene in the USA.

There are well recognized issues in case management of severely emotionally disturbed children which are equally applicable to children with ARND.

There may be multiple providers who do not communicate with each other, leading to duplication and fragmentation.

Example:

It is not uncommon for a child to be removed from birth parents because of concerns about parenting and then placed in a no. of different foster placements due to the inability to manage the child's behaviors. The alcohol use of the birth mother in pregnancy has not been documented or the information passed from the obstetrician, midwife or even public health nurse to the social worker.

The birth mother has a long history of psychiatric and addictive problems and is under specialist addictive counseling services. When she is pregnant no information is passed on to the maternity services. When the mother delivers no information is available on her long standing psychiatric and addictive problems and the infant is removed from care because she cannot cope.

The infant is brought to a GP or pediatrician for primary care. The infant is not growing and is labeled Failure to Thrive and given increased nutrition. The child continues to have developmental growth problems but the antenatal history is not available from the hospital.

A teenage UK girl with ARND is hospitalized because of intermittent and escalating suicidal thoughts and acts i.e., putting laces around neck. The hospital labels the patient as a typical 'child in care' and minimizes the neurodevelopmental component, which includes marked expressive/receptive language impairments to her illness. The 'child in care' is seen as a 'catch all' for suicidal depressed teenagers who are traumatized and felling hopeless and helpless. This unfortunately invalidates the foster parents who had nurtured the child from 12 months old, although she has a Full Care Order as the birth mother could not cope. The psychiatrist and psychologist diagnose Borderline Personality Disorder in the patient, which in many ways blames the patient and invites a certain intolerance to her lack of progress in talk therapy, which she actually does not process properly. The new social worker decides to take over the active management from the foster parents and contradicts their therapeutic alliances in the community. The teenager is confused, upset, with marked mood dysregulation, and now is receiving higher and higher dosages of differing atypical neuroleptics from the in- patient psychiatrist.

Multiple Alcohol Generations

A transgenerational perspective is recommended in order to address effectively the social as well as the biological factors that influence ARND.

The rule of thumb in the transgenerational management of ARND should be:

> 'Always think multi-generations, multi-system and multi-modal and remember that alcohol is at the core of the problem.'

Clinicians who see ARND patients are not dealing simply with the so-called 'identified patient.'

Alcohol dependence and abuse weave their way through different races, cultures and generations, so patients presenting in the clinician's office frequently bring the legacy of previous generations with them and are a harbinger of generations to come. Documentation of these intergenerational alcohol and offspring characteristics has recently been reported from northern France (Lemoine et al., 1992).

Clinical Vignette for Scoring Using the CASII Instrument

A 23-month boy was assessed for possible effects of prenatal alcohol exposure. His birth mother disclosed that she drank wine steadily for the first 5 months of her pregnancy, then stopped as she would become nauseous when she drank.

There was no history of intellectual disability in either birth parent. He was born at term in a local maternity hospital but at birth his weight was low for his gestational age. His temperament was difficult to settle in infancy, and this temperament persists. He was removed from his birth home at 5 months because of concerns about neglect, and the birth mother's return to alcohol addiction postnatally. He is still with his first foster placement.

He was monitored closely by a health visitor, and his height and weight indicated a marked Failure to Thrive up to 12 months. Since 12 months of age, his weight remained at the 25th percentile, but his height was still below the 10th percentile, (his birth parents were normal or above average height). The health visitor documented delays in gross and fine motor skills, as well as early language difficulties. She could not test the hearing properly because of sensory reactivity to sound and light in the examining room.

The 23 month old boy had little spontaneous play with few vocalizations, and was incapable of co-operative or imitative play, as he was too sensory seeking and distracted by his surroundings. Formal assessment of sensory motor function showed auditory, visual, olfactory, tactile and co-ordination problems.

He had no classic FAS facial dysmorphology, but had microcephaly. He also had global developmental delay with early features consistent with ARND, presenting

Regulatory Disorder (sensory stimulation seeking/impulsive). (Same story in a different 24-month girl).

This Is a Clinical Vignette for Scoring on the CASII Instrument

Shannon, 12 and half years old.

She had been drinking since 11 years old when she was expelled from school because of violent behaviors. She lived in a particularly dangerous neighborhood of the city, and had no support except a maternal aunt who lived nearby.

She had a history of binge drinking exposure in pregnancy and her birth mother had died of liver cirrhosis when she was 10 years old. She had been brought up by her mother's older sister from 3 years of age because of alcohol abuse and violence in the family home. She was very affectionate and adored the family dog Mollser.

There is an unproven story that she had been abused by a former boyfriend of her mothers.

She was a good student when she was in the mood, and was strong willed and brooked no challenges, and had a real talent for singing and dancing.

She had a 16-year-old boyfriend who was a great drinker himself, and sang a mean song or two. She was not yet sexually active.

She wanted to get on the X Factor and become a star, but could never make time for the auditions, as she was too disorganized, and impatient.

She had never had a psychiatric assessment, and had no medical problems in her early childhood.

There are many stories such as Shannon's.

Children grow up in homes where the transgenerational legacy of alcohol is ever present.

In the Irish context this becomes almost an accepted norm, not unlike certain communities in Canada and, USA and Australia.

Grandparents, great grandparents have stories about 'alcohol fueled' escapades.

They are told in rambling mythical family narratives, songs and tall tales of adventure and almost always have a hint of anti-authority.

Where the transgenerational legacy of trauma, victimization, colonization sits embedded in these alcohol-washed stories still remains to be unraveled. There is now an international reckoning related to historical trauma; its transmission through what Carl Jung called the 'collective unconscious'. We are to-day part of what we were many centuries ago. Part of us has still not let go of that need to rebel against the oppressor and dampen our 'psychic pain'.

A country such as Ireland is old but still very new. Seems a contradiction, but the reality is that the new Republic, free of colonization, is only 90 years old. And still the northern part of the country remains 'colonized' in some people's language, and 'united/part of the union' in other people's minds. You cannot step into the here and now of clinical assessment of ARND without casting an eye to the past.

Another Transgenerational Alcohol Story

A six year old Irish boy, Sean, received many services since birth but still was unmanageable.

In addition to being short and underweight, He had a small head, and hypoplasia of the corpus callosum was documented at 2 years of age with MRI of the brain. He now had major expressive and receptive language problems.

No syndrome could describe his disorder, but a misplaced hospital neonatologist examination had noted facial dysmorphology. A number of years later a social worker contacted a child psychiatrist to assess the child for dysmorphic ARND because of his small stature and 'funny looking face.'

The 26-year-old mother was overwhelmed, but not surprised, when a possible dysmorphic ARND (FAS) was made. She had never been asked about alcohol use during her pregnancy, but now freely readily admitted to binge drinking, 6 or more beers a night, in the first and second trimester.

As the story continued, her own 48-year-old mother (maternal grandmother) had a severe psychiatric undiagnosed disorder, and had been an alcoholic who drank throughout her pregnancy with Sean's mother. So Sean's mother had a neurotoxin created craving for alcohol from an early age due to the possible effects of prenatal alcohol exposure in utero.

Now what if Sean in the clinical case example above had been a girl rather than a boy – a girl who started craving alcohol at 10 years of age and drifted into binge drinking, unprotected sex, and pregnancy at 15 years of age? Another cycle in this family's sad legacy would have repeated itself.

Current clinical experience in Ireland and the UK as well, as recent studies in France, provide more than their fair share of these types of transgenerational alcohol stories. For example, in a recent clinical consultation case in Ireland the paternal grandmother of two children with ARND had become their primary parent.

The interaction between ARND and negative environment has been called a 'double jeopardy' effect by Olson and colleagues 2009. It has been described as a case of 'double jeopardy' because the adverse environment kindles insecure attachment, disorganized attachment, but also exposes the child to possible early traumatic events, either directly or indirectly, i.e., witness of domestic violence.

Clinical Vignette for Scoring Using CASII Instrument

A 14 year old adopted Russian girl has significant history of prenatal alcohol exposure throughout pregnancy. Her adoptive Irish parents were both exhausted and at the end of their tether. She lived in a good upper middle class small town housing estate.

She is first assessed for ARND at 13 years of age., and presents no facial dysmorphology. Although she had clear dysmorphological features in earlier age photographs at 3, 5 and 8 yrs. old.

She has had WISC III, verbal 60 -69 and performance 60 -69 when 8 years old. However when she was tested 5 years later with WISC IV her cognitive functioning had decreased in both verbal and performance domains, verbal, 50, performance 54.

She also had delayed language development and a recent CELP 4 placed her at > 0.1 percentile for pseudo word decoding, sentence and word recognition expressively and receptively.

She has a long history of impulsive aggressive behaviors in school with peers and teachers related to her academic and social disconnection in the school setting. She had been on the waiting list for a special needs school for a year.

She has been treated with methylphenidate 20 mgs for the last year by local CAMHS child psychiatrist with no improvement in function and possible increase in aggression. She has what was well described as some visual and auditory hallucinations when taking the methylphenidate.

Her blood sugar was borderline low, as was her thyroid function indices.

She had few friends in school and did not identify any adult figure as a 'significant other'.

Clinical Vignette for Scoring with the CASII Instrument

A 16 year-old Irish teenage girl, now living in a residential home, had been binge drinking weekly for 3 1/2 years. She reported being pregnant a year ago, but losing the pregnancy in the first few months. She did not follow-up at the maternity hospital, but became involved with child and adolescent psychiatry after a serious, self-harm overdose of aspirin, and a short crisis hospitalization in a pediatric hospital.

She was found to have been prenatally exposed to alcohol. Hospital and school records revealed a history of developmental delay, academic school failure with particular problems in Mathematics and spelling. The school had not carried out any formal academic tests because her school attendance had been inconsistent. She had been labeled as having ODD. The hospital school assessments showed clear evidence of dyslexia, dyscalculia and poor working memory. As she had no dysmorphic facial features, she was diagnosed with ARND.

She presented a clinical picture of a combination of Disruptive Mood Dysregulation Disorder with some emotional incontinence, that had not responded to previous individual insight-orientated psychotherapy in the community.

In conversation with professionals, she described having had a craving for alcohol from as early as 9 or 11 years of age, and said that she had started drinking continuously at 12 1/2years old.

She also reported a sexual assault episode 4 weeks before her overdose. The A. and E. hospital which treated her had verified sexual assault, but would not fully believe her story because she had a learning disability, and could not consistently remember the details of the sexual assault. Child protection services in the hospital were contacted by the hospital social worker working with the consultation liaison child and adolescent psychiatrist, and the community child protection services in the teenager's residential group home area were contacted as the perpetrator was a well-known, violent, teenage boy who was in care, and lived near the home.

She was the subject of an interim custody agreement between social services and her birth mother, who was still alcohol dependent, and may herself have had ARND due to her own prenatal alcohol exposure.

On the positive side she responded to carbamazepine, and her mood became much more settled with no explosive episodes in over 3 months.

With the epidemic of underage drinking in Ireland and the UK, this type of case could become a 'new norm'.

How could services protect this vulnerable teenager with ARND, protect her from an unplanned, possibly alcohol exposed pregnancy, and approach/support her birth mother's home environment?

Effective management in this case would have to begin with 'joining up' of child and adult services in obstetrics, developmental pediatrics, psychiatry, social service and addiction services.

This Is a Vignette for Scoring Using the CASII Instrument

For example: ICD 10 Diagnostic Formulation

Axis I: Described a 12-year-old Irish boy in a foster home placement who had a confirmed history of prenatal alcohol exposure and clinical features of ARND.

Recent clinical assessment established there was no evidence of Attachment Disorder; the boy has been in same foster home placement since 12 months of age and was well attached to his foster parents. Hyperkinetic disorder (or you could say ADHD), Inattention/Impulsive subtype

Axis II: Evidence of complex learning disorder with specific spelling disorder and specific disorder of arithmetic skills [assess using the Wechsler Intelligence Scale for Children (WISC),

Wechsler Individual Achievement Test (WIAT), evidence of language disorder with problems in expressive and expressive language

Clinical Evaluation of Language Fundamentals (CELF) identified problems in social communication disorder with problems in social cognition and social communication (Coggins et al., 2008, Greenbaum et al., 2009)

Axis III: 13-point difference between verbal IQ (=89) and performance IQ (=76) assessed WISC IV

Axis IV: ARND, evidence of Specific Developmental Disorder of Motor Function with Developmental Coordination Disorder, showing gait and truncal ataxia.

Axis V: Early psychosocial stressor of separation from birth parents at 1 year

Axis VI: Level of functioning 50/100 as in school.

What extra information is need for scoring on CASII?

In a similar way, the *DSM IV –TR Formulation,* made mental health professionals to code anxiety, mood or psychotic disorder due to general medical condition of prenatal alcohol exposure with clinical evidence of ARND.

'Cognitive disorder not otherwise specified (NOS)' was the best DSM IV –TR descriptor of the learning disorder associated with ARND, along with such psychiatric diagnoses as ADHD or Mood Disorder, and provided the option for mental health professionals to diagnose this disorder as 'secondary to dysmorphic ARND (FAS) or non-dysmorphic ARND'.

As with the ICD, the DSM's five-axis structure supports the same diagnostic descriptive approach.

(NOW we are in the era of DSM V).

For Example: *This is a Clinical vignette for scoring with CASII instrument*

Axis I: A 9-year-old Polish/Irish girl with Mood Disorder and Intermittent Explosive Disorder with history of prenatal alcohol exposure and clinical evidence of ARND.

Axis II: A verbal IQ of 75 and a performance IQ of 82 identified; subtests showed reading disorder, writing disorder, mathematics disorder and working memory at 2nd percentile, using WISC IV

Axis III: Evidence of Developmental Coordination Disorder; also left eye strabismus and ventricular septal defect, both recognized Alcohol Related Birth Defects (ARBD) (Stratton et al., 1996, O'Malley 2008)

Axis IV: Psychosocial stressor of continual school failure with no special needs support in school identified

Axis V: Level of functioning 40/100 as currently out of school, Patient needs VABS.

What extra information is needed to score the CASII?

This clinical vignette is for scoring in CASII instrument

A 38-year-old single mother with a history of manic depression and domestic violence in a common law relationship, delivered an infant exposed to alcohol.

The infant girl with a slow to warm temperament from birth, continuing into early childhood.

The birth mother could not cope with basic parenting, and had to strop breast feeding because her baby girl would not suck properly.

Later at 2 to 3 years of age the young child became unmanageable with temper tantrums, explosive episodes and periods of severe anxiety.

The mother saw a number of psychologists with her girl between ages 4 and 5 years. Her girl was prescribed play therapy which did not work.

She was then assessed by the local CAMHS team a number of times between 6 and 9 years of age.

At this stage the young girl's behavioral profile was attributed to a range of diagnoses including ADHD, Oppositional Defiant Disorder (ODD), Autistic Spectrum Disorder, possible Psychotic Disorder and inconsistent/inadequate parenting, with poor attachment between the mother and child going back to early childhood.(the last diagnosis being the most destructive to the mother).

A prescription of Concerta made the problems worse, and a subsequent switch to biphasic, Equasym did not make any substantive difference.

The mother became depressed, and overwhelmed, but sought a further opinion, recognizing that the alcohol in pregnancy that she took in response to severe manic depression and domestic violence might be related to her child's unusual behaviors. Her feelings of guilt had prevented her from disclosing this in previous assessments, but neither had the CAMHS professionals questioned her about the possibility of her daughter's prenatal alcohol exposure.

This gave rise to a hypothesis of prenatal alcohol, linked to a presentation consistent with non-dysmorphic ARND, being suggested. Cognitive testing with WISC IV was done and showed a 14 point split between Verbal and Performance IQ, with Performance, being higher, in the average range.

This conceptualization fitted the child's developmental psychiatric profile, and afforded an opportunity for a more specialized multimodal treatment programme, including sensory integration, language therapy, and a specialized school placement.

This led to the Dimensional conceptualization of the ARND, developmental psychiatric disorder.

Finally, the child psychiatrists contacted the mother's adult psychiatrist, with her permission, and this lead to enhanced communication between the mother and her psychiatrist.

She, as well, had a change in her psychotropic medication which helped.

A family therapist was contacted, and began to do instrumental family function with mother and child which was appreciated and quite successful.

A year later the child was in a specialized school and much happier. She was receiving language therapy every 2 weeks, and her social communication skills were improving.

THE SYSTEMS OF CARE APPROACH TO MANAGEMENT. AN UPDATE. 2020

The intervening 5 years have welcomed the introduction of a new Systems of Care Instrument from American Academy of Child and Adolescent Psychiatry, AACAP.

This is the Early Childhood Service Intensity Instrument, ECSII., which is available through the AACAP membership and has a standardized training on line.

Unfortunately, the reality is that many countries do not have the basic organized or adequately-funded early intervention services or resources. Nevertheless, the usage of a clinical instrument such as ECSII in either Community-based services, or more appropriately in obstetric/neonatology hospital-based services will lead to a greater appreciation of the need and the true value of wrap-around multidisciplinary service provision for the under 5 populations. (AACAP 2019).

At a personal level, the more years in which I work with children affected by prenatal alcohol the more it has become patently obvious that systems of care need to re-align for the under 5 populations and their birth, foster or adoptive families. This is especially true for the families bathed in transgenerational alcohol with all its global neurodevelopmental and social sequelae.

The critical distinction between a 3-year-old with NDPAE who has either a Regulatory Disorder, Hyperresponsive or Regulatory Disorder Sensory Seeking/Impulsive informs the suitable 'wraparound care' at many levels. It also anticipates the service intensity need as the clinical phenotype of the NDPAE changes through the following years., impacting both the child and the parent.

The clinical examples given in my 2014 book for the CASII are still very much valid, and have been tested in the last few years for cultural sensitivity in Ireland (Although they utilized the DSM IV R diagnostic formulation these clinical vignettes remain valid).

Field training and testing in 2018 with ICP, a community-based health care organization in Naas Co. Kildare, has shown that it has immediate clinical utility in patients with NDPAE as it identifies through a standardized multi –dimensional clinical scale the complexity of level of care needed for optimum management success.

Many of the consultation patients whom I have seen in Ireland were in the more service- intense, levels 4, 5 and 6 of care. The practical problem in Ireland was that these types of patients needed to be transferred to the UK or USA for suitable and safe level of care provision. On the positive side the introduction of CASII as a regular triage assessment tool in the community could help medical administrators locally and nationally in directions to allocate appropriate mental health funds. (this situation became a common 'double-bind 'for Native American and First Nations communities in Canada and USA as they had to spend scarce health dollars to send patient s with NDPAE/FASD out of the community for level 4 to 6 care provision).

A new clinical vignette shows the potential transgenerational use of CASII and ECSII.

A 19-year-old Polish young man with NDPAE has a long history of academic school failure and has been expelled from school 3 times because of violent episodes. His birth mother died of cirrhosis of the liver when he was 9 years old and he was not allowed to go to the funeral as he was in acute residential care. He started abusing alcohol at 12 years of age and left school at 16 years of age with no national examination qualification. When he was 5 years old and EEG was read as abnormal, but no follow-up was done until recently when it showed complex partial seizure disorder. At that time his explosive episodes had included auditory and visual, hallucinations as an aura,

He is now the father of a 10-month old daughter and the UK born mother was 16 years at the birth of the child. The birth mother has probable NDPAE but is undiagnosed. Her family have a long history of alcohol dependence, and she has a younger sister in care.

The 19-year-old wants custody of his child and had threatened the birth mother. The social service involved with the young man do not want to release information on his potential risk to the child protection workers because of data protection concerns.

The infant has been exposed to alcohol in pregnancy and has a difficult to settle temperament with sleep wake and feeding problems. Her birth mother is having difficulty in parenting her daughter.

A court case is set in the near future.

CASII and ECSII instruments could inform decision making for culturally sensitive and culturally appropriate wrap- around services in many child and/or adolescent community or hospital based mental health service providers.

Chapter 12

POSTSCRIPT (2014 BOOK)

Co-occurring developmental psychiatric disorders in patients with ARND should always be considered in relation to the brain dysfunction that can be caused by the prenatal alcohol exposure (Archibald et al., 2001, Bookstein et al., 2005, Mattson et al., 1996, Riley et al., 1995, Sowell et al., 2007, 2008, O'Leary et al., 2011). For example the association between brain circuits and structural brain damage has been well established in relation to such problematic conditions as antisocial personality disorder (Raine et al., 2001).

The prenatal alcohol effect on the developing corpus callosum, frontal lobes, hippocampus and cerebellum all have potential effects on executive function decision making, impulsivity and memory which must be incorporated in the diagnostic understanding of the patient's clinical presentation. (Pine et al., 2012).

The developmental psychiatric disorders within ARND are the entry to management, but the child, adolescent or even adult must always be seen within their family, community and/or cultural context.

There are changes in the attitude and knowledge regarding the long term consequences and developmental psychiatric disorders related to prenatal alcohol exposure occurring worldwide.(Streisguth & O'Malley 2000, Lambin 2011, Elliott 2013, Rich and Novick Brown 2013).

Now Australia, Europe as a whole, and back in the USA the DSM V has introduced a new diagnostic category Neurodevelopmental Disorder (Prenatal Alcohol Exposure), ND (PAE). Thus in the USA this will mean that ARND is now a billable condition through the medical insurance companies (with a code, 315.8), and so will be diagnosed, treated and hopefully open the doors for intervention research, initially in the USA and maybe in Canada as it also uses the DSM V classification system. Thus ND (PAE) now sits in the area of Specific Other Neurodevelopmental Disorders.

Table 13. Percentages of psychiatric disorders found in children, adolescents and adults with ARND, dysmorphic and non dysmorphic, in certain research and clinical populations

Percentage Psychiatric Disorders in Population				
Study and cohort details	**ADHD/ADD**	**Depression/ Mood disorder**	**Anxiety Disorder**	**Addiction**
Streissguth et al., 1996, n=417, 6 to 51 years old, parent/patient report	60 percent	20 percent	20 percent	
O'Malley 2001, n=51, 3 to 33 years old, psychiatric examination	58 percent	44 percent		
O'Malley 2011a, n=59, infancy to 20 years old, psychiatric examination	60 percent	20 percent		
Famy et al. 1998, n=25, adults, Structured Clinical Interview for DSM-IV, I and II	58 percent	44 per cent	20 percent	60 percent
Chun et al., 2001 n=25 Adults, Structured Clinical Interview for DSM IV, I & II		52 percent	72 percent	52 percent
O'Malley KD 2011b Developmental Psychiatric Assessment n= 59 Infancy to 20 years' old		20 percent	12 percent*	
O'Malley KD 2011b Adults, N ==29 Psychiatric Assessment and Pt/family Report		65 percent		65 percent

*ASD.

In the UK a recent multi-author book on Fetal Alcohol Spectrum Disorders edited by Barry Carpenter, Carolyn Blackburn and Jo Egerton sets a new template for interdisciplinary perspectives on approaching such patients especially from a learning or educational view. (Carpenter et al., 2013).

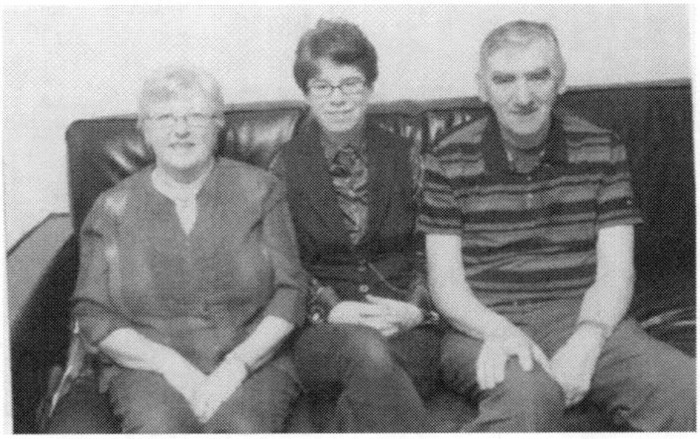

Charlene and foster parents Joan and Ralph.

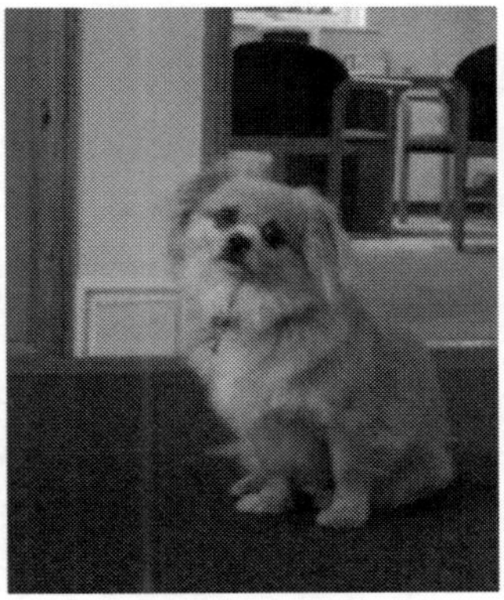

Mollyo the therapy dog.

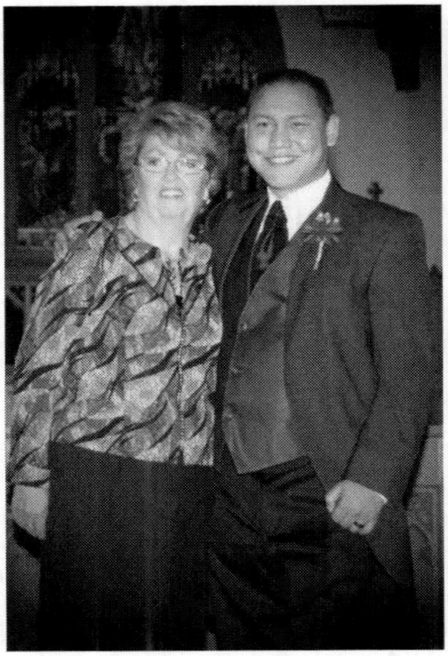

Randy Mc Donald and adoptive mother Nanci.

Hello,

My name is Charlene Marshall. I am 23 years old and have Fetal Alcohol Syndrome and Asperger's Disorder.

I was fostered when I was 5 days old and I maintained contact with my birth family up to the present day.

I have lived with my foster family my whole life but I am going to start my story at my early teens as it was probably the most important part of my life so far.

When I turned 13, my mum & dad started sending me to horse riding lessons. It was to get me out of the house & get me interacting with other people as I was very anxious around people but I found the horses very calming & it helped me to socialize more. I even worked with the stables over the summer for about 5 years or so & I have continued to ride up to the present day.

I found school very difficult as I would have found it very hard to concentrate if the rest of the class was very disruptive, although I was allowed to go to another classroom to finish my work in peace. I finished school with 5 GCSE'S. After I left school at16, I wanted to do animal care as I loved animals, especially horses. I did an Animal Care Course at the Belfast Metropolitan College & after a year I got my first Diploma in Animal Care. Dog grooming is now my part-time job after starting work placement in 2009 & I have never looked back. I had started off just washing & drying dogs & now I teach the trainees & cut the dogs hair as well. After having sensory issues to notice dryers & barking dogs & touch water from the shower & vibrations from the clippers, I have come a long way. I never thought I'd be able to put a scissors near a dogs face.

The hardest part of my life so far was in August 2007 just after I got my first Diploma in Animal Care. I was due to visit my mother that morning & I had never felt so happy in my entire life. The doorbell rang; it was my mother's best friend. She asked if she could speak to mum & dad so I called them down. After she left, mum & dad called me in & then I was hit with the worst news I had ever heard. My mother died in her sleep. I didn't think I'd ever be happy again. Even to this day I haven't been to her grave as I can't bear it. When my mum died I lost contact with my siblings, she was the one who kept me in touch with them. There were 3 things which helped me through it. My family who I love so very much, my friends who I couldn't live without & getting some pet rats for my 18th birthday. Daniel, named after the British ice skater, Daniel Whiston & Scooter (because he was very fast). These 2 rats became part of the family. I will never forget them. They helped me through the toughest part of my life as they gave me something else to focus on, as I was grieving. I no longer have Daniel & Scooter as they passed away in 2010 but I have a wonderful Cocker spaniel "Misty," who is nearly 4.I, have made some very good friends through my lessons over the years & we like to meet up occasionally to go for movie nights or dinner. I have also joined an Autistic social group, which meets up once a month & that is going very well. Work is going very well & we are busier than ever! I have got back in contact with my sister from my birth family & have a new wee niece. I never thought I would be the way I am today if it wasn't for all the support, my friends, which includes Dr O'Malley & my family, especially Joan & Ralph have given me. I would never have got this far.

Thank you all very much.

Nanci (McDonald- McLennan) Heninger
Calgary, Alberta, Canada.

During the early 80's I had been a foster parent to a number of newborn babies & in December 1982 our family was approached & asked to adopt a baby boy, brought to Ontario from Saskatchewan, where we were living at the time. He apparently had been born to a native woman, who specifically asked that he be placed off his Reserve, out of the province & into a good Christian home.

We later came to the knowledge that this child was so difficult to handle that he was placed in 5 different foster homes between birth & 2 months of age when he was finally placed with us. Within 2-3 days I realized this child was not functioning normally & spent the next 10 years trying to understand what was wrong. He rarely slept for more than an hour or 2 & was unable to function without immediate gratification.

We asked the professionals specifically about FAS. At the time we were assured that it wasn't the case.

Yet years later confirmation of prenatal exposure to alcohol was revealed. The mother drank in early pregnancy, but with further study we came to understand that even a short exposure to alcohol in the womb could indeed affect the developing foetus.

10 years after his adoption & moving to Calgary, Alberta, our then Pediatric Physician referred our son to Dr. Kieran O'Malley. Our son was a troubled child expelled from school in Grade 1. He was also bullied by other children, likely due to his poor communication & poor age appropriate functioning skills. He was placed in special classes in school. He saw Dr O'Malley until 2006 when he moved back to Ireland, & then Randy continued with the family doctor, Dr Bill Hanlon, who was familiar with the situation.

However late in his teens he was not accepted for interventions or assistance through the adult system, which deemed him not disabled, under their definition. Eventually he was accepted 3 years later. However during those 3 years his lifestyle & functioning lead him down many difficult roads.

The system itself being flawed created many further disadvantages, resulting in many trials & difficulties. With no appointed guardian to make decisions & keep him safe, he became his own guardian. He took himself off all his medications & refused to co-operate with any of his doctors & resorted to smoking pot as a medication for his anxiety and impulsiveness.

He finally met a lady, (Kerry) older than him who had several children whom he wanted to have a permanent relationship with. They had a child together & during that time she seemed somehow to know how to handle him. Somehow he managed to settle down & was married in October 2012.

Today he has his daughter with him as well as having taken custody of his biological son from a previous relationship. The blended family has helped him to mature & today his focus is on being a good husband & father, working 2 jobs, as well as participating in many worthwhile endeavors providing assistance to those in need in his community.

Randy Mc Donald, now aged 31 years old.

I have had jobs in which I have been the Director of Marketing/Management/PR/Sales for a local television Show. Also a Personnel Assistant to some of Calgary's top income earners in a Condo & have been at the same 2 jobs for the last 3 years.

I finished a Movie as the Extras Special Effects Make-up Artist, which I am credited for in the movie, it is called the "Dead Mile."

I am now working on helping company create a mobile Theater showing of 2D/3D movies, to show to small towns in Alberta.

There is not a lack of talent coming from me or intelligence.

Postscript. An Update for NDPAE, 2020

The intervening 5 years have not brought a wealth of psychiatric morbidity studies on NDPAE but one new case series was presented at an International FASD meeting in London in 2016 (O'Malley 2016).

1. Russian Adopted Children in Ireland with NDPAE.

N=22

Gender male 17, female 5

Age range: 2 ½ to 19 yrs.

Ethnic Russian 19, Ukrainian 3

Early adoption, (under 5 years old) 17

Late adoption (over 5 yrs. old) 5

Psychiatric Disorders

ADHD; 12

ADD: 7

Mood disorder: 6

ASD/SCD: 7
PTSD: 7
Conduct disorder/antisocial behavior: 3
Alcohol abuse/dependence: 3
Identity Disorder: 3

A number of patients had co morbid diagnosis.

Neurological Problems

Developmental Co-ordination Disorder, (including gait and truncal ataxia). 11
Sensory disorders: 8
Seizure disorder: 2
Sleep problems: 8
Microcephaly: 7

A number of neurological problems were seen co-morbidly. Late adoption was seen as most problematic.

NB. One interesting clinical fact was the reaction of my therapy dog Molly, a Tibetan spaniel, who refused to approach 3 males (as she sensed danger in approaching these individuals). Later 2 of these patients were assessed for forensic risk and one needed treatment in UK (previously mentioned under animal therapy section).

2. Only recently a review of 23 clinical research studies showed the link between neurodevelopmental disorder and prenatal alcohol exposure with no safe amount of alcohol in pregnancy (Manklak et al. 2020).

Patient Stories

Shannon's Story

I have known Shannon since 2009, when I saw her in my Belfast consultation office. Her birth mother sadly died of acute alcohol related causes when she was only 3 years old.

However, the steadfastness of their joint physical and emotional scaffolding and consistent affection of her foster parents Margaret and Charlie, and her own innate resilience, have sustained her through the trials and tribulations of her life. At one stage she needed carbamazepine for mood dysregulation stabilization, mis- understood as ADHD, and this had mixed success, but better than she felt ! It did help her a bit through a bad patch. It also highlighted the challenge psychiatric diagnostic veracity in medication usage with this alcohol- acquired brain injury condition. However it was only a wee part of her story which shows the importance of school support in early life.

Hello my name is Shannon. I am the youngest of a big family. growing up was quite a struggle for me, although I had many brothers and sisters, could turn to them as we were all separated, our parents were too sick, could'nt cope with us all.

I had started out in many different foster placements, I cannot remember much about back then though I would only have been a baby.

I came to live with Margaret and Charlie when I was about 10 months old again I cannot remember much of then.

I do remember all the happy memories, one of my first memorys is when i get my first pet I got a dog,a little chihuahua, and we named him Tyson. I can remember starting school, but Margaret was not well and was going through surgery, so me and Tyson made her a get well soon video for her to watch when she came home of me getting ready for my first day of school so she never missed anything.

School started out great, I loved it. I love painting and drawing. It was a way for me to make more friends, not that we were ever short on kids with Margaret and Charlie fostering. I used to make a lot of new friends, but would be sad when they all had to leave or move on to other places, you create a lot of strong bonds when you have things in common or can relate to other people going through struggles too.

School started to get a lot harder for me around the end of primary school. Teachers would blame me for being an attention seeker, and being a class clown, when in reality I was just trying to get some extra help.as I could not keep up with anything.

I would suffer from anxiety attacks, and through them, I would end up with a sick stomach and would endure a migraine headache that felt like someone had a hammer to my head.

If I had got my medicine just in timer all of this could have been prevented, but my teachers looked at me as a nuisance and instead of helping me try to get my medicine from my parents they just let me play until it was too late, in most cases I couldn't even get off the bathroom floor I was that ill and weak.

Secondary school started out okay I thought to myself now that I am a bit older the teachers would take me a little more seriously, this was not the case for us all. I started to get badly bullied, kids could tell I was different. The anxiety started even worse, I was prescribed medication for it, but it just tended to make me drowsy and didn't mix well with me having to do school work and keep up everything. I found it hard to manage with everything.

My attendance slipped a lot, Margaret and Charlie would constantly be getting warning off the school that my attendance would need to pick up. It created a lot of friction and tension at home too, but mum knew I was trying my hardest. As time went on things got more difficult for me, I tried keeping up with everything at school, there was talk about statementing* me and getting me and assistant but I did'nt want that; it was just another way for the kids to see me as being different, and I never wanted that.

I wanted to be treated like I was just one of them, but I knew under the surface I was not.

When I was about 15 or 16 I was getting ready for school one morning, and I just said to my parents," I don't want to go top that school" and it started a huge fight that ended up with me moving out of on my own to Derry. I always tried to keep in contact with Margaret and Charlie and tried to come up and down some weekends to see them.

I am going to be 22 now next month and boy does the time fly. My whole life has been a rollercoaster with a lot of ups and downs but the two people who have stuck by me are still there, but I am now in a happy relationship. will hopefully be starting college now to study to work with kids with special needs, because I don't want other kids to experience things like I have. I want to try to help and make a difference.

*Statementing' is the Educational process in the UK of applying for extra educational support for the pupil.

Other Patient/Family Stories

I was hoping to include 2 other clinical stories of Adopted children from Russia living in Ireland with NDPAE. Unfortunately, the 'stigma' of the condition inhibited the adoptive parents and the adolescent and/or young adult with NDPAE from telling their stories.

Chapter 13

EPILOGUE

THE KNOTTED CORD. (2014 BOOK)

This book encapsulates 25 years of professional psychiatric practice dealing with children, adolescents and young adults, and their families who had experienced the trials and tribulations of a 'not it' disorder, namely Alcohol Related Neurodevelopmental Disorder.

Probably it could only have been written in Ireland the small island of little room where there is a potent Celtic cocktail of alcohol romance, stigma and ethical dilemmas which seem to immobilize medical professionals and politicians alike.

Its spiritual guiding light comes from the Native American literary scholar and humanitarian Michael Dorris who died suddenly in April 1997, but who first offered the umbilical cord as the metaphor for transgenerational alcohol and its long lasting effects.

It was probably no accident, in the collective unconsciousness of transgenerational alcohol that his mother Mary Bessy was of Irish stock. Just as alcohol pervaded the lives of his three adopted Native American children, so it pervaded his own life and sadly also his death.

This is a suitable time to acknowledge and remember him.

A Song for Michael Dorris

Let not his voice
Be the sound of a guitar
With a broken string;
No, let his voice
Soar on eagles' wings

And drift as a yellow raft
In blue water…

Kieran D. O'Malley, April 14th 1997(published in *Watch for the Rainbows*, 2001)

This is a personal professional perspective grounded in a specific geographic area, but I know its thrust the avoidance of transgenerational alcohol issues has universality from the aboriginal communities in Australia and the Western Cape of South Africa, to the Upper East Side of Manhattan and the leafy suburbs of Calgary. It is written in the vain hope that Governments, Public Health doctors, Obstetricians, Psychiatrists and Medical Alcohol Specialists will wake up and smell the coffee (alcohol actually!) and see what is before their eyes in plain view.

Finally, the clinical journey has always been rewarded by the simple privilege of being allowed to enter people's unique life stories and dreams where you need to tread softly. The stories are not all doom and gloom; in fact, many are inspiring in so many ways. The first book that I wrote with Frances Kapp in 2001, 'Watch for the Rainbows' deliberately captured the joy, humour, spontaneity, fearlessness, creativeness, multiple musical, artistic and manipulative wood and metal sculpting talents within these special groups of children and adolescents.

Nothing has really changed since I moved back across the pond. Only now they are more rambunctious, but they still remain 'in the moment'!

I will end my Epilogue by giving voices to those voiceless amidst the world's cacophony;

"I wish that I could go back in time and tell my mother and father not to drink if they want a baby"
(A 10 year old girl),

"I wish that I could have my mother back again"
(A 12 year old boy whose mother died two years previously of alcohol related liver problems at the age of 35 years).

"I wish that I could think better at school"
(A 9-year-old boy who was failing academically when in a mainstream class with 30 pupils.)

"I wish that M 'would be called my mother in the future"
(A 8-year-old Russian adoptive boy speaking of his adoptive Irish mother)

"I wish that I could speak my feelings better"
(A 8 year old girl suspended from school because of unexplained defiant behavior).

"I was never told my drinking in my pregnancy would harm my baby"

(A birth mother, more than one, who has had a child removed with suspected ARND, reporting what her alcohol counselor had not said when she was pregnant).

"I wish that I had been told the history of my son's exposure to alcohol in pregnancy as I would have got help much sooner"

(An adoptive father of a 16-year-old Russian boy).

My 25-year experience with this clinical population has taught me many things about medicine, and life, and resilience.

I suppose in the final analysis I do not subscribe to a Beckettian, or in some ways a Michael Dorris, nihilistic world view, but to more of a humanistic pragmatism mingled with a tincture of time.

I was involved with Randy Mc Donald and his mother Nanci for well over 10 years at a time when he was an impulsive, anxious teenager with pervasive disruptive mood dysregulation and posed multiple challenges in therapy.

He is now 31 years old, married and a father. This is what he wrote to me on January 6th 2014.

"What has helped me most in life with my disability is learning who I am and how I think and what works. Every person is unique in their own special way and no book or training will teach you how to deal with every person. I have spent my life making my weaknesses my strengths and using my creativity to overcome any difficulty which has arisen in my life.

If any advice I could give another person with ARND is to learn to believe in yourself, never give up on yourself and always push your limitations as with time you will overcome different problems as you get to know yourself. You are not alone in the feeling of frustration of not being able to think clear or not understanding your thoughts, doing things which are impulsive which are potentially destructive in your life and the pain which with this, but understand with help of others and structure and understanding yourself it will get better."

THE KNOTTED CORD. AN UPDATE, 2020

I have a wish that medical, nursing professionals, psychologists, social worker's addiction counsellors and/or probation officers who reach this point in the book will appreciate the complexity of this transgenerational alcohol "orphan" condition, which has become a modern-day Gordian Knot.

Thirty years of working Internationally with individuals with NDPAE and their families has taught me that there are *4 Nodal points of Intervention.*

The 1st Nodal Point Is the Parent/Infant Dyad

This involves a parallel process of adult and pediatric health professionals addressing the pregnant alcohol/substance abusing mother's possible medical, psychiatric, addictive and or developmental problems.

Therefore, it is at this clinical juncture where the obstetrician, midwife, and perinatal psychiatrist roles are crucial. Thus, supporting a simultaneous process of treating both the pregnant mother and her infant-in-utero is paramount in the world of transgenerational alcohol dependence.

In parallel the usage of neuroprotective agents during the alcohol/substance exposed pregnancy can address the fetal/infant medical needs. The obstetrician, neonatologist and developmental pediatrician all have crucial roles. The separate development of the interpersonal world of the infant has been studied and mapped by clinical researchers such as Daniel Stern and Elfrain Bleiberg (Stern, 1983, Bleiberg, 2001,) and the confluence of environmental adversity and biological vulnerability are critical mediating factors to self-expression and self- realization.

i. The "at risk" alcohol abusing pregnant mother is identified, but as well her delivery of a child with NDPAE is a potential marker for her premature death due to alcohol–related medical causes. The trauma of losing a birth child is ever present.
ii. The "at risk" infant is identified as having the potential global neurodevelopmental disorder NDPAE. The trauma of being separated/abandoned by the birth mother is ever present.
iii. The challenge of engaging in the parent/infant or young child dyad is the ultimate challenge of NDPAE in which the vulnerable parent is attempting to manage the vulnerable child, and they weave a disorganized attachment dance which is both warm and secure but chaotic!

The 2nd Nodal Point Is the Entry of an Infant/Child or Adolescent into State Care

The prevalence of medical, psychiatric and developmental problems in this population has already been well documented. The research and clinical experience has shown that attachment therapy alone is not enough to ameliorate all these co-morbid problems.

So, the placement of a child in state care should trigger a 'soon as possible' holistic developmental pediatric child psychology/child psychiatry assessment.

Misdiagnosis and non-diagnosis of children with NDPAE are rife in the state care population (Chasnoff et al., 2015).

Standard behavioral management/operant conditioning techniques are not a good fit for these children with the global neurodevelopmental disorder of NDPAE. (you only have to appreciate the pervasive deficits in working memory and processing to witness the clinical mismatch). Foster parents need strategies for the management of children with neurodevelopmental disorders and not only behavioral disorders. (see Appendix the Knotted Cord 2014).

Finally, systems of care evaluations such as the child adolescent service intensity instrument, CASII, or the early childhood service intensity instrument ECSII, are both very useful way of assessing the current service need and probable, deficits between the child or adolescent's clinical needs and the State Care service which is being provided. (The CASII is portable and has been tested in Ireland) (AACAP 2019).

A Parallel Process Should Be Utilized for the Birth Mothers of the Children Who Are Taken into State Care

This involves a perinatal psychiatrist or adult psychiatrist with particular expertise in addictive disorder. As well, a hidden disability in the birth parents in the world of transgenerational diagnosed NDPAE itself) see Henshaw et al., 2019.

The hidden psychiatric disorders associated with NDPAE (or FASD) are seen in all ethnic populations .re4cent work in Russian adoptive children with FASD (NDPAE) showed ADHD most prominent diagnosis with 50% showing emotional Control problems, using the KIDDIE –SADS Assesment (Barras et al. 2016). The confluence of Reactive Attachment Disorder, PTSD and FASD or NDPAE are key components in assessing this unique adoptive population (O'Malley 2012).

Also hidden are growth trajectory problems have been demonstrated in treatment of ADHD symptoms with methylphenidate, but lisedexamphetamine as well.

Adolescents with NDPAE commonly enter into State Care, mostly Residential due to a break-down of placement in foster home or adoptive Home. Sadly, the lack of recognition of their longstanding neurodevelopmental disorder, and sometimes pervasive scapegoating at home, or even bullying in school, may precipitate this state care intervention. Many countries espoused a health and social care department, but the truth is that country/state care remains the" poor cousin" when it comes to adequately researched, funded and planned service (Holfon et al., 2013, O'Higgins et al., 2015).

Suicidal risk is a particular issue for adolescents removed from longstanding homes, and is still not fully recognized in this brain- injured, impulsive population who have severe deficits in problem solving, and emotional control. The epigenetically kindled risk of alcohol craving and dependency complicate this developmental period of life in the adolescent with NDPAE.

The 3rd Nodal Point of Intervention Is on the Expulsion or Suspension of a Child or Adolescent from School

This should be an opportunity for another holistic pediatric/child or adolescent psychiatric assessment. This provides a chance to unearth a n individual with an unknown global neurodevelopmental disorder such as NDPAE.

Learning disability services in many places are 'frozen' in an under 70 IQ paradigm, and the presence of a non- IQ driven global neurodevelopmental disorder such as NDPAE challenges this old formula of educational services. The co-morbid psychiatric disorders which are so prevalent with NDPAE need informed service provision from developmental pediatricians and child/adolescent psychiatrists sometimes need added learning disability knowledge.

Adolescents out of school because of acute destructive or self -destructive behaviors should have an urgent clinical risk asseesmemnt.as impulsive suicide risk is a specific problem in individuals with often undiagnosed NDPAE (Huggins et al. 2008).

Children with Conduct disorder can be assessed for possible neurodevelopmental origins to the condition (Bolhuis 2019).

The impact of brain biology on emerging Conduct Disorder and Antisocial Personality Disorders has been long established (Siever et al., 1991, Raine et al., 2000, Blair 2003).

This fundamental research, coupled with increasing new scientific studies, form a template for understanding the roots of such behaviors in individuals with NDPAE (Bolthius 2019).

It also continues to challenge the pervasive nihilistic attitude to management of this type of personality disorder. (0'Malley PP 1999).

4th Nodal Point. Family Functioning and Stress in NDPAE

I could not end this update by neglecting to acknowledge the multi- faceted impact of parenting a child or adolescent with FASD, or NDPAE has on their family.

This is an intervention point that changes with the age and placement of the child. Sometimes it is the stress of parenting a child or adolescent with NDPAE which leads to Social Service Care placement due to lack of basic Disability or Psychiatric services and lack of effective therapy available.

The source of pervasive Compassion Fatigue can be analyzed into four broad categories.

i. The physical health needs of their child or adolescent
ii. The mental health or psychiatric disorders present in the child or adolescent.
iii. The financial burden of care- giving on the family

iv. The emotional stress of care -giving on the family.

(Gelo & O'Malley 2003)

The Compassion Fatigue, or self-compassion in the parents contributes to complicated family dynamics such as Scapegoating of the patient with NDPAE, or a pervasive Double Bind communication which can immobilize families. Biddle and colleagues studied biological parents and non- biological parents, and cited shame and guilt as issues for biological parents, and blame and pride with non- biological parents. However, the authors did not factor in the complexity of diagnosis, accessibility to treatment, success of treatment or financial cost of treatment which are all key factors in FASD or NDPAE. (Biddle et al. 2020)

Clinical Examples:

i. A family of 4 with 2 adopted adolescents with NDPAE functioned a 4 families of 1, due to the pervasive Double Bind Communications which severely affected family functioning.
   This can be an issue in Birth families and their extended families, due to the split in recognizing the effect of alcohol and its potential collateral damage to succeeding generations. On the one hand alcohol in women as seen as liberating and empowering with no serious consequences, but on the other hand Sobriety is also celebrated as emancipating.
   (Catastrophe TV show 2015-, Working Moms TV show 2017-, McKowen 2020)
   Family Therapy intervention was critical with a family education and/or Reflecting Team useful modalities.
ii. I have seen 30 to 40 families in which the child with NDPAE has been Scapegoated and Blamed for negative family interactions.
   Age, Gender and Ethnic Group were not seen as important determining variables, but the phenomenon appeared much more commonly if the child with NDPAE was placed in an adoptive or foster family with pre-exiting natural children
   Family Therapy was the useful approach in all these cases.

In truth, no-one in the family system is to blame for these destructive family functioning dynamics. This is because the continued lack of recognition of FASD or NDPAE in the general medical community creates its own Double Bind for the carers, often invalidating their calls for help and understanding. In many ways these destructive family dynamics just mirror the equally destructive dynamics of the Larger Medical

System, which continue to be subtly influenced by the denial and minimization disinformation created by the alcohol industry machine. (Bateson et al. 1963, Figley 1995).

Conclusion

Dr. Li Wenliang, the Chinese ophthalmologist who exposed the extent of the coronavirus epidemic and died prematurely at 34 years, famously said:

> "A healthy society should not only have one kind of voice."

In the world of transgenerational alcohol, where the message is carefully crafted by alcohol industry "groupspeak," his statement is quietly prescient.

Appendix

PRACTICAL STRATEGIES FOR MANAGING CHILDREN/ADOLESCENTS WITH NEURODEVELOPMENTAL DISORDERS INCLUDING FAS OR ARND (NOW NDPAE)

Kieran D. O'Malley and Michele Savage

INTRODUCTION

This document has been over 6 years in gestation since the first author's (KOM) return to Ireland from the USA in 2006, and the continuation of his psychiatric consultation work with children exposed to alcohol in pregnancy. Although Ireland has one of the highest rates of per capita drinking in the EU (12 liters), and over 50% of Irish drinkers have a binge drinking pattern, as well as one of the highest under 14 yrs. drinking (18.9%) in the world (Byrne 2013), the prevalence of children and adolescents with Fetal Alcohol Spectrum Disorders (FASD) still remains an unknown figure in this country (O'Malley 2011). This is also a known problem in a number of children adopted into Ireland from Russia or Romania with no quantification of their exposure to prenatal alcohol being available. Recent HSE estimates of the overall cost of problem alcohol usage in Ireland give a figure of €3.7 billion. There is no mention of the financial cost of Fetal Alcohol Spectrum Disorders in this 2013 HSE Study Notwithstanding the reluctance to acknowledge the effect of prenatal alcohol exposure on the developing fetus, the truth remains that the island, North and South, has a significant number of undiagnosed children, adolescents and probably young adults with dysmorphic Fetal Alcohol Syndrome or non-dysmorphic Alcohol Related Neurodevelopmental Disorder, the latter being likely to be the more prevalent condition. Foster parents and Social workers on the island of Ireland are progressively being sensitized to, and educated in, the chronic complex management problems of FASD (Orakwue et al., 2012).

The strategies mapped out in this document were initially pilot tested with 12 patients (South and North Ireland) and their families (5 with FAS, 7 with ARND), diagnosed by the first author (KOM). The ages of the patients ranged from 3 ½ years to 17 years. One patient had had prenatal heroin exposure as well as prenatal alcohol exposure.

The strategies were well received, and deemed helpful, and suggestions include adding 'Neurodevelopmental Disorders' at the beginning to decrease stigma to birth mothers, as well as placing the 'General Principles' at the start of the document not after the Transition and Environment sections. No child or adolescent complained about the strategies.

Co-author Michele Savage, a foster parent with experience of children with ARND and co-founder of FASD Ireland was instrumental in making the strategies immediately useful and practical. The strategies have been informed by a wealth of information from the USA and Canada, where FAS and ARND are recognized diagnoses and where there are many FASD diagnostic clinics. (Stratton et al., 1996, Streissguth 1997, Tanner Halverson 1997, Kulp 2004, O'Malley 2008, Densmore 2011, Malbin 2012, ADD WareHouse 2011).

The basic premise of management of children or adolescents with FAS or ARND continues to be a 'Systems of Care' approach in which the patient/client is seen within the context of his/her caring environment first, but remembering that it is the specific neurodevelopmental disorder related to the alcohol exposure and NOT the face that is the kernel to understanding diagnosis and management.

These strategies are therefore part of a 'multimodal' treatment model whereby the child or adolescent is also receiving Cognitive testing WPPSSI or WISC IV to assess basic cognitive functioning (including dyslexia or dyscalculia), OT (for Developmental Co-ordination Disorder/Dyspraxia or Sensory integration issues,), speech and language Therapy (for expressive and receptive language problems of a Social Communication Disorder variety, often misunderstood as Autism) and frequently medication. Medication is particularly useful but as well problematic in this population of patients as 'acquired organic brain injury' due to prenatal alcohol exposure is at the core of the complex developmental psychiatric presentation. (O'Malley 2010). Patients with FAS or ARND present clinical phenotypes such as Regulatory Disorders (under 3 yrs), ADHD, ASD/Asperger's Disorder, Mood Instability or Intermittent Explosive Disorder which can, and do, respond to careful choice of medication (Streissguth 1997, Kulp 2004, O'Malley 2008, 2011, Densmore 2012).

Usually forgotten is the legacy of physical abnormalities due to prenatal alcohol exposure called Alcohol Related Birth Defects (ARBD) with structural effects on the developing heart, kidney, eye, ear, and skeletal systems. It is here that a basic pediatric assessment is essential as a starting point in medical/holistic management (Stratton et al., 1996).

Finally children or adolescents with FAS or ARND can never be treated in isolation or lack of recognition of their primary rearing environment. Thus co-occurring clinical problems such as early onset Post Traumatic Stress Disorder (PTSD) due to direct or indirect exposure to violence, or Reactive or Disorganized Attachment Disorder due to problems in attachment with multiple care givers (as in sharing parenting arrangements between foster and birth families) must always be considered as contributing to the clinical presentation.

It is the authors' hope that this document can become standard of initial care for every newly diagnosed patient, whether child or adolescent, with FAS or ARND in Ireland. The instrument is meant for parents/caregivers, but also for social workers and teachers to help them in management of these complex patients it is also envisioned that formal testing, both of Parenting Stress and of Child/Adolescent Adaptive Functioning (Preferably using the Vineland II) will be performed after the implementation of the Strategies document in their care.

The instrument is aimed for clinical usage from preschool/nursery age children to late adolescence. The first 2 pages of the instrument are presented, but the full instrument is available from either of the co-authors.

UPDATE 2020

This clinical instrument has been given to all parents of newly diagnosed patients with NDPAE whom I have seen over the last 5 years, and also has been given to their schools. It has proven helpful and supportive in offering a script of management different from standard behavioral management which generally does not work well with NDPAE.

The Guiding Principles, Environment, Transitional Periods, Pervasive Developmental or Autistic features and Sexually Inappropriate Behavior have proven the most useful parts of the instrument.

GENERAL GUIDING PRINCIPLES

1) Begin by emphasizing a strengths-based approach to learning rather than identifying and addressing the child's learning weaknesses, thus developing a success rather than failure orientation approach to the learning environment;
2) Identify and emphasize what is theirs to them: "This is your chair, desk, pencil";
3) When child feels angry acknowledge the anger and then go on;
4) Reduce any peer competition in classroom or home environment as much as possible;

5) Help the child/young person to see the value of doing a task/game, whether successful or not;
6) 'Catch them' being good, doing things right, and praise them (but remember that the child may not be able to successfully repeat the deed or behavior or apply it in another setting/activity/domain);
7) Stop at key points in teaching lesson to determine student's understanding;
8) Telling stories i.e., children with FASDs often 'confabulate' or fill in the blanks of stories because of their memory problems. It is better to gently clarify and confront the untruths/inconsistencies in the story and re-direct the child to a more coherent story;
9) From age 12-13, school educational programming should also focus on daily self-care, communication, and day-to-day functioning/survival skills;
10) Preschool curriculum should emphasize readiness skills such as increasing attention span, compliance with requests, sitting in a seat, listening;
11) Work with behavior momentum (teenagers) i.e., encourage and acknowledge continuation of positive success in the school situation;
12) Careful use of sensory stimulation, as some children may be hyper –responsive to auditory, visual or other stimuli and so can become overwhelmed;
13) Teach drugs/alcohol refusal skills (teenagers). This is very important as prenatal alcohol exposure has been shown to increase the biochemical and structural vulnerability of the developing pre-teen and teenage brain to alcohol dependence;
14) Teach generalization of skills (teenagers) i.e., money management or even simple social skills management can be taught at school and to be introduced in the home/community environment later;
15) Living and working with neurologically impaired children can be very stressful. It is important to have a respite plan in place to regularly follow for your own physical/mental health as parents, whether birth, adoptive or foster;
16) *Brevity in the delivery of instructions, coupled with persistence in delivering these instructions, is a key element in dealing with these children at all ages.

1. Environment

The environment should be structured and predictable.

1.1. Well defined areas;

1.2. Preferential seating explores the possibility of using individual pods for individual tasks work requiring very focused concentration;

1.3. Get child involved i.e., teacher to engage the child in active learning;

1.4. Remove extraneous and distracting material pinned on walls, dangling from ceilings, etc.);

1.5. Opaque glass in windows (or line with opaque uncolored adhesive contact paper) at child-height level;

1.6. Tell child to put head down on their folded arms on the desk, (lama transit), when over stimulated;

1.7. Have separate daily timetable for each day in flip-chart mode, or daily programmer;

1.8. Use same staff consistently;

1.9. Do not change teacher's teaching position often;

1.10. Whiteboard screen may cause sensory overload for some students;

1.11. Separate student by having frame around desk to decrease distractibility.

2. Transitional Periods

2.1 Visual time cues – Pictorial class schedule with moving indicator showing where class is in the daily routine schedule;

2.2. Verbal early warning system – "we are going to change to … in 10 mins., 5 mins., 2 mins.;

2.3. Song or music/rhythm tone cues for academic talks;

2.4. Egg timer (can use different colors for different times) clearly defines end of lesson or activity;

2.5. Puppet Play (where age appropriate);

2.6. Assess for frustration tolerance, i.e., see what irritates the child;

2.7. Adapt tasks/materials accordingly for frustration tolerance, i.e., decrease time at task, or adjust number of sums (task-load) for individuals.

3. Helping with Organizational Skills

No structure =No function.

3.1. Parents/carers to help children get clothes and bag ready for school the night before;

3.1.1. Sort major tasks/assignments from less significant ones (remembering that developmental capacity is not necessarily in line with chronological age).

3.2. Give assignments with consistent follow up i.e., pupil receives regular feed-back;

3.3. Morning review of the daily programme;

3.4. Calendars, notebooks/assignment books which are all used as tools of organization;

3.5. Color code lesson segments;

3.6. Plain cover (pastel color not strong or neon) – a different one for each subject, i.e., yellow = maths;

3.7. Work sheets go on a giant paper clip or in an A4 plastic envelope;

3.8. Give direct instruction in thinking skills i.e., use single words for verbal cues;

3.9. Teach organizational skills i.e., use of notebook or assignment book;

3.10. Teach analyzing and synthesizing skills i.e., planning skills and how to use color code for planning and identifying a task;

3.11. Provide a schedule for activities;

3.12. Anchor points to define times i.e., visual cue or sound/voice cue;

3.13. Provide visual lists for work assignments;

3.14. Sequence after special activity i.e., clear transition plan after each task/assignment;

3.15. Short tasks with clear terminal objectives - Explicit, concrete, brief, carefully defined directions, broken down into segments/steps if necessary;

3.16. Give adequate time to organize material and between activities, extra time to complete tasks, but ensure that child has adequate time to eat lunch and avail of movement break in yard at break-time, i.e., need to build in some flexibility in task or assignment work in order to relieve frustration/anxiety building up.

4. Helping with Attention Problems

4.1. Use ear phones or ear plugs (to screen out background noises);

4.2. Use red or pink highlighters not yellow or neon;

4.3. Use a study carrel/organizer;

4.4. Use visual cues to start and stop – Green to start, Red to indicate the end of task;

4.5. Use eye contact, say child's name, or gently touch shoulder to alert the distracted pupil (be aware of possible hypersensitivity to sensory stimuli);

4.6. Outline to increase comprehension i.e., Picture outlines instead of written ones, series of comic/cartoon boxes;

4.7. Reduce, and then speed up speech tempo;

4.8. Vary loudness, inflection/quality of voice;

4.9. "Focus" words – key words used over and over to "grab" attention;

4.10. Novelty is an excellent attention getter i.e., singing the alphabet, sums tables, etc.;

4.11. Present new topic to increase curiosity;

4.12. Control classroom interruptions i.e., do not let classroom disruptions go on for too long, e.g., greater than 5 minutes;

4.13. Give brief, simple anticipatory explanations of inattention in classroom or home, i.e., getting distracted when eating breakfast before school;

4.14. Describe/compare objects, events, details to help child's understanding of situation.

4.15. Ask child to repeat your directions – to ensure awareness and/or comprehension and not just the rote verbal memory of words;

4.16. Slowly and gradually increase sustained attention i.e., table top exercise, jigsaws, short stories (with pictures);

4.17. Random participation i.e., use a flexible work task schedule to help if pupil bored with current task, so switch to a different, maybe more' hands on' task;

4.18. Omit key words from rhymes;

4.19. Focus attention with uncomplicated unfussy pictures/objects;

4.20. Child completes several items, then check to ensure they understand task i.e., give one item, and then check if completed and give a second item. Some children can do 2 stage commands.

5. Helping to Control Impulsivity

5.1. Child can have fidgets at hand to self-calm, i.e., chewing pen or hand held 'squeezy' or even small ball;

5.2. Complete directions before handing out materials;

5.3. Tell child to slow down in answering questions;

5.4. Broken record interruptions – Use same words every time;

5.5. Turn taking - Use tangible object for example a Talking Stick/Puppet;

5.6. Require that they explain their answers i.e., ask the pupil to break down into simple words the task/assignment they are being asked to do;

5.7. Ask answer-hogs/keeners to help – Get them or the 'enthusiastic/keen students' to help classmates by waiting until 3 other people can answer the question for a specific lesson (give them time to show their knowledge too). This will take the pressure off the student who processes answers slower;

5.8. Teach the skill of five deep breaths and/or counting to five or ten to reflect upon a situation before acting.

5.9. Teach the language to reflect upon a situation before acting i.e., help the pupil register the situation in real time, a form of 'mindfulness'.

5.10. Teach a rhyme or set of words for repeating silently to help child not flare up on provocation;

5.11. Familiarize students with 'mindfulness' as a self-awareness strategy (for older pupils), i.e., stop the impulsive student in the here and now and have them think and reflect on their negative action, (an egg-timer could be used).

6. Decreasing the Hyperactivity

6.1. If medication is needed, better to start the day with medication, and then chase the behavior later;

6.2. Limit type/number of situations encountered at one time;

6.3. Anticipate - know danger signs/situations. Build mindfulness and relaxation into programme;

6.4. Teach substitute behaviors when child can't keep hands off others starting with recognizing boundaries i.e., help the child recognize that he/she is too close or too loud for other children;

6.5. Protect from over stimulation. Control TV and avoid computer games, especially in the evening (Avoid having Nintendo/Playstation, X Box in the school);

6.6. Have a respite plan in place for when child is overwhelmed;

6.7. Teach appropriate ways to respond to overwhelming stimuli i.e., recognize and identify disturbing/over arousing stimuli, or alternatively have child go to a quiet place or use a soothing toy to calm himself/herself;

6.8. Reduce/control complexity of assigned tasks;

6.9. Teach yourself to monitor each child, when they are over-stimulated or under-stimulated;

6.10. Ask child what she/he thinks works in calming them;

6.11. Child to self-monitor i.e., practice mindfulness;

6.12. Involve child in drawing up a plan for avoiding escalating or for de-escalating (i.e., proactive and reactive. They know what helps soothe them. This is especially good for older children;

6.13. Help child get back under control if necessary;

6.14. Provide lessons which emphasize manual/physical expression;

6.15. Avoid long periods of desk work, i.e., give physical movement breaks;

6.16. Sensory cushion for the child with sensory hyper responsiveness may sometimes be useful for whole class;

6.17. Don't keep child in from recess. Short breaks during the day;

6.18. Aggression as physiology i.e., child may have organic brain dysfunction, including seizure disorder which makes aggression part of his/her make-up. This is very important to consider in children with FASD.

7. Recognizing Pervasive Developmental or Autistic Features

7.1. Boundaries issues outward and inward i.e., be sensitive to proprioceptive issues in the child such as need to ground themselves in a physical space, so need to touch feel space that they are working in i.e., desk, immediate surroundings, even classroom boundaries;

7.2. Social and pragmatic use of language issues may be lower because of inattention and distractibility, i.e., child may misunderstand verbal and non-verbal directions from the teacher showing a basic lack of social awareness and social understanding of even simple situations;

7.3. Child will often misunderstand changes in tone of voice and especially more subtle censoring such as sarcasm;

7.4. Medication may have a role in helping social responsiveness by increasing visual and auditory attention to social cues, and so make the child more connected;

7.5. Medication may as well worsen a child's performance and behavior by increasing focus so much that the child becomes 'hyper-focused' on small details, say specific numbers or colors, and so perseverates about them.

7.6. Medication may bring a change in the nature of a child and create a disconnected schizoid personality change.

7.7. A calming toy such as a squeezable ball/tennis ball is useful to decrease acute anxiety especially in social interactions (have the child or teenager keep it with them)

7.8. Calming odors such as geranium, coral sage or lavender, depending on personal preference, can be used in small vials kept in mother's purse. Useful for addressing acute anxiety in social situations such as shopping Centre/airport.

8. Helping to Establish Routine and Discipline

8.1. Be firm, but supportive

8.2. Redirect negative behavior i.e., distract the child with visual or auditory cues

8.3. Ignore negative behavior when possible, so the child does not receive positive re-enforcement for negative attention

8.4. Specifically labelling any unacceptable behavior as it occurs will draw attention and endorse that behavior;

8.5. Teach other words to use rather than swearing;

8.6. Reward the children who remember the appropriate skills;

8.7. Make "My Choice" cards (reward individualized choices);

8.8. Take a reinforcement survey, i.e., see which positive affirmations work;

8.9. Use a classroom "quiet chair," but not outside classroom as child often does not remember why outside the classroom because of working memory problems;

8.10. This is not the "great debate" – Don't argue/renegotiate consequences when dealing with;

8.11. Reduce lag time between tasks, but be flexible due to child's probable anxiety or frustration;

8.12. Guide to solutions i.e., Leave problems solved as much as possible;

8.13. Behavior management i.e., specific strategies to cope with specific identified behaviors;

8.14. Past behavior is a valuable guide i.e., (unless new/chronic stressors are a factor);

8.15. Negative behavior may be a symptom of unidentified and/or unmet needs (or unidentified and/or undeclared problems at home in yard). However it is essential to remember that FASD are organic brain dysfunction conditions;

8.16. Consultations with families to help at home and with school liaison work in behavior management and through Individualized Educational Plans (IEP);

8.17. Collaboration with families on joint management strategies, using consulting psychiatric/psychological specialists as appropriate.

9. Increasing Self Esteem

9.1. Recognize successes every day;

9.2. Positive incentives for finishing tasks or assignments;

9.3. Encouragement is as good as praise;

9.4. Recognize partially correct responses;

9.5. Encourage use of positive self-talk – "I can do this";

9.6. Give attention to children who are behaving appropriately;

9.7. If a child is discouraged over repeated mistakes, stress they are just getting another chance;

9.8. Have child write about something they know;

9.9. Have peers model behavior i.e., use peer modelling in teaching certain skills especially social skills;

9.10. Model alternative behaviors (teacher);

9.11. Model, rehearse social skills (teacher/pupils), in dyads or small groups;

9.12. Have child tell the class about something they know i.e., a special interest such as identifying different makes of cars;

9.13. Test knowledge not attention span;

9.14. Avoid asking WHY? questions. Use how, who, what, where, as 'Why?' often provokes defensive responses in these children because of their basic cognitive disconnection in processing of information.

10. Recognizing Sexually Inappropriate Behaviors

10.1. This is the area of behavioral problems which is most avoided;

10.2. It is essential to have the child, where age- or developmentally- appropriate, write down details of the SIB episode/s, guided by an adult (parent);

10.3. It is important to have a medical doctor, child psychiatrist or psychologist verify the episode/s as soon as possible;

10.4. It is important that the local social service child protection services are notified as soon as possible;

10.5. The professional working with the child should make sure that the relevant organizations are informed i.e., nursery, day care, playschool or school;

10.6. Therapy should use a cognitive reality approach with clear list of inappropriate behaviors and situations and a clear list of steps to avoid a repeat of these situations, i.e., no contact with young children without adult present;

10.7. Education of social boundaries, i.e., clears definition on people whom you are allowed to touch/hug (parents), and strangers who you must keep 'at a distance';

10.8. Sometimes a verbal or written apology, especially if child of a relative or close neighbor is involved in the episode. (Always have parent present with child if apology given to reduce risk of misunderstanding);

10.9. The victim/perpetrator model does not really fit for patients with FASDs as they are often in advertent victims and inadvertent perpetrators, i.e., they may behave or dress in such a way as to attract unwanted attention, but are unaware of this, or they may impulsively become involved in inappropriate behaviors with younger peers without any malicious intent.

11. Helping with Memory Problems

11. Acknowledging that brain damage from prenatal alcohol exposure impairs working memory, the processing of information, the ability to navigate social situations and his formulation of planning decisions (executive functioning):

11.1. Repeat and restructure continually;

11.2. Chunk work into manageable pieces;

11.3. Use short sentences (e.g., 'Books into bags', 'pencils onto desks';

11.4. Teach one concept at a time (pace);

11.5. Ask child to repeat information just heard;

11.6. Have child physically perform sequential activities;

11.7. Teach memory strategies focused on basic living skills;

11.8. Show pictures/objects for 30-60 seconds and then ask questions about them;

11.9. Ask child for repetition of instructions of material in a form other than the one you just used;

11.10. Make a one-page visualization of the lesson;

11.11. Make subject matter meaningful to the child;

11.12. Have older children take notes on verbal directions;

11.13. Play memory games (picture or number cards upside down on desks, half-pack, build up);

11.14. Groups of 4 or so, small group learning modules for older children i.e., 'I went to the shops and bought some ------, next child says I went to the shops and bought some ----- and some #####' and so on, incrementally.

12. Helping with Reading Problems

12.1. Underline key words;

12.2. Use large print/talking books;

12.3. Play letter/word bingo;

12.4. Rewrite directions at a lower reading level;

12.5. Figure ground confusion – Avoid "busy" pages i.e., (cover pictures with a page if necessary);

12.6. Use cognitive mapping, i.e., sequence the steps of the learning task or assignment;

12.7. Make a Pictionary dictionary;

12.8. Use materials with simple illustrations;

12.9. Put paper strip under line;

12.10. Have child verbally repeat or paraphrase the material he or she has read;

12.11. Tape record stories so child can listen and read along;

12.12. Use a color dot at left hand and another at right. Use arrows showing direction;

12.13. Stress related or inferential reading. Prepare by a series of questions to think about while they read;

12.14. Avoid phonics to teach reading, unless processing skills are adequate.

13. Helping with Mathematics Problems

This is another key to understanding many of the deficits in the learning disability in FASDs, as they pervade deductive reasoning, logic, and ultimately executive functioning and decision making

13.1. Work on number concepts not just rote counting;

13.2. Use a calculator, number line, abacus;

13.3. Spend extra time on decimal points in maths, spelling etc. because of inattention to detail;

13.4. Put math problems with same process on single line or sheet;

13.5. Make operation symbols extra-large, bolded or color coded (make a list of and group number operations as expressed in 'story' sums;

13.6. Domino worksheets;

13.7. Give child multiples of one digit problems when they complain about "baby stuff";

13.8 Provide practice of math facts with a computer that gives immediate feedback (in the school or at home) to the child;

13.9. Spend extra time on money concepts and making change;

13.10. Find opportunities for child to apply math to real life i.e., give example of going to the shop with a fixed amount of money and buying certain food items, and bringing back correct change;

13.11. Use abacus to count numbers, add, subtract (for a more robust kinesthetic memory).

14. Educational and Service Needs of Professional Staff Involved in Care of Children/Adolescents with Neurodevelopmental Disorders Especially FAS or ARND

14.1. Staff should have basic training in general child/adolescent psychiatry disorders, learning disorders, and developmental disorders;

14.2. Awareness of the child's Functional Ability not just being related to IQ level;

14.3. Awareness of sensory integration issues and their importance to management of children with FAS or ARND, especially the younger ones;

14.4. Awareness of language delay not just as expressive language but also in receptive understanding, especially in social communication problems, which incorporate social awareness and cognition;

14.5. Awareness of the pervasive effect of low working memory on every day class function;

14.6. Awareness of the positive and negative effects of medication on classroom functioning;

14.7. Ideally have access to a FASDs curriculum.

(Adapted from ADD WareHouse 2011, Densmore 2011, Kulip 2004, Malbin 2012, O'Malley 2008, Tanner Halverson 1997)

Published Irish Foster Carers Association News, Summer 2013, No 57, pages 19-20.

References

References (2014 Book)

Key References

Carpenter B, Blackburn C, Egerton J. (2014) *Fetal Alcohol Spectrum Disorders. Interdisciplinary Perspectives.* Routledge Publishing, London.

Driscoll CD, Streisguth AP, Riley EP. (1990) Prenatal alcohol exposure: Comparability of effects in humans and animal models. *Neurotoxicity and Teratology:* 12, (3),231-237.

Additional References

Abate P, Paeta M, Spear NE, Molina JC (2008). Fetal learning about ethanol and later ethanol responsiveness: evidence against safe amounts of prenatal alcohol exposure. *Exp. Biol. Med.,* 233 (2) 139-154.

Abidin RR. *Parenting Stress Index Manual.* 2nd ed. Charlottesville: Pediatric Psychology Press 1986.

Adnams CM, Soreur P, Kolberg WO et al., (2007). Language and literacy outcomes from a pilot intervention study for children with fetal alcohol spectrum disorders in South Africa. *Alcohol,* 41, 403-414.

Adudabo, S. and Cohen, D. (2011). *Prenatal Alcohol Use and Fetal Alcohol Spectrum Disorders: Diagnosis, assessment and new directions in research and multimodal treatment,* Oak Park, IL: Bentham On Line Publishing.

Alexander FG Selesnick ST (1965). The History of Psychiatry. *An evaluation of psychiatric thought from prehistoric times to the present.* 341-345.

Althoff RR. Dysregulated children reconsidered. *J Am Acad Child Adolesc Psychiatry* 2010; 49: 302-4.

Altink ME, Slaate-Willense DIE, Ronnelse NNJ, et al.(2009). Effects of maternal and paternal smoking on attentional control in children with and without ADHD. *Eur Child Adolesc Psychiatry,* 18; 465-75.

Althoff, R.R. (2010). 'Dysregulated children reconsidered', *Journal of the American Academy of Child and Adolescent Psychiatry,* 49: 302-4.

American Psychiatric Association. (200) *Diagnostic and statistical manual of mental disorders,* 4th ed., text revision. Washington, DC.

American Psychiatric Association (2013). *Diagnostic and Statistical Manual of Mental Disorders* (5th edn) (DSM-V), Arlington, VA: APA.

And Thinking Of (2014). *2nd poetry collection,* Kieran Darragh O'Malley, Original writing.ie.

Anum EA, Springel EH, Shriver MD, Strauss JF (2009). *Genetic contributions to preterm birth.* Paed. Res, Vol. 65, 1-9.

Archibald, S.L., Fennema-Notestine, C., Ganst, A., Riley, E.P., Mattson, S.N. and Jernigan, T.L. (2001). 'Brain dysmorphology in individuals with severe prenatal alcohol exposure', *Developmental Medicine and Child Neurology,* 43: 148-54.

Astley SH, Clarren SK. (2000). Diagnosing the full spectrum of fetal alcohol exposed individuals: introducing the 4-digit diagnostic code. *Alcohol,* 35: 400-410.

Astley SJ, Clarren SK .(2001). Measuring the facial phenotype of individuals with prenatal alcohol exposure: Correlations with brain dysfunction. *Alcohol Alcohol,* 36: 47-59.

Astley SJ, Aylward EH, Olson HC, Kerns K, Brooks A, Coggins TE, Davies J, Dorn S, Gendler B, Jirikowic T, Kregel P, Maravilla K, Richards T (2009). Magnetic resonance imaging outcomes from a comprehensive magnetic resonance study of children with fetal alcohol spectrum disorders. *Alcoholism: Clin. & Exp. Res.* 33, 1671-1689.

A Sun's Eye (2013). 1st poetry collection, Kieran Darragh O'Malley, Originalwriting.ie.

Baer, JS, Sampson, PD, Barr, HM, Connor, PD, Streissguth, AP. (2003). A 21-year longitudinal analysis of the effects of prenatal alcohol exposure on young adult drinking, *Archives of General Psychiatry,* 60:377-85.

Baren Cohen S, Ring, HA, Ballimore ET, Wheelwright, S, Ashwin C, Williams SCR (2000). The amygydala theory of autism. *Neuroscience and Biobehavioural Reviews.*24, 3355-3344.

Barker DJP, Martyn CN, Osmond CN, Hales (1993). Growth in utero and serum cholesterol concentration in adult life. *British Medical Journal,* 307, 1524-15327.

Barr, HM. and Streissguth, AP. (2001). Identifying maternal self-reported alcohol use associated with fetal alcohol spectrum disorders, *Alcoholism: Clinical and Experimental Research,* 25: 283-7.

Barr, HM, Bookstein, FL, O'Malley, KD, Connor, PD, Huggins, J. and Streissguth, AP. (2006). Binge drinking during pregnancy as a predictor of psychiatric disorders on the

Structured Clinical Interview for DSM-IV in young adult offspring, *American Journal of Psychiatry,* 163:1061-5.

Barry S, Kearney A, Daly S, Lawlor E, Mc Namee E, Barry J (2006). The Coombe Women's Study of Alcohol, *Smoking and Illicit Drug Use.* (1987-2005, Dublin, Ireland).

Bearer CF (2001). L1 adhesion molecule signal cascades. Targets for ethanol developmental neurotoxicity. *Neurotoxicity,* 27 (6) 625-633.

Bearer CF (2001). Markers to detecting drinking during pregnancy. *Alcohol Res Health,* 25: 210-8.

Beauchaine JP, Gutzke-Kopp L, Meach AK (2009). Polyvagal theory and developmental psychoapathogy: emotion dysregulation and conduct problems from pre-school to adolescence. *Biological Psychology,* 74(2) 174-184.

Bell AW, Ehrhardt E (2002). Regulation of placental nutrient transport and implications for fetal growth. *Nutrition Research Reviews.* Vol. 15(2) 211-230.

Benhke M, Smith VC (2013). Prenatal substance abuse: short and long term effects on the exposed fetus. Committee on Substance Abuse, *Committee on Fetus and Newborn.* Pediatrics; Vol.131, No3, March 1st, 1009-1024.

Benini R, Ben Amour IM, Shevell MI (2012). Clinical clues to differentiating inherited and non-inherited ataxias. *J Paediatr. Jan.* 160, 152-157.

Bertrand, J. (2009). Interventions for children with fetal alcohol spectrum disorders (FASD): overview of findings for five innovative research projects, *Research in Developmental Disabilities*, 30: 986-1006.

Blumstein A, Farrington DO, and Mortea SD (1985). *Delinquent Careers: Innocence, Desistance and Persistence in an Annual Review of Research,* Vol. 6.

Bond NW, Di Gusto EL. (1976). Effects of prenatal alcohol exposure on open field behavior and alcohol preference in rats. *Psychopharmacologia,* 46: 163-5.

Bonthius D, Woodhouse J, Bonthius NE, Taggrad DA, Lothman EW (2001). Reduced seizure control and hippocampal cell loss in rats exposed to alcohol during brain growth spurt. *Alcohol Exp Clin Res.,* 25, (1) 70-82.

Bookstein FL, Sampson PD, Streissguth AP, Connor PL (2001). Geometric morphometrics of corpus callosum and subcortical structures in fetal alcohol effected brain. *Teratology:* 4, 4-32.

Bookstein, FL, Sampson, PD, Connor, PD. and Streissguth, AP. (2002). Midline corpus callosum is a neuroanatomical focus of fetal alcohol damage, *The Anatomical Record,* 269: 162-74.

Boyadjieva NI, Sarkon DK (2010). Role of microglia in ethanol's aptoptic action on hypothalamic neural cells in primary cultures, *Alc. Clin. Exp. Res.*, 34 (11) 1835-1842.

Brain (2005). E*ditorial on Normal Gescwind's classic 1965 papers on Disconnexion syndromes in animals and man.* Vol. 128, (10) 2217-2218.

Bremner JD, Randall P, Scott TM, Bronen RA, Selby JP, Southwick SM, Delaney RC, Mc Carthy G, Charney DB, Innis RB (1995). MRI –based measures of hippocampal volume in patients with PTSD. *Amer. J Psychiatry,* 152, 973-981.

British Medical Association Board of Science (2007, June). *Fetal Alcohol Spectrum Disorders: A Guide for Professionals.* Publisher: BMA, London.

Browne N (1952). *The Mother and Child Scheme,* March/April, Ireland.

Brown TE. (2010). A new model of understanding ADHD: Implications for patient care, January 29th, *Lilly National Meeting on Topics in Psychiatry,* Westbury Hotel, Dublin, Ireland.

Brown, TE. (ed.) (2009). *ADHD Comorbidities: Handbook for ADHD complications in children and adults.* Arlington, VA: American Psychiatric Press.

Burd L, Selfridge R, Klug M, Bakko S. (2004). Fetal alcohol syndrome in the United States corrections system. *Addict Biol,* 9: 177-8.

Byrne, C. (2008). Psychopharmacology basics for FASD. *Workshop Presentation, 3rd National Biennial Conference on Adolescents and Adults with Fetal Alcohol Spectrum Disorder,* 9-12 April, Vancouver, British Columbia.

Byrne, S, (2013). *"The Irish drink problem is hidden in plain sight, and it's escalating."* Evening Herald, Comment, Monday February 25th, Ireland.

Carlson GA, Findling RL, Post RM, et al. AACAP (2009). Research forum-advancing research in early-onset bipolar disorder: Barriers and suggestions. *J Child Adolesc Psychopharmacology;* 19: 3-12.

Carlson, GA, Findling, RL, Post, RM, Birmaher, B, Blumberg, HP, Correll, C, Delbello, MP, Fristad, M, Frazier, J, Hammen, C, Hinshaw, SP, Kowatch, R, Leibenluft, E, Mayer, SE, Pavulrui, MN, Dineen Wagner, K. and Tohen, M. (2009). 'Advancing research in early-onset bipolar disorder: barriers and suggestions', *Journal of Child and Adolescent Psychopharmacology,* 19: 3-12.

Carmichael-Olson H, Feldman JJ, Streissguth AP, Sampson PD, Bookstein FL (1998). N europsychological deficits in adolescents with fetal alcohol syndrome. Clinical findings. Alcoholism. *Clin. & Exp. Research,* 22, 1998-2012.

Carpenter B, (2012). *21st Intercountry Adoption Conference,* Plenary Talk, Education Issues in FASD, Cork, Jan 21st.

CASII (2005) Child and Adolescent Service Intensity Instrument, Users Manual, March, version 1.2, American Academy Child Adolescent Psychiatry, USA

Castellanos RH, Seguin JR, Vitano F, Parent S, Tremblay RE (2013). Impact of a 2 year multimodal intervention for disruptive 6 year old olds on substance use in adolescence: randomized controlled trial. *Brit J Psych* 203 (3) 188-195.

CDC, FAS: Guidelines for Referral and Diagnosis (CDC, HHS, NOFAS) (2005). *3rd Printing. National Center Birth Defects and Developmental Disabilities, Centers* for Disease Control and Prevention, Department of Health Human Services, and NOFAS, USA.

Ceccanti M, Spagnolo PR, Tarani L, et al. (2007). Clinical delineation of fetal alcohol spectrum disorders (FASD) in Italian children: Comparison and contrast with other racial/ethnic groups and implications for diagnosis and prevention. *Neuroscience Biobehavioral Rev, 31*: 270-7.

Centers for Disease Control (CDC). *Fetal Alcohol Syndrome: Guidelines for referral and diagnosis.* (2004). In coordination with National Task Force on Fetal Alcohol Syndrome and Fetal Alcohol Effect, American Academy of Pediatrics, American College of Obstetricians and Gynecologists, March of Dimes, and National Organization on Fetal Alcohol Syndrome (NOFAS).

Chess S (1971). Autism in children with congenital Rubella. *Journal of Autism and Developmental Disorders.* 1(1), 33-47.

Chess S and Thomas A (1977). *Temperament and Development.* New York. Brunner/Mazel.

Child Welfare Information Gateway. (October 2001). Understanding the effects of maltreatment on early brain development. *Bulletin for professionals. US Department of Health and Human Services,* Administration on Children, Youth, and Families, Children's Bureau.

Chudley AE, Conry J, Cook JL, Loock C, Rosales T, le Blanc N (2005, March 1) Fetal Alcohol Spectrum Disorder: Canadian Guideline for Diagnosis. *Can. Med. Assoc. Journal,* 172 (5 supplement).

Chudley AE (2009). Fetal Alcohol Spectrum Disorders across The Lifespan. *Proceedings from IHS Development Conference*. 37-41, Edmonton, Canada.

Clarren SK, Smith DW (1978a). *The Fetal Alcohol Syndrome.* Lamp, 35, 4-7.

Clarren SK and Smith DW (1978b). The Fetal Alcohol Syndrome: A review of the world literature. *New England Journal of Medicine.* 298:1063-1067.

Clarren SK, Astley, SJ, and Bowden DM (1988). Physical Anomalies and Developmental Delays in Nonhuman Primate Infants Exposed to Weekly Doses of Ethanol During Gestation. *Teratology* 37:561-569.

Clark E, Lutke J, Minnes P, Ouellette-Kuntz H. (2004). Secondary disabilities among adults with fetal alcohol spectrum disorder in British Columbia. *J FAS,* 2: 1-12.

Coggins, TE, Timler, GR, and Olswang, LB (2008). Identifying and treating social communication deficits in school-age children with fetal alcohol spectrum disorders, in KD. O'Malley (ed.) *ADHD and Fetal Alcohol Spectrum Disorders* (FASD). New York, NY: Nova Science.

Coles CD, Platyman KA, Ruskind –Hood CL, Brown RT, Falek A, Smith JE (1997). A comparison of children affected by prenatal alcohol exposure and attention deficit hyperactivity disorder. *Alc. Clin. Exp. Res*. 1, 150-161.

Coles C (2009). *IHE Consensus Developmental Conference. FASD: Across the Lifespan. Management Strategies.* Westin Hotel, Edmonton, Alberta, Canada.

Coles CD, Kable JA, Toddeo E (2009). Math performance and behavior problems in children affected by prenatal alcohol exposure. Intervention and follow-up. *Journal of Developmental and Behavioural Pediatrics.* 30, 7-15.

Coles CD & Zhihao L (2012). *Functional neuroimaging in the examination of effects of prenatal alcohol exposure.* Neuropsychology Review, in press.

Cox JL, Holden JM, Sagovsky R. Detection of postnatal depression. Development of the 10-item Edinburgh Postnatal Depression Scale. *Brit J Psychiatry* 1987; 150: 782-6.

Cox JL, Holden JM, Sagovsky R. (1987). Detection of postnatal depression. Development of the 10-item Edinburgh Postnatal Depression Scale. *Brit J Psychiatry,* 150: 782-6.

Cronin J, Mc Coy S, O'Malley KD, Walsh S, O'Sullivan R (2012). *A review of acute mental health presentations in a tertiary care paediatric emergency department.* Paediatric Emergency Medicine, submitted.

Cross JC, Watson ED (2013). Mutation in folate metabolism cause epigenetic instability and transgenerational effects on development. *Cell,* 155 (1) 81 DOI.

Cummings EM, Davies, PT, Campbell SB (2000). *Developmental psychopathology and Family Process. Theory, Research and Clinical Implications.* The Guilford Press, London, New York.

DC: 0 to 3R Classification (2005). Washington DC: Zero to Three Press, USA.

Denham S (1998). Emotional development in young children. Guilford Press, New York.

Densmore, R. (2011). *FASD Relationships: What I have learned about fetal alcohol spectrum disorder,* Altoma, Manitoba: Freisen Corporation.

Dominguez HD, Chotro MG, Molino JC (1993). Alcohol in amniotic fluid prior to caesarian section delivery. Effects of subsequent exposure to drug's odor upon alcohol responsiveness. *Behav. Neural Biology,* 60, 129.

Dou X, Menkori CE, Shannugasudaeraj S, Miller KW, Charness ME (2011). Two alcohol binding residues interact across a domain interface of the L1 neuronal cell adhesion molecule and regulate cell adhesion. *The Journal of Biological Chemistry,* 286, 16131-16139.

DSM 5 Symposium (2012). The making of DSM S. Part 1. *AACAP, 59th annual meeting* Oct 25th, San Francisco.

Dreosti IE. (1993). Nutritional factors underlying the expression of fetal alcohol syndrome. *Ann NY Acad. Sci,* 678: 193-204.

Dufour-Rainfray D, Vourc'h P, Tourlet SB, Guilloteau D, Chalon S, Andres CR (2011). Fetal exposure to teratogens Evidence of genes involved in autism. *Neuroscience & behavioral review,* 35(5) 1254-1265.

Dumaret, AC., Cousin, M. and Titran, M. (2009). Two generations of maternal alcohol abuse: impact on cognitive levels in mothers and their children, *Early Childhood Development and Care,* 9: 1-11.

Economic and Social Research Institute (ESRI), (2012). *Perinatal Statistics Report,* Ireland.

Edelsohn GA (2012). Ethics and research with vulnerable children. *Journal of Amer, Acad. Child & Adolesc. Psychiatry,* Vol 51, No. 6, 566-567.

Edwards B (2011). Legal issues in FASD, *AACAP symposium,* Chair: Susan Rich at AACAP/CAACP annual meeting Oct. Toronto, Canada.

Elias, S., Coughlan, B. and O'Malley, K.D. (2013, in press) *Fetal alcohol spectrum disorders, children, parents and cares living with the disorder: a mixed methods approach.*

Elliott E. (2013). Fetal Alcohol Spectrum Disorders. *Australian Perspectives, Chapter 23, 288-293 in Fetal Alcohol Spectrum Disorders.* Eds Carpenter B, Blackburn C, Egerton J, Routledge Publishing, London, New York.

EL –Sheikh M, Kouros CD, Erath S, Cummings EM, Keifer P, Staton L (2009). *Marital conflict and children's externalizing behavior: Interactions between parasympathetic and sympathetic nervous system.* Monographs of the Society for Research in Child Development. Wiley, Blackwell, Boston, Oxford.

Famy, C, Streissguth, AP, and Unis, AS (1998). Mental illness in adults with FAS, *American Journal of Psychiatry,* 155; 552-4.

Fast, DK, Conry, J, and Loock, CA (1999). Identifying fetal alcohol syndrome among youth in the criminal justice system, *Journal of Developmental and Behavioral Pediatrics,* 20: 370-2.

Feldman R (2009). Parent-infant synchrony and the construction of shared timing, physiological processes, developmental outcomes and risk conditions. *Journal of Child Psychology & Psychiatry,* 48, 329-354.

Ferrer L, Galofne E (1987). Dendritic spine anomalies in fetal alcohol syndrome. *Neuropaediatrics,* 18, 161-163l.

Fetal Alcohol Spectrum Disorders Center for Excellence, Substance Abuse and Mental Health Services Administration (SAMHSA). *Fetal Alcohol Spectrum Disorders by the Numbers.* March 6, 2010. www.samhsa.org.

Fitzgerald, M (2010). *Violent and Dangerous to Know. Nova Science Publishers,* New York. Available at www.amazon.com.

Fitzgerald M (2013). Editor, *Recent Advances in Autistic Spectrum Disorders,* www.intechopen.com.

Flak AC, Su S, Bertrand J, Denny CH, Kesmodel US, Cogswell ME (2013). The association of mild, moderate and binge prenatal alcohol exposure and child neuropsychological outcomes: a meta analysis. Alcoholism: *Clinical and Experimental Research.*doi.10 1111/acer 12214, on line.

Fombonne E (2002). Is exposure to alcohol during pregnancy a risk factor for Autism. *J Autism Dev. Disord.* 32(3) 243.

Fraiberg S, Adelson E, Shapiro, V (1975). Ghosts in the nursery. A psychoanalytic approach to the problems of impaired infant/mother bond. *J Amer. Acad. Child Psychiatry,* 14 (3) 387-421.

Gahagan S, Sharpe TT, Brimacombe M, et al. (2006). Pediatricians' knowledge, training, and experience in the care of children with fetal alcohol syndrome. *Pediatrics;* 118: 657-68.

Gardner H Spiegelman D., Baka S (2011). Perinatal and neonatal risk factors for autism: A comprehensive meta analysis. *Pediatrics,* Vol. 128, No2. 344-355.

Geller B, Zimerman B, Williams M, Delbello MP, Frazier J, Beringer L (20O2) Phenomenology of pre-pubertal and early onset adolescent bipolar disorder: examples of elated mood, grandiose behaviors, decreased need for sleep, racing thoughts, hyper-sexuality. *J of Child Adol. Psychopharmacology:* 12 (1) 3-9.

Geschwind N (1965). Disconnexion syndromes in animals and man. *Brain,* 88, 237-294, 585- 644.

Giarratano G (2006). Genetic influences on preterm birth. MCN. Amer. *J Matern. Child Neurol., Paed. Res;* Vol. 31, 167-175.

Gilberg C, Gilberg CI (1983). Infantile autism. A total population study of reduced optimality in the pre, peri and neonatal period. *Journal of Autism and Developmental Disorders,* 32(4) 153-166.

Glancy GD, Knott TF (2002a, Dec 13-18) Part I: the Psychopharmacology of Long-Term Aggression-Toward an Evidence-Based Algorithm. *Canadian Psychiatric Association Bulletin,* Psychiatry and the Law.

Glancy GD, Knott TF (2002b, Dec 19-24) Part II: The Psychopharmacology of Long-Term Aggression-Toward an Evidence-Based Algorithm, *Canadian Psychiatric Association Bulletin.* Psychiatry and the Law.

Glazer D (2000). Child abuse and neglect and the brain. *A review. J. Child Psychol. & Psych.,* 41, 97-116.

Goffman E (1963). *Stigma. Notes on the Management of Spoiled Identity.* Simon and Shuster Publishers, NY.

Goldman SK (1999). *The conceptual framework for wraparound: definition, values, essential elements and requirements for practice* in BJ Burns & SK Goldman (eds) Promising practices in wraparound for children with severe emotional disturbance and their families (1998 series, Vol. 4) Washington DC, Center for Effective Collaboration and Practice, American Institute for Research.

Goodlett CR, Horn KH (2001). Mechanisms of alcohol induced damage to the developing nervous system. *Alcohol Research and Health,* Vol. 23, No 3, 173-184.

Goodlett, CR, Horn, KH and Zhou, FC (2005). Alcohol teratogenesis: mechanisms of damage and strategies for intervention, *Experimental Biology and Medicine,* 230: 394-406.

Gore, A (2006). An Inconvenient Truth. *The planetary emergency of global warming and what we can do about it.* Rodale Press, Pennsylvannia, USA.

Grant T, Youngblood Pedersen J, Whitney N, Ernst C. (2008). In O'Malley KD, ed. ADHD and fetal alcohol spectrum disorders (FASD), 2nd printing, Nova Science Publishers,

New York, *The role of therapeutic intervention with substance abusing mothers: Preventing FASD in the next generation.* Chapter 5, 69-93.

Grant, TM, Huggins, JE, Sampson, PD, Ernst, CC, Barr, HM. and Streissguth, A.P. (2009). Alcohol use before and during pregnancy in western Washington, 1989-2004: implications for the prevention of fetal alcohol spectrum disorders, American *Journal of Obstetrics and Gynecology*, 200 (3): 278.e1-8.

Green JJ (2004). The effects of ethanol on the developing cerebellum and eyeblink classical conditioning. *Cerebellum,* 3(3) 178-187.

Greene T, Ernhardt CB, Ager J, Sokol R, Martier S, and Boyd T (1991). Prenatal Alcohol Exposure and Cognitive Development in the Preschool Years. *Neurotoxicology and Teratology,* Vol. 13, pp. 57-68.

Greenbaum, RL, Stevens, SA, Nash, K, Koren, G, and Rovet, J. (2009). Social cognitive and emotion processing abilities of children with fetal alcohol spectrum disorders: a comparison with attention deficit hyperactivity disorder, *Alcoholism: Clinical and Experimental Research,* 33: 1656-70.

Gurvitz TV, Shenton ME, Pitman RK (1995). Reduced hippocampal volume on magnetic resonance imaging in chronic posttraumatic stress disorder. *Paper presented at Annual Meeting of International Society on Traumatic Stress Studies, Miami.*

Hagerman, RJ (1999). Neurodevelopmental Disorders: Diagnosis and treatment, Oxford: Oxford University Press., 3-47 Hannigan J, Randall S (1996). Behavioural pharmacology in animals exposed prenatally to alcohol. In Abel, EL, editor, *Fetal alcohol syndrome. From mechanism to prevention.* CRC Press, 191-213, New York,

Hannigan, JH, O'Leary-Moore, SK, and Berman, RF (2007). Postnatal environmental or experimental amelioration of neurobehavioural effects of prenatal alcohol exposure in rats, *Neuroscience and Behavioural Review,* 31: 202-11.

Handley, E, and Chassin, L (2009). Intergenerational transmission of alcohol expectancies in a high-risk sample, *Journal of Studies on Alcohol and Drugs,* 70 (5): 675-82.

Harris J (1995). *Developmental Neuropsychiatry,* Volume 1 and Volume 2, Oxford University Press.

Haycock PC. (2009). Fetal alcohol spectrum disorders: the epigenetic perspective. *Biology of Reproduction,* 81: 607-17.

Henshaw, C, Cox, J, and Barton, J (2009). *Modern Management of Perinatal Psychiatric Disorders,* London: Royal College of Psychiatrists.

Hobson RP (1989). Beyond Cognition. A theory of autism. In Dawson G, ed. Autism, *nature, diagnosis and treatment.* 222-448 Guilford Press, New York,

Hosenbocus S, Chahal R (2012). A review of executive function deficits and pharmacological management in children and adolescents. *J Can Acad. Child Adolesc. Psychiatry,* 21, No.3, 23-29,

Howlin, P, Charman, T, and Ghazziuddin, M (eds.) (2011). *The Sage Handbook of Developmental Disorders,* London: Sage.

Hoyme, HE, May, PA, Kalberg, MA, Kodituwakku, P, Gossage, JP, Truijillo, PM, Buckley, DG, Miller, JH, Aragon, AS, Khaole, N, Viljoen, DL, Jones, KL, and Robinson, LK (2005). A practical clinical approach to diagnosis of fetal alcohol spectrum disorders: clarification of the 1996 Institute of Medicine criteria, *Pediatrics,* 115: 39-47.

H.S.E. (2013). Study *on Costs to Society of Problem Alcohol Use in Ireland.*

Ibsen H (1881). *Ghosts,* Doubleday Anchor Publications, New York.

Jokela M, Keltikaugas-Jarvinen L, Kivinaki M, Pattanen EM, Roatu R, Lehtinaki T (2007). Serotonin receptor 2A gene and the influence of childhood maternal nurturance on adult depressive symptoms. *Archives of General Psychiatry,* 64, 356-360.

Jones KL, Smith DW, Ulleland CN, Streissguth AP (1973a). Pattern of malformation in offspring of chronic alcoholic mothers. *Lancet;* 1: 1267-71.

Jones KL, Smith DW (1973 b) Recognition of the fetal alcohol syndrome in early infancy. *Lancet;* 2: 999-1001.

Jones KL and Smith DW (1975). The Fetal Alcohol Syndrome, *Teratology,* 1975,12: 1-10.

Jones KL, Robinson LK, Bakhireva LN, et al. (2009). Accuracy of the diagnosis of physical features of fetal alcohol syndrome by pediatricians after specialized training. *Pediatrics* 2009; 118: 1734-9.

Jung CG (1959). *Archetypes and Collective Unconscious.*

Kagan J (1999). Human Development. *Two Forms of Discontinuity.* 42, 257-259.

Kapp F ME, O'Malley KD (2001). *Watch For The Rainbows. True stories of educators and caregivers of children with Fetal Alcohol Spectrum Disorders.* Publishers Frances Kapp Education, Calgary, Canada,

Karr-Moore R, Wiley MS (1999). Ghosts from the nursery. *Tracing the roots of violence.* USA.

Kodituwakku, PW, and Kodituwakku, EL (2011). From research to practice: an integrative framework for the development of interventions for children with fetal alcohol spectrum disorders, *Neuropsychology Review,* 21; 204-23.

Kelly K (2009). *Legal Issues in FASD, Power Point Presentation,* Youth Offenders Centre, Belfast, N. Ireland.

Knitzer J (1982). *Unclaimed Children.* Children's Defense Fund, Washington DC, USA.

Koren G, Nulman J, Chudley A, Locke C. Fetal alcohol spectrum disorder*, Can Med Assoc. J* 2003; 169: 1181-5.

Kraemer, GW, Moore, CF, Newman, TK, Barr, CS, and Schneider, ML (2008). Moderate fetal alcohol exposure and serotonin transporter gene promoter polymorphism effect neonatal temperament and limbic-hypothalamic-pituitary-adrenal axis regulation in monkeys, *Biological Psychiatry,* 63: 317-24.

Kulp, J (2004). Our Fascinating Journey. *2nd Edition, Better Endings. New Beginnings.* Publisher, Brooklyn Park, MN, USA.

Kvigne VL, Leonardson GR, Borzelleca J, Neff-Smith M, Welty TK. (2009). Characteristics of children whose siblings have fetal alcohol syndrome or incomplete fetal alcohol syndrome. *Pediatrics;* 123: e526-33.

Lambin D (2011). SAFFRANCE, *2nd International Colloquium,* Strasbourg, Dec 14th & 15th.

Lingford Hughes A (2013). *Updates in pharmacology and pharmacotherapy of harmful alcohol use and dependence.* Plenary talk, All Ireland Psychiatrists Meeting, Malahide, Dublin, November 8th.

Laufer BI, Mantha K, Kleiber ML, Diehl EJ, Addison SM, Singh SM (2013). Long-lasting alterations in DNA Methylation and nc RNA underlie the effects of fetal alcohol exposure in mice. *Disease and Mechanisms,* 6, 977-992.

Laufer BI, Kleiber ML, Diehl EJ, Kapalanga J Singh SM (2013a). *The pre-clinical spectrum: Low to moderate fetal alcohol exposure leaves life long epigenetic marks,* IN PRESS.

LeDoux J (2000). Emotion circuits in the brain. *Annual Review of Neuroscience,* 23, 155-184.

Lattmore Keri A, Donn SM, Kaciroti N, Kemper AR, Neal CR, Vazquez DM.(2005). Selective serotonin reuptake inhibitors (SSRI) use during pregnancy and effects on the fetus and newborn: A metal analysis. *J Perinatology,* 25: 595-603.

Learnpediatrics. sites.olt.ubc.ca (2013). FASD Fetal Alcohol Spectrum Disorder.

Lee R, Coccaro E (2001, Feb) The Neuropsychopharmacology of Criminality and Aggression. *Canadian Journal of Psychiatry,* vol. 46, 35-44.

Lemoine P, Harousseau H, Borteyru JP, Menuet JC. (1968). Children of alcoholic parents: Abnormalities observed in 127 cases. *Selected Translations of International Alcoholism Research (STIAR).* Rockville, MD: National Institute on Alcohol Abuse and Alcoholism 1968. (Translation from the French of: Les enfants de parents alcooliques: Anomalies observées, à propos de 127 cas. Ouest Medical, Paris), 21: 476-82.

Lemoine, P, and Lemoine, PH (1992). Avenir des enfants de mères alcooliques (Étude de 105 cas retrouvés à l'âge adulte) et quelques constatations d'intérêt prophylactique (Outcome in the offspring of alcoholic mothers (study of 105 adults) and considerations with a view to prophylaxis), *Annales depédiatrie,* Paris, 39: 226-35.

Leonard P, O'Neill C, Kelly B (2013). *Capacity and Asssociated Législation symposium, All Ireland Psychiatrists Meeting, Malahide*, Dublin, November 8th.

Löser H, Bierstedt T, Blum A. (1999). Fetal alcohol syndrome in adults: Long-term observations on 52 patients. (Alkoholembryopathie im erwachsenenalter: Eine langzeituntersuchung). *Deutsche Medizinische Wochenschrift* 1999; 124: 412-8.

Lewis M (2000). Self conscious emotions: Embarrassment, pride, shame and guilt. In M Lewis & JM Haviland –Jones (eds), *Handbook of Emotions,* Guilford Press, New York, 563-573.

Little RE, Streissguth AP, Guzinski GM, et al. (1985). An evaluation of the pregnancy and health program: *Alcohol Health Res World,* 10: 44-53, 75.

Little JF, Hepper PG, Dornan JC (2002). Maternal alcohol consumption during pregnancy and fetal startle behaviour. *Physiology Beh,* 76: 691-4.

Lord C, Mulloy, C Wendelboe M., Schopler E (1991). Pre and perinatal factors in high functioning females and males with autism. *J autism Dev Disorder,* 21 (2)197-209.

Lord C Kim SH, Dimartino A (2011). Autism Spectrum Disorders. General Overview. Chapter 14, Editors Howlin P, Charman T, Ghaziuddin M, *The Sage Handbook of Developmental Disorders,* Published London, California, New Delhi, Singapore.

Lorney LH, Stein AD, Kahm HS, Van der Pal-de Bruin K, Blauw CJ, Zybert PA, Sasser ES (2007). Cohort Profile: The Dutch Winter Families Study. *International journal of epidemiology,* Vol.36, Issue 6, 1196-1204.

Lucas A (1991). Programming by early nutrition. *Ciba Foundation Symposium.* 156, 38-50.

Lupton C, Burd L, Harwood R. (2004). Cost of fetal alcohol spectrum disorders. *Am J Med Genet,* 127C:42-50.

Mahabin S, Chatterjee D, Garlin R (2013). Strain dependent neurochemical changes induced by embryonic alcohol exposure in zebra fish. *Neurotox. Teratol.* Nov. 10th.

Malbin D. (2012). Fetal Alcohol/Neurobehavioral Conditions. Understanding and application of a brain –based approach. *A collection of information for parents & professionals.* 3rd Edition, FASCETS Inc. Portland, USA.

Malone K (2013). *Suicide study Results,* Irish Times, May 21st, Ireland.

Marian M, Bornstein Mh (2009). Dynamics of emotion regulation in infants of clinically depressed and non-depressed mothers. *Journal of Child Psychology & Psychiatry*, 50, 11, 1410-1418.

Matthews R, Thorn M, Giorgi C (2013). Vested interests in addiction research and policy. Is the Alcohol Industry delaying Government action on alcohol health warning labels in Australia? *Addiction;* 108 (11) 1889-1896.

Mattson, SN, Riley, EP, Sowell, ER, Jernigan, TL, Sobel, DF, and Jones, KL (1996). A decrease in the size of the basal ganglia in children with FAS, *Alcoholism: Clinical and Experimental Research, 20*: 1088-93.

Mattson SN, Calarco KE, Lang AR (2006). Focused and shifting attention in children with heavy prenatal alcohol exposure. *Neuropsychology,* 20, 361-369.

Mattson, SN, Crocker, N, and Nyguen, TT (2011). Fetal alcohol spectrum disorders: neuropsychological and behavioural features, *Neuropsychology Review.* 2: 84-101.

May PA, Brook L, Gossage JP, et al. (2000). Epidemiology of fetal alcohol syndrome in a South African community In the Western Cape Province. *Am J Public Health;* 90: 1905-12.

May PA, McCloskey J, Gossage, JP. (2002). Fetal alcohol syndrome among American Indians: epidemiology, issues, and research. In Mail PD, Heurtin-Roberts S, Martin

SE, Howard J, eds. Alcohol use among American Indians: multiple perspectives on a complex problem. *National Institute on Alcohol Abuse and Alcoholism Research Monograph No. 37.* Bethesda, MD: National Institute on Alcohol Abuse and Alcoholism.

May PA, Fiorentino D, Gossage JP, et al. (2006). Epidemiology of FASD in a province in Italy: prevalence and characteristics of children in a random sample of schools *Alc Clin Exp Res* 30: 1562-75.

May PA, Gossage JP, Marais AS, et al. (2007). The epidemiology of fetal alcohol syndrome and partial FAS in a South African community. *Drug Alc Dep;* 88: 259-271.

May PA, Gossage JP, Kalberg WO, et al. (2009). Prevalence and epidemiologic characteristics of FASD from various research methods with an emphasis on recent in-school studies. *Dev Dis Res Rev;* 15: 176-192.

Manteueffel MD (1996). Neurotransmitter function: changes associated with in utero alcohol exposure. In: Abel EL (ed.) *Fetal alcohol syndrome: from mechanism to prevention.* CRC, New York, pp 171-189.

Mantha K, Kleiber M, Singh S (2013). Neurodevelopmental timing of ethanol exposure may contribute to observed heterogeneity of behavioural deficits in mouse model of Fetal Alcohol Spectrum Disorders. *Journal Biomedical & LIfe Sciences,* Vol. 3, No.1 Feb., 85-99.

Mc Cord R (2013). The Mother and Child scheme-*The role of Church and State Irish History on line,* 19th June.

Mc Gee CL, Sconfield AM, Roebuck –Spencer TM, Riley EF, Mattson SN (2008). Children with heavy prenatal alcohol exposure demonstrate deficits on multiple measures of concept formation. *Alcoholism, Clin & Exp Research.*32, 1588-1597.

Meewise, ML, Reitsma, JB, De Vries, GJ, Gersons, BPR, and Olff, M (2007). Cortisol and post traumatic stress disorder in adults: systematic review and meta-analysis, *British Journal of Psychiatry,* 191: 387-92.

Mick, E, Biederman, J, Farone, S, Sayer, J, and Kleinman, S (2002). Case-control study of ADHD and maternal smoking, alcohol use and drug use during pregnancy, *Journal of the American Academy of Child and Adolescent Psychiatry,* 41: 378-85.

Milberger, S, Biederman, J, Farone, SV, Chen, L, and Jones, J (1996). Is maternal smoking during pregnancy a risk factor for attention deficit hyperactivity disorder in children? *American Journal of Psychiatry,* 153: 1138-1142.

Mongan D, Mc Cormick PA, O'Hara S, Smyth B, Long J (2011). Can Ireland's increased rates of alcoholic liver disease morbidity and mortality be explained by per capita alcohol consumption? *Alcohol and Alcoholism,* April 2011, on line.

Moore, TE, and Green, M (2004). Fetal alcohol spectrum disorder: a need for closer examination by the criminal justice system, *Criminal Reports,* 19: 99-108.

Motherrisk (2013). *The Hospital for Sick Children,* Toronto, Canada.

Mukarjee R, Hollins S, Turk, J (2006). Psychiatric comorbidity in fetal alcohol syndrome. *Psychiatric Bulletin.* 30, 194-195.

Mukherjee, RAS, Hollins, S, and Turk, J (2008). Fetal alcohol spectrum disorder, *Journal of the Royal Society of Medicine,* 99: 298-302.

Mukarjee RA, Hollins S, and Curfs L (2012). Fetal Alcohol Spectrum Disorders: Is it something we should be more aware of? *J R. Coll. Physicians Edin.* 42:143-150.

MurphyDJ, Mullaly A, Cleary BJ, Fahy T, Barry J (2013) Behavioural change in relation to alcohol exposure in early pregnancy and impact on perinatal outcomes –a prospective cohort study. *BMJ Pregnancy and Childbirth* 13:18 on line wwwbiomedical
central.com/1471-2393/13/8.

Murray, L, Arteche, A, Fearon, P, Halligan, S, Goodyear, I, and Cooper, P. (2011). 'Maternal postnatal depression and the development of depression in offspring up to 16 years of age', *Journal of the American Academy of Child and Adolescent Psychiatry,* 50 (5): 460-70.

My World Survey/Headstrong/*UCD Dept. of Psychology* (2011). National Survey of Youth Mental Health, Dublin, Ireland.

Nanson J (1992). Autism in Fetal Alcohol Syndrome: a report of 6 cases. *Alcoholism: Clin & Exp. Res.* Vol. 16, 3, 558-565.

Nash LM (1997). Fertile Minds, June 9th, Time Magazine.

National Institute on Alcohol Abuse and Alcoholism (NIAAA, 2000 June). Highlights from Current Research: 10th Special Report to the U.S. Congress on Alcohol and Health from the Secretary of Health and Human Services. *US Department of Health and Human Services,* Public Health Service, National Institutes of Health.

National Scientific Council on the Developing Child (2004). *Children's emotional development is built into the architecture of their brains.* Helen Keller School for Social Policy and Management, Brandeis University, USA.

Nguyen TT, Riley EP (2013 2014). The effects of prenatal alcohol exposure on brain and behaviour. Chapter 18, 219-240, in Fetal Alcohol Spectrum Disorders. *Interdisciplinary Perspectives.* (eds. Carpenter B, Blackburn C, Egerton J) Routledge Publishers, London, New York.

Novick Brown, N, O'Malley, KD and Streissguth, AP (2011). FASD: diagnostic dilemmas and challenges for a modern transgenerational approach, in S.A. Abudato and S. Cohen (eds) *Prenatal Alcohol Use and Fetal Alcohol spectrum Disorders: Diagnosis, assessment, and new directions in research and multimodal treatment,* Oak Park, IL: Bentham On Line Publishing.

Oberlander, T.F., Gingrich, J.A. and Ansorge, M.S. (2009). Sustained neurobehavioral effects of exposure to SSRI antidepressants during development: molecular to clinical evidence, *Clinical Pharmacology and Therapeutics,* 86: 672-7.

O'Casey S (1926). *Juno and The Paycock,* Samuel French publishers.UK.

O'Connor TG, Rutter M. (2000). Attachment disorder behavior following early severe deprivation: extension and longitudinal follow up. *J Am Acad Child Adol Psychiatry*, 38: 703-12.

O'Connor MJ, Shah, B, Whaley, S, Cronin, P, Gunderson B, Graham J (2002). Psychiatric illness in a clinical sample of children with prenatal alcohol exposure. *Amer. J. Drug & Alcohol Abuse,* 28 (4) 743-754.

O'Connor MJ, Paley B (2009). Psychiatric conditions associated with prenatal alcohol exposure. *Developmental Disabilities Review,* 15,☹ (3), 225-34.

Oesterheld JA, Kofoed L, Tervo R, Fogas B, Wilson A, Fiechtman H (1998). Effectiveness of methylphenidate in Native American children with fetal alcohol syndrome and attention deficit hyperactivity disorder. A controlled pilot study. *Journal of Child & Adolesc. Psychopharmcology*. 8, 39-48.

O'Leary –Moore SK, Ponnell SE, Godin EA, Sulik KK (2011). Focus on: Magnetic Resonance based studies on FASD in animal models. *Alcohol Research and Health.* Vol 34, No 1.

Olson HC, Ohlemiller MM, O'Connor MJ, et al. (2009). A call to action: Advancing essential services and research on fetal alcohol spectrum disorders. *A report of the national task force on fetal alcohol syndrome and fetal alcohol effects.* March 2009.

O'Malley KD (1997). *Medication therapy's role for FAS*. Iceberg, 7; 1-4.

O'Malley, KD (2001). Medication in FASD: uses in primary, secondary and tertiary prevention. *Presentation to the National FAS Conference, Centers for Disease Control and Prevention,* 27-28 April, Atlanta, USA.

O'Malley, KD (2003). Youth with comorbid disorders, in A.J. Pumariega and N.C. Winters (eds) *The Handbook of Child and Adolescent Systems of Care: The new community psychiatry,* Hoboken, NJ: Jossey-Bass.

O'Malley KD (2006) Fetal Alcohol Spectrum Disorders. Iinvited Plenary. Alaska Psychiatric Conference April 23rd. Girdwood.

O'Malley KD (2007). *The Politics and Ethics of Health Care Delivery,* Social Science Journal, USA.

O'Malley, KD (Ed.) (2008). *ADHD and Fetal Alcohol Spectrum Disorders (FASD). 2nd edition, Nova* Science Publishers. New York, NY.

O'Malley, KD (2010). Fetal Alcohol Spectrum Disorders, in I.P. Stolerman (ed.) *Encyclopedia of Psychopharmacology*. Berlin, Germany: Springer Verlag.

O'Malley KD (2011a) Fetal Alcohol Spectrum Disorders, Chapter 24, in in P. Howlin, T. Charman and M. Ghazziuddin (ed.) *The Sage Handbook of Developmental Disorders.* 479-496, London, California, New Delhi, Singapore.

O'Malley, KD (2011b) Psychiatric review of 95 to 100 transgenerational patients with FASD, Ireland 2006-2011. *Plenary talk to the 4th International Conference on FASD,* 3-6 March, Vancouver.

O'Malley KD (2011c) ADHD and FASD. From animal research to clinical experience. Invited talk, *International CADDRA meeting Toronto,* October 16th.

O'Malley KD (2013). Developmental psychiatric disorders in children, adolescents and young adults with Fetal Alcohol Spectrum Disorders. A transgenerational approach to diagnosis and management., Chapter 19, 241-261 in *Fetal Alcohol Spectrum Disorders. Interdisciplinary Perspectives.* editors, Carpenter B, Blackburn C, Egerton J, Routledge Publishing, London, New York.

O'Malley KD (2013A) Alcohol Related Neurodevelopmental Disorder. ARND. in JP Stolerman (ed.) *Encyclopedia of Psychopharmocology,* Springer. Verlag Publishers, Berlin, Heidelberg, Germany.

O'Malley KD and Barr HM (1998). *Fetal Alcohol Syndrome and Seizure Disorder.* Letter to editor, Can J Psychiatry.

O'Malley KD, Hagerman RJ (1998). Developing clinical practice guidelines for pharmacological interventions with alcohol-affected children. In: *Centers for Disease Control & National Institute of Alcohol Abuse and Alcoholism* (eds.) Proceedings of a special focus session of the Interagency Co-ordinating Committee on fetal alcohol syndrome, Chevy Chase MA, USA, Sept 10-11, pp 145-177.

O'Malley KD, Koplin B, Dohner VA (2000). Psychostimulant response in Fetal Alcohol Syndrome, *Can J. Psychiatry,* 45, 90-91.

O'Malley, KD, and Mukherjee, R (2010). Fetal alcohol syndrome/alcohol related neurodevelopmental disorder (Syndrome sheet), Bourne End, Buckinghamshire: *Society for Study of Behavioral Phenotypes*. [Online at: http://www.ssbp.org.uk/site/images/stories/ssbp/downloads/Foetal_alcohol.pdf; accessed: 21.1.13].

O'Malley, KD, and Nanson, J (2002). *Clinical implications of a link between fetal alcohol spectrum disorder and attention-deficit hyperactivity disorder,* Canadian Journal of Psychiatry, 4: 349-54.

O'Malley KD, Rich S (2012). Clinical implications of a link between Fetal Alcohol Spectrum Disorders (FASD) and Autism or Asperger's Disorder- A neurodevelopmental frame for helping understanding and management. Chapter 20, in *Recent Advances in Autism Spectrum Disorders,* Vol. 1 (Fitzgerald M. Editor). www. intechopen.com.

O'Malley KD & Streissguth AP (2006). *Clinical intervention and support for children aged zero to five years with fetal alcohol spectrum disorders and their parents/caregivers.*, revised 2006, in Tremblay RE, Barr RG, Peters RdeV (eds.) Encyclopedia on early childhood development (on line) Montreal, Quebec, Canada, Center of Excellence for Early Childhood Development, available at earlychildhoodca/documents/OMalley-Streissguth.

O'Malley KD, and Storoz, L (2003). Fetal alcohol spectrum disorder and ADHD diagnostic implications and therapeutic consequences, Expert Review of Neurotherapeutics, 3 (4): 477-89.

Orphan Drug Act, *US Congress; Designation of Drugs for Rare Diseases or Conditions;* SEC. 526 [360bb].

Orakwue, N, McNicholas, F, and O'Malley, KD (2010). Fetal alcohol spectrum disorders: The Irish perspective, *Irish Journal Psychological Medicine,* 27: 223-7.

Orakwue N, (2012). Alcohol. The Teratogen. Paediatric Grand Rounds, with a clinical case presentation of an ARND teenage patient and his family by Dr. Kieran D. O'Malley, *Child & Adolescent Psychiatrist,* May 12th, Our Lady's Children's Hospital Crumlin, Dublin.

Orakwue, N, Curran, L, Savage, M, O'Malley, KD (2012). Fetal Alcohol Spectrum Disorders. Pre-Training Evaluation: What the Irish Social Workers are saying. *The Irish Social Worker,* 17-21.

Padmunabhan N, Dongxin J, Geary-Joo C, Wu X, Ferguson-Smith AC, Fung E, Bieda MC, Synder FF, Gravel RA.

Page, K, (2008). Adult neuropsychology of fetal alcohol spectrum disorders, Chapter 7, in K.D. O'Malley (ed.) *ADHD and Fetal Alcohol Spectrum Disorders,* 121-142, New York, NY: Nova Science.

Paponastasion E, Stone JM, Shergill S (2013). When the drugs don't work: the potential of glutaminergic antipsychotics in schizophrenia. *Brit J Psych.* 202 (2) 91-93.

Pasamanick B, Knoblock H, Lilienfeld AM (1956). Socio-economic status and some precursors of neuropsychiatric disorders. *Amer. J Orthopsychiatry,* 26, 594-601.

Pasamanick B, Knoblock H (1996). Retrospective studies on the epidemiology of reproductive causality: Old and new, *Merrill-Palmer Quarterly of behavior and Development,* 12, 7-26.

Pembrey ME. (2002). Time to take epigenetic inheritance seriously. *European J Hum Genet,* 10: 669-71.

Pennington BF (2009). *Diagnosing Learning Disorders. A Neuropsychological Framework.* 2nd Edition, The Guilford Press, London, New York.

Pine, D, Regier, DA, Chmura Kraemer, H, Fisher, P, and Shaffer, D, (2012). 'Symposium 21: the making of DSM 5 (Part 1)'. *Presentation to the American Academy of Child and Adolescent Psychiatry 59th Annual Meeting,* San Francisco, 25 October.

Pumariega A (2003). Cultural Competence in systems of care for children's mental health. Chapter 5 in The Handbook of Child and Adolescent Systems of Care. *The New Community Psychiatry* (Eds. Pumariga AJ, Winters NC,) Jossey –Bass publishers, USA.

Purges SW (1996). Physiological regulation in high risk infants. A model for assessment and potential intervention. *Development and Psychopathology.* 8, 43-58.

Raine, A, Lencz, T, Bihrie, S, Lacasse, C, and Colletti, P (2000). Reduced prefrontal gray matter volume and reduced autonomic activity in antisocial personality disorder, *Archives of General Psychiatry,* 57: 119-127.

Rayoguru P, Cooper M (2013). Role of dietary supplementation in attention deficit hyperactivity disorder. *Brit J Psych.* 202 (6) 398-399.

Reyes, E, Garcia, KD and Jones, BC (1985). Effects of maternal consumption of alcohol on alcohol selection in rats, *Alcohol,* 2: 323-6.

Rich SD (2005). *Fetal Alcohol Syndrome: Preventable Tragedy. Psychiatric News, Residents' Forum.* Volume 40, Number 9, Page 12.

Rich SD, Sulik KK, Jones KL, Riley EP, Chambers C (2009, Nov). Fetal Alcohol Spectrum Disorder: A Paradigm for Neurodevelopmental Formulation and Multidisciplinary Treatment. *Presented at the American Academy of Child and Adolescent Psychiatry Annual Conference,* Honolulu, Hawaii.

Rich SD & O'Malley KD (2012). A neurodevelopmental formulation for the psychiatric care of Fetal Alcohol Spectrum Disorders. *Journal of psychiatry and the Law,* Accepted.

Rich SD & Novick Brown N (2013). *New DSM code should benefit clinicians, researchers.* December 18th, Psychiatric News.

Riley, EP, Mattson, SN, Sowell, ER, Jernigan, TL, Sobel, DF, and Jones, KL (1995). Abnormalities of the corpus callosum in children prenatally exposed to alcohol, *Alcoholism: Clinical and Experimental Research,* 19: 1198-202.

Riley EP, McGee CL (2005). Fetal Alcohol Spectrum Disorders: an overview with emphasis on changes in brain and behavior. *Experimental Biology and Medicine,* 230, 357-365.

Rosett HL, Weiner L, Edelin KC. Treatment experience with pregnant problem drinkers. *J Am Med Assoc.* 1983: 249; 2029-33.

Rumbull CWH, Bloomfield FH, Oliver MH, Harding JE (2009). Differential periods of a peri-conceptual undernutrition have different effects on growth, metabolic and endocrine status in fetal sheep. *Paed. Res. Vol.* 66, No.6, 605-613.

Russell J (1997). Autism is an executive disorder. Oxford University Press, New York.

Salee, FR, Lyne, A, Wigal, T, and McGough, JJ (2009). Long term safety and efficacy of guanfacine extended release in children and adolescents with attention-deficit/hyperactivity disorder, *Journal of Child and Adolescent Psychopharmacology,* 19: 215-26.

Salinger JD (1945). *The Catcher in the Rye.* Bantam Books, New York.

Sanz EJ, De las Caevas C, Kioru A, Bate A, Edwards R (2005). Selective serotonin reuptake inhibitors in pregnant women and neonatal withdrawal syndrome: a database analysis. *Lancet,* Vol. 365, Issue 9458, 482-487.

Sartorius N (2007). Stigma and Mental Health. *Lancet,* Vol. 370, Issue 9590, 810-811.

Sartorius N, Stuart H (2013). *Reducing the Stigma of Mental Disorders, College of Psychiatrists of Ireland Academic Meeting,* November 22nd.

Savage, DD, Rosenberg, MJ, Wolff, CR, Akers, KG, El-Emawy, A, Staples, MC, et al. (2010). 'Effects of a novel cognition-enhancing agent on fetal ethanol induced learning deficits', *Alcoholism: Clinical and Experimental Research,* 34 (10): 1793-802.

Screiber, ML, Moore, CF, Gajewski, LL, Larson, JA, Roberts, AD, Converse, AK, and De Jesus, OT (2008). Sensory processing disorder in primate models: evidence from a longitudinal study of prenatal alcohol and prenatal stress effects, *Child Development,* 79 (1):100-13.

Shaw P, Kaboni NJ, Lerch JP, Eckstarand K, Lenroot R, Gogtoy N, Greenstein D, Closen L, Evans A, Rapoport JL, Giedd JN, Wise SP (2008). Neurodevelopmental trajectories of the human cortex. *Journal of Neuroscience,* April 2nd, 28(14) 3586-3594.

Siegel D (2012). The Developing Mind, 2nd edition. *How relationships and the brain interact to shape who we are*. Amazon.com, USA.

Sifneos P (1973). The prevalence of 'Alexithymic' characteristics in psychosomatic patients. *Psychotherapy and Psychosomatics,* 22:225-262.

Sigman D (2011). *Alcohol Nation. How to protect our children from to-day's drinking culture.* amazon.co.uk.

Sinha, R. and O'Malley, S.S. (1999). Craving for alcohol: findings from the clinic and the laboratory, *Alcohol and Alcoholism,* 34: 223-30.

Singh SP, Pullen GL Srivenugopal K, Yuan XH, Synder AK (1992). Decreased glucose transporter 1 gene expression and glucose uptake in fetal brain exposed to ethanol. *Life sciences,* 51, 527-536.

Smith, DW (1981). Fetal alcohol syndrome and fetal alcohol effects, *Neurobehavioral Toxicology and Teratology,* 3: 127.

Smith DW (1970). *Recognizable patterns of human malformation; genetic, embryologic, and clinical aspects.* 1st ed. Philadelphia: WB Saunders. USA.

Smith DW, Fetal Alcohol Syndrome and Fetal Alcohol Effects. *Neurobehavioral Toxicology and Teratology* 1981; 3: 127.

Sokol RJ, Delaney-Black V and Nordstrom B (2003, Dec 10). *Fetal Alcohol Spectrum Disorder JAMA,* Vol 290, No. 22 (2996-2999).

Solomon M, Hessl D, Chiu S, Olsen E, and Hendren R (2009, March 1). Towards a Neurodevelopmental Model of Clinical Case Formulation. *Psychiatric Clinics of North America.* 32(1): 199–211.

Sowell ER, Thompson PM, Mattson SN, et al. (2001). Voxel-based morphometric analyses of the brain in children and adolescents prenatally exposed to alcohol. *Neuroreport.* 12: 515-523.

Sowell, ER, Lu, LH, O'Hare, ED, McCourt, ST, Mattson, SN, O'Connor, MJ, and Bookheimer, SY (2007). Functional magnetic resonance imaging of verbal learning in children with heavy prenatal alcohol exposure, *Neuroreport,* 18: 636-9.

Sowell, E., Johnson, A., Kan, E., Lu, L.H., Van Horn, J.D., Toga, A.W. et al. (2008). Mapping white matter integrity and neurobehavioral correlates in children with fetal alcohol spectrum disorders. *Journal of Neuroscience,* 28 (6): 1313-19.

Spohr HL, Willms J, Steinhausen HC. (2007). Fetal alcohol spectrum disorders in young adulthood. *J Pediatr;* 150: 175-9.

Steinmetz G (1992). The Preventable Tragedy. Fetal Alcohol Syndrome. *National Geographic Magazine.*

Stratton, K, Howe, C, and Battaglia, F (eds.) (1996). *Fetal Alcohol Syndrome: Diagnosis, epidemiology, prevention, and treatment*, Washington, DC: National Academy Press.

Strategic Task Force on Alcohol (2004). Ireland.

Steinhausen HC, Willms J, and Spohr HL (1993, Sept). Long-Term Psychophathological and Cognitive Outcome of Children with Fetal Alcohol Syndrome. *Journal of the American Acad. of Child & Adoles. Psychiatry,* 32:5, 990-994.

Streissguth AP, and LaDue RA (1987). Fetal Alcohol Teratogenic Causes of Developmental Disabilities. In S. Schroeder (Ed.), *Toxic Substances and Mental Retardation,* Washington, DC: American Association on Mental Deficiency, pp. 1-32.

Streissguth AP, Aase JM, Clarren SK, Randels SP, LaDue RA, Smith DF (1991), April 17). Fetal Alcohol Syndrome in Adolescents and Adults, *Journal of the American Medical Association,* Vol 265, No. 15, p. 1961-1967.

Streissguth, AP, Barr, HM, Kogan, J, and Bookstein, FL (1996). Understanding the Occurrence of Secondary Disabilities in Clients with Fetal Alcohol Syndrome (FAS) and Fetal Alcohol Effects (FAE): Final report to the Centers for Disease Control and Prevention (CDC). Seattle, WA: University of Washington.

Streissguth A, Barr H, Kogan J, Bookstein F. (1997). In: Streissguth, AP, Kanter J, eds. *The challenge of fetal alcohol syndrome: Overcoming secondary disabilities.* Seattle, University of Washington Press, 23-39.

Streissguth AP, Kanter J eds. (1997). *The challenge of fetal alcohol syndrome: Overcoming secondary disabilities.* University of Washington Press, Seattle, USA.

Streissguth, AP, (1997). *Fetal Alcohol Syndrome: A guide for families and communities,* Baltimore, MD: Brooks.

Streissguth, AP, and O'Malley, KD (2000). Neuropsychiatric implications and long-term consequences of fetal alcohol spectrum disorders, *Seminars in Clinical Neuropsychiatry,* 5: 177-90.

Streissguth AP, Connor PD (2001). Fetal alcohol syndrome and other effects of prenatal alcohol: developmental cognitive neuroscience implications. Chap 32. In: Nelson CA, Luciana M (Eds.) *Handbook of developmental cognitive neuroscience. Massachusetts Institute of Technology, Cambridge,* USA, pp 505-518.

Streissguth AP, Bookstein, FL, Barr, HM, Sampson, PD, O'Malley, K, and Kogan Young, J (2004). 'Risk factors for adverse life outcomes in fetal alcohol syndrome and fetal alcohol effects', *Journal of Developmental and Behavioral Pediatrics,* 25: 228-38.

Streissguth AP, Bookstein FL, Barr HM, Kogan J, O'Malley KD, et al. (2004). Risk factors for adverse life outcomes in fetal alcohol syndrome and fetal alcohol effects. *J Dev Behav Ped;* 25: 228-38.

Sulik KK, Johnston MC, Webb MA (1981). Fetal Alcohol Syndrome: Embryogenesis in a Mouse Model. *Science,* 214:936-38.

Sullivan, A. (2008). Fetal alcohol spectrum disorders in the adult: vulnerability, disability or diagnosis – a psychodynamic perspective, in KD O'Malley (ed.) *ADHD and Fetal Alcohol Spectrum Disorders* (FASD), 215-245, New York, NY: Nova Science.

Tanner Halverson, P, (1997). *Strategies for parents and caregivers of children with FAS or FAE,* Www. nofas.org/main/strategy.htm, USA.

Terr L (2003). Childhood Traumas. *An Outline and Overview. FOCUS,* 1, 322-334.

Tchurikov NA. (2006). Molecular mechanisms of epigenetics. *Biochemistry* (Moscow) 70: 406-23.

The Health of Irish Students (2005). *Health Promotions Unit,* Dept. of Health and Children, Ireland.

Thompson RA, LAgalutta (2005). Feeling and understanding: early emotional development. in K Mc Cartney & D. Phillips (eds.) *The Blackwell Handbook of Early Childhood Development.* Blackwell Press, Oxford, UK.

Times of Malta (2014) 'Minimum price of alcohol would cut UK deaths.' Reuters, Feb 11rh

Tomkins DM, Sellen EM (2001). Addiction and the brain: The role of neurotransmission in the cause and treatment of drug dependence. *CMAJ,* 164, 817-824.

Treit S, Lebel C, Baugh L, Rasmussen C, Andrew G, Beaulieu C (2013). Longitudinal MRI reveals altered trajectory of brain development during childhood and adolescence in Fetal Alcohol Spectrum Disorders. *J of Neuroscience,* June 12th, 33 (24) 100098-10109.

Tronick E (2009). *The neurobehavioural and socio-emotional development of infants and children.* Norton, Publishers, New York, London.

Turk, J (2007). Behavioural phenotypes: their applicability to children and young people who have learning disabilities, *Advances in Mental Health and Learning Disabilities,* 1: 4-13.

Turk J (2009). *Behavioural Phenotypes in Relation to ADHD. ADHD in Practice.* Vol 1. No.3, 4-8, UK.

Turk J (2012). Behavioural Phenotypes. *Royal College of Learning Disability Psychiatrists residential meeting,* Manchester, September 27th.

Uber R, Mc Guffin P (2009). The moderation of the serotonin transporter gene of environmental adversity in the aetiology of mental illness: review and methodological analysis. *Molecular Psychiatry,* 12, 1-16.

U.S. Surgeon General (Feb 21, 2005). Releases Advisory on Alcohol Use in Pregnancy: Urges women who are pregnant or who may become pregnant to abstain from alcohol.

http://www.surgeongeneral.gov/pressreleases/sg02222005.html. US Department of Health and Human Services, Office of the Surgeon General.

Van der Polk BA, Mc Farlane AC Welsaeth L (1995). *Traumatic Stress: The effects of overwhelming experience of mind,* body and society.

Velez, M, and Jansson, LM (2008). The opoid dependent mother and newborn dyad: non pharmacological care, *Journal of Addiction Medicine,* 2 (3): 113-20.

Vidal, BV (2012). Sensory processing in children with fetal alcohol spectrum disorders (session 52). *Presentation to the Second European Conference on FASD, Barcelona,* 21-24 October.

Vocci FJ, Acri J, Elksahef, A (2005). Medication Development for Addictive Disorders: The State of the Science. *Am J. Psychiatry,* 162, 8, 1432-1440.

Warren K, Floyd L, Calhoun F, Streissguth AP, O'Malley KD et al. Consensus Statement on FASD (2004). *National Organization on Fetal Alcohol Syndrome,* April 7. Washington DC, USA.

Warren KR, Li TK (2005). Genetic polymorphisms: impact on the risk of fetal alcohol spectrum disorders. *Birth Defects Res. A Clin. Mol. Teratol.,* 73 (4) 195-203.

Waterland RA, Jirle RL (2003). Transposable Elements: Targets for Early Nutritional Effects on Epigenetic Gene Regulation. *Molecular and Cellular Biology.* Aug, 5293-5300.

Watson RR (1992). *Alcohol and Neurobiology: Receptors, Membranes and Channels.* CRC Press, Baca Raton FL, 1-203.

Weiss B (2000). Vulnerability of children and the developing brain to neurotoxic hazards. *Environmental Health Perspectives.* Vol. 108, supplement 32, 375-381.

Weitch SD, Patterson J, Shaw R, Stewart-Brown S (2009). Family relationships in childhood and common psychiatric disorders in later life: systematic review of prospective studies. *Brit J Psych.* 194, 392-398.

Weitzman M, Rosenthal DG, Liu YH (2011). Paternal depression symptoms and child behavioral or emotional problems In the United States. *Paediatrics,* Vol 128, nbo6, 1126-1134.

Werner, EE (1986). Resilient offspring of alcoholics: a longitudinal study from birth to age 18. *Journal of Studies on Alcohol,* 47: 34-40.

Wernicke K (1995). The Aphasia symptom complex. A Psychological study on an anatomical basis. (1875). IN *Paul Elins, Reader in History of Aphasia,* John Benjamin Publications, 69-89.

Wilens, TE (2009). Combined pharmacotherapy in pediatric psychopharmacology: friend or foe? *Journal of Child and Adolescent Psychopharmacology,* 19: 483-4.

Wilhelm – Benartzi CS, Houseman EA, Maccani MA, Poage GM, Koestler DC, Langevin SM, Gagne LA, Banister CE, Padbury JF, Marsit J (2012). European Birth Cohorts for Environmental Health Research. *Environ. Health Perspect.* 120, (2), 296-302.

Winnicott DW. (1967). In: Lomas P, ed. *The predicament of the family: A psychoanalytical symposium*. London, Hogarth Press: 26-33.

Wozniak, J, and Biederman, J (1996). 'A pharmacological approach to the quagmire of comorbidity in juvenile mania', *Journal of the American Academy of Child and Adolescent Psychiatry,* 35: 826-8.

World Health Organisation (2004). *International Statistical Classification of Diseases and Related Health Problems 10th Revision* (ICD-10), Geneva.

Wright CJ, Dennery PA (2009). Manipulation of gene expression by oxygen: A primer from bedside to bench. *Ped Res.* Vol. 66, No.1. 3-10.

Yehuda R, Teider MH, Seckl JR, Grosman RA Morris A, Bierer CM (2007). Parental posttraumatic stress disorder as a vulnerability for low cortisol in offspring of holocaust survivors. *Arch Gen Psychiatry,* Sept. 64(9) 1040-8.

Zero to Three (2005). *Diagnostic Classification of Mental Health and Developmental Disorders of Infancy and Early Childhood* (revised edn), Washington, DC: Zero to Three.

References for the Knotted Cord. Transgenerational Alcohol. An Update 2020

Key References

Ford, T, Vostanis, P, Meltzer, H, & Goodman, R. (2007). Psychiatric disorder among British children looked after by local authorities: Comparison with children living in private households. *British Journal of Psychiatry*, 190(4), 319-325. doi:10.1192/bjp.bp.106.025023

Glaser D. Child abuse and neglect and the brain--a review. J Child Psychol Psychiatry. 2000 Jan;41(1):97-116. Erratum in: *J Child Psychol Psychiatry* 2000 Nov;41(8):1076. PMID: 10763678.

Henshaw, C, Cox, J, Barton, J. (2019). *Modern Management of Perinatal Psychiatric Disorders*, 2nd Revised edition. Amazon Kindle.

Kamara, D. & Beauchaine, T. (2019). *A Review of Sleep Disturbances among Infants and Children with Neurodevelopmental Disorders*. 10.1007/s40489-019-00193-8.

Roos LE, Distasio J, Bolton SL, Katz LY, Afifi TO, Isaak C, Goering P, Bruce L, Sareen J. (2013). A history in-care predicts unique characteristics in a homeless population with mental illness. *Child Abuse Negl*. doi:10.1016/j.chiabu.2013.08.018. Epub 2013 Sep 27. PMID: 24080062.

Sempik J, Ward H, Darker I. Emotional and Behavioural Difficulties of Children and Young People at Entry into Care. *Clinical Child Psychology and Psychiatry*. 2008;13(2):221-233. doi:10.1177/1359104507088344.

Waite, J, Heald, M, Wilde L, Woodcock, K, Welham, A, Adams, D, Oliver, C. The importance of understanding the behavioural phenotypes of genetic syndromes associated with intellectual disability, *Paediatrics and Child Health*, Volume 24, Issue 10, 2014, Pages 468-472.

Additional References

American Academy of Child and Adolescent Psychiatry, AACAP (2019) Early Childhood Service Intensity Instrument. (ECSII), 1.1 ed. USA.
www. aacap.org.cp-products
www.aacap.org/ecsii
www.aacap.org/casii

Adolphs R (2001) The neurobiology of social cognition. Current Opinion in Neurobiology, 11, 211-239.

Adolphs R (2009) The social brain. Neural basis of social knowledge. Annual Review of Psychology, 60, 693-716.

Anderson V, Beauchamp MH (2012) Developmental Social Neuroscience and Childhood Brain Insult. Theory and Practice. The Guilford Press, New York, London.

American Psychiatric Association, APA (2013) Diagnostic Criteria to the DSM 5, Desk Reference.

Aros S, Mills JL, Inquez G., Avila A, Conley MR, Troendle J, Cox C, Cassorlz (2011). Effects of prenatal ethanol exposure on postnatal growth and the insulin-like growth factor axis. Horm. Res. Peaediatr. Mar., 75(3) 166-173.

Astley SJ, Bailey D, Talbot C, Clarren S (2000) FAS Primary prevention through FAS diagnosis. Identification of high risk mothers through diagnosis of their children. *Alcohol and Alcoholism.* Vol. 35, Issue 5, 499-508.

Astley, S. (2000). Fetal Alcohol Syndrome (FAS) Primary Prevention through FAS Diagnosis: I. Identification of High Risk Birth Mothers through the diagnosis of their children *Alcohol and Alcoholism,* 35(5), 499-508. doi: 10.1093/alcalc/35.5.499.

Barr HM Bookstein FL, O'Malley KD, Connor PD, Huggins JE, Streissguth AP (2006). Binge drinking during pregnancy as a predictor of psychiatric disorders on the structured clinical interview for DSM –IV in young adult offspring. *Am. J Psychiatry,* 163, 1061-1065.

Bayley Scales of Infant and Toddler Development, 3rd edition. Pearson Clinical.

Beardslee WR (2019) Master Clinician Review: Parental Depression and Family Health and Wellness: What clinicians can do and reflections on opportunities for the future. *J Am Acad.Child Adolescent Psychiatry,* 58(8) 759-767.

Bearer CF, Swick AR, O'Riordan MA, Cheng B (1999) Ethanol inhibits L1 mediated neurite out growth in postnatal rat cerebellar cells. *J.Biol. Chem.* 274(19) 12364-12370.

Bearer CF, Welman KA, Tong M, Mooney SM (n 2015) choline ameliorates deficits in balance caused by acute neonatal ethanol exposure. *Cerebellum,* Aug 14, (4), 413-20.

Bell CC, Chimata R. NDPAE associated with prenatal exposure to alcohol, Chicago, USA, Power point presentation.

Bell SH, Stade B, Reynolds JM, Rasmussen C, Andrew G, Hwang PA, Corlen P (2010) Fetal Alcohol Spectrum Disorder linked to high prevalence of Epilepsy. *Alcoholism: Clin Exp. Res.*

Bhatia S, Drake DM, Miller L, Wells PG (2019) Oxidative stress and DNA damage in the mechanism of fetal alcohol spectrum disorders. Special Issue. *Fetal Alcohol Spectrum Disorders,* Vol 111, Issue 12, 714-748.

Bleiberg E (2001) Treating Personality Disorders in Children and Adolescents. *A Relational Approach.* The Guilford Press, New York, London

Bolhuis K (2019) Editorial: Conduct Disorder as a neurodevelopmental condition: White matter brain microstructure and the importance of gender, callous traits and development. *Journal Amer. Acad. Child Adolesc. Psychiatry* Vol 58, No 123, 1154-1156.

Bond NW, Di Gusto (1976) Effects of prenatal alcohol consumption on open field behavior and alcohol preference in rats. *Psychopharmacologia.* 46, 163.

Boronat S, Vicente M, Lainez E, Sanchez-Montanez S, Vasquez E, Martinez-Ribat L, Del Lapo M (2017) Seizures and electro-encephalopathy findings in 61apients with Fetal Alcohol Spectrum Disorders, *Eur. J. Med Genet.,* January, 60(1)72-78.

British Psychological Society (2016) *Psychological therapies and people who have intellectual disabilities.* Ed. Nigel Beail published Royal College of Psychiatrists, UK.

Brown J, Oberoi P, Lang-Mc Gee J, Warnick Judge Tony, Winkauf E, Herrick S (2015) *A review of criminal justice system for professionals.* FASD. FASD and confabulation, www. sofoceanindien.org/en/home.

Brown Novick N (2008) Sexually inappropriate behaviors in patients with Fetal Alcohol Spectrum Disorders, Chapter 9, 179-196, in *ADHD and FASDs,* 2nd Ed, Editor O'Malley KD, Nova Science Publishers New York.

Burd L (2012) *FASD: Diagnosis informed Care*. University of North Dakota. USA.

Buxton B (2005) *Damaged Angels.* Carroll and Graf Publishers, NY.

Calarusso CA (1987) Mother is that you? *The psychoanalytic study of the child.* Eds. Solnit AJ, Neubauer PB, VOL. 42, New Haven Press, USA.

Carelli RM, Wightman RM (2004) Functional micro circuitry in the acccumbens underlying drug addiction: insights from real-time signaling during behavior. *Current Opinions in Neurobiology,* 14, 763-768, www.sciencedirect.com.

Carmichael Olson H (2006) The Families Moving Forward Project. *Promising research helps families raising children with FASD. Iceberg Newsletter.* Univ. of Washington. USA, www.fasiceberg.org/newsletter.htm.

Carpenter B, Blackburn C, Egerton J Eds. (2014). *Fetal Alcohol Spectrum Disorders. Interdisciplinary Perspectives,* Routledge Publishers, London, New York.

Catastrophe British TV series started 2015, Sharon Horgan and Rob Delaney originators.

Catterick M, Curran L (2014) Understanding fetal alcohol spectrum disorders. *A guide for parents, carers, professionals,* Amazon. co.uk.

Chasnoff I, Wells A, King l (2015) Missed diagnosis in foster and adopted children with prenatal alcohol exposure. *Pediatrics,* vol. 138, no 2, 266-271.

Chudley AE (2010) Genetic factors contributing to FASD: In *Fetal Alcohol Spectrum Disorder: Management and Policy Perspectives of FASD.* 1ST Edition. Eds. Riley EP, Clarren S, Weinbergh J Jonsson E, Weilheim Germany, Wiley –VCH Verlag Publishers.

Church M Watts s (2007) assessment of Mental Capacity. A flow chart guideline. *Brit J Psych. Bulletin,* Vol 31, issue 8, doi 10/1192/pb.bp 106.011353.

Ciccetti D Ganniban J Barnett D (1991) Contributions from the study of high risk populations to understanding the development of emotion regulation, In J Garber & K Dodge Eds. *The development of emotion regulation and dysregulation,* pp 15-48, Cambridge University Press, New York.

Ciccietti D, Richters JE (1997) Examining the conceptual and scientific underpinnings of research in developmental psychopathology. *Development and Psychopathology,* 9, 189-191.

Cook JL, Green LR, Lilley CM, Anderson SM, Baldwin ME, Chudley AE et al. (2016) A guideline for diagnosis across the lifespan. *CMAJ,* Feb 16, 188(3) 191-97.

Corito V, Ceccanti M, Coccurello R, Ferraguti G, Ciafre S, Tirossa MF (2019) Nerve Growth Factor and Brain Derived Neurotrophic Factor alterations by prenatal alcohol exposure. *Current Neuropharmacology,* Vol. 17, Issue 4. *DNA Research* 15(4) August, doi 10. 2174/1570159x1566617082510138.

Coles C (1994) Critical periods for prenatal alcohol exposure: evidence from animal and human studies. *Alcohol Health and Research World.* Vol 18, issue 1, 22.

Crawley J Smith W Murphy M (2013) *Atlas of the Great Irish Famine.* Publishers Cork University Press.

Cummings EM, Davie P Simpson K (1994) Marital conflict, gender and children's appraisal and coping efficacy as mediators of child adjustment. *Journal of Family Psychology,* 8, 141-149.

Cummings EM, Davies PT, Campbell SB (2000) *Developmental Psychopathology and Family Process. Theory, Research and Clinical Implications.* Publishers The Guilford Press, New York, London.

Darlington R, Margo J, Sternberg S, Borks BR (2011) *Teenage girls' self esteem is more than skin deep-through the looking glass*. Demos, London.

Davies R, Butler N, Goldstein H (1972) *From birth to seven The National Children's Bureau.* Longmans, UK.

Deltour L, Ang HL, Drester G (1996) Ethanol inhibition of retinoic acid and synthesis as a potential mechanism for development of Fetal Alcohol Syndrome. *FASEB Journal,* 10, 1050-57.

Densmore R (2011) FASD Relationships. What I have learned about Fetal Alcohol Spectrum Disorder, Publishers Dory Spirit Books. Salmon Arm, BC, Canada.

Duke University (2016) Understanding Fetal Alcohol Spectrum Disorders–Rise. Duke University, Chapter 3, Neurotransmitter systems important in neuropsychological and behavioral effects of prenatal alcohol exposure.

Eberhart JK, Harris LA (2013) Understanding variability in ethanol teratogenicity. *Proceedings Maternal Academy of Sciences.* PMAS, USA, April 2nd, 110, 14, 5285-5286.

Emhart CB, Sokol RJ, Martier S, Martin P, Nadler D, Ager JW, Wolf A (1987) Alcohol teratogenicity in the human: A detailed assessment of specificity, critical periods and threshold. *Am J Obstet. Gynaecol.,* Jan. 156(1) 33-9.

Elliott E, Payne J, Morris, Haan E, Bower C (2008) Fetal Alcohol Syndrome: a prospective surveillance study. *Archives of Diseases in Children,* 93, 732-737.

Elliott EJ (2014) Fetal Alcohol Spectrum Disorder Australian Perspectives. Chapter 23, 294-305, in FASD. *Interdisciplinary Perspectives.* Eds. Carpenter B, Blackburn C, Egerton J, Routledge Publishers., London, New York.

Ellsoff T (2014) Neurodevelopmental Disorder Prenatal Alcohol Exposure (NDPAE) Smart Speech Therapy. USA.

Ernak G (2015) *Emerging Medical Technologies*. World Scientific, ISBN 978-981-4675-80-2.

FASD-HUB. Australia. (2019) Brain Structure and Neurology.updated10/10/19.

FASDHub.org.au/understanding-FASD/What-is-FASD/brain impairment –in FASD.

Flynn EP (2000) Issues in Health Care Ethics, Chapters 1, Ethical decision making in the health care context, and 16, Roles of the Courts, Government and Professional Societies in Health Care Ethics., Prentice –Hall Publishers. New Jersey, USA.

Gill I, O'Malley KD (2015) Motor and Sensory issues in FASDs, Poster presentation, AACAP Annual meeting, Oct. San Antonio, USA.

Glick M, Zigler E (1992) Premorbid competence and the course and outcomes of psychiatric disorders Chapter 22, 497-513. Risk and Protective factors in

Developmental Psychopathology. Eds Rolf J, Masten AS, Ciccetti D, Neuchterlein KH, Weintrub S, Cambridge University Press, Cambridge UK, New York, USA.

Goodlet CR, Horn KH (2000) Mechanism of alcohol –induced damage to the developing nervous system. Pubs. NIAAA, NIH, GOV. USA.

Golden J (1999) An argument that goes back to the womb. The demedicalisation of Fetal Alcohol Syndrome. (1973-1992). *Journal of social history.* Volk 33, no2, 269-298.

Govorko D, Bekdash RA, Zhong C, Sakar DK (2017) Male germline transmits fetal alcohol effect on hypothalamic proopiomelanocortin gene across generations. *Biol. Psychiatry.* 72(5) 378-88.

Gray R, Henderson J (2006) Review of the fetal effects of prenatal alcohol exposure. Report to, the Department of Health. National Perinatal Epidemiology Unit, Oxford. (www.npeu.ox.ac.uk/alcoholreport).

Granato A, Dering B (2018) Alcohol and the developing brain. Why neurons die and how survivors change *Int. J. Mol. Sci.* 19, 2992-3004.

Gubitosi –Klug R, Larimer CG, Bearer CF (2007) L1 cell adhesion molecule is neuroprotective of alcohol induced cell death. *Neurotoxicology,* 28(3) 457-462.

Hannigan JH (1996) What research with animals is telling us about alcohol-related neurodevelopmental disorder. *Pharmacol Biochem Behav,* 55(4) 488-499.

Haltigan JD (2019) Editorial: Putting Practicality into "p": Leveraging General Factor Models of Psychopathology in Clinical Intervention. *Journal American Academy of Child and Adolescent Psychiatry,* Vol. 58, No 8, August, 751-753.

Hawkes S (2013) Gender and Global Health: Evidence, Policy and Inconvenient Truths. *Lancet,* Vol. 381, May 18th, 1783-1787.

Haycock PC (2009) Fetal Alcohol Spectrum Disorders. The Epigenetic Perspective. *Biology of Reproduction.* doi 10.1095/biolreprod.108.074690, May 27th.

Heljmans BT, Tobi EW, Stein AD et al. (2008) Persistent epigenetic differences associated with prenatal exposure to alcohol. *Proc Nat. Acad. Sci.*, 105, 17046-49, USA.

Hibiel BJ, Guttorsonsson U, Ahlstron S et al. (2009) The 2007 ESPAD report on substance use among students at 35 European countries. The Swedish Council on Alcohol and Other Drugs.

Hobson RP (1993) The intersubjective domain: Approaches from developmental psychopathology. *Journal of the Psychoanalytic Association,* 41(Suppl.), 167-192.

Holfon S, friendly M (2013) *Inclusion of young children with disabilities in regulated child care in Canada.* Occasional Paper No 27. Child Resource and Research Unit, Canada.

Huggins JE, Grant T, O'Malley KD, Streissguth AP (2008) Suicide Attempts among adults with fetal alcohol spectrum disorders: Clinical considerations. *Mental Health Aspects of Developmental Disabilities,* Vol 11, No 2, 1-9.

Ipsioglu OS, Smith S, Berger M, Salmon A, Rauscher A, Stockler SD, Weinberg, J (2016) Is iron supplementation a 'disruptive intervention'? Sleep-wake behaviors and iron deficiency in prenatal alcohol exposure (PAE) –from animal research to clinical implications. Session 51, European FASD meeting, 4th European Conference, Royal Holloway Hospital, London September 12-14th.

Jan JE, Asante KO, Conry JL et al. (2010) Sleep health issues for children with FASD: clinical considerations. *International Journal of Pediatrics* http://www.nchi.nlm.nih.gov/pmc/articles/PMC2913852/November.

Johnston AD (2013) *Drink: The intimate relationship between women and alcohol.* Fourth Estate Publishers, USA.

Jones KL, Smith DW (1973) Recognition of the fetal alcohol syndrome in early infancy. *Lancet,* 2; 999-1001.

Kadouceur CD (2012) Amygdala response to emotional faces: A neural marker of risk for Bipolar Disorder? *J. Am acad. Child Adolesc, Psychiatry,* Vol 51, No 3, 235, -237.

Kannabiran M, Pearson R, Narayan G (2007) *Perinatal Psychiatry. BMA Careers.* March 3rd, 75-76.

Kellerman T (2010) Prenatal alcohol and the Brain. NIAAA Publication. FAS and the brain (updated from 2003). USA.

Kelly K (2018) Personal communication re FASD legal advocacy, Seattle.

Kinada M, Hara N, Kawnchi S, Kagawa N, Nago T, Ikeda Y (2017) Mechanism underlying neuro-inflammation and neurodevelopmental toxicity in the mouse neocortex following prenatal exposure to ethanol. *Scientific Reports,* 7, Article no. 49345.

Kolko D (2002) *Handbook on fire-setting in children and youth.* Academic Press.

Kristjanson, A., Wilsnack, S., Zvartau, E., Tsoy, M., & Novikov, B. (2007). Alcohol Use in Pregnant and Nonpregnant Russian Women. *Alcoholism: Clinical and Experimental Research,* 31(2), 299-307.doi:10.1111/j.1530-0277.2006.00315.

Krueger RF, Kotov R, Watson D (2018) Progress in achieving quantitative classification of psychopathology, *World Psychiatry,* 17, 282-293.

Larsen JK, Brand N, Bermond B, Hijman R (2003) Cognitive and emotional characteristics of alexithymia. A review of neurobiological studies. *Journal of Psychosomatic Research,* 54, 533-541.

Le Strat Y, Ramoz N, Shuman G et al. (2008) Molecular Genetics of alcohol dependence and related phenotypes. *Current genomics.* (9) 444-457.

Linask KK (2015) Folic acid supplementation in animals with prenatal alcohol exposure. Tallinn, Estonia, Conference on FASD.

Lingford-Hughes A (2020) Can neuroscience influence national policy on addiction and should it do so? Distinguished Lecture, Royal Society Medicine, London, March 19th.

Lussier AA, Weinberg J, Kabor MS (2017) Epigenetic studies of fetal alcohol spectrum disorders: where are we now? *Epigenomics,* Vol 9, No 3. On line doi.org /10.2217/epi-2016-0163.

Malbin D (1997) Personal Communication, Portland, Oregon USA.

Manlak l, Jones T, Ijaz S, Edwards HB, Savoic J, Leach V, MooreTHM, Van Hinke S, Lewis SJ, Donovan JL, Smith GD, Fraser A, Zuccalo L (2020) Evidence of effects of prenatal alcohol exposure on offspring birth weight and neurodevelopment from systematic review of 23 quasi –experimental studies. *Int J. epidemiology,* Jan 29th, doi.org/10.1-093/ice/dyz272.

Manically R, Carlucci E, Palminiello S, Saso L (2011) Oxidative stress and brain diseases. Biomarkeand analytic methodologies. *Indian Journal of Biotechnology.* Vol. 10, 395-403.

Martinez Frias, Bernejo E, Rodriquez –Pinilla E, Luis Frias J. (2004) Risk for congenital anomalies associated with different sporadic and daily dose of alcohol consumption during pregnancy: A case control study. *Clinical and Molecular Teratology,* Vol. 70, Issue 4, 194-2000.

Mason S Zhou FL (2015) Editorial. Genetics and epigenetics of fetal alcohol spectrum disorders, *Front Genet,* April 16th, 6, 146.

Matlow JN, Aleksa K, Lubetsky A, Koren G (2012) The detection and quantification of ethyl glucuride in placental tissue and placental perfusate by head space solid mass micro extraction coupled with gas chromatography –mass spectroscopy. *J Popl. Ther. Clin. Pharmacol.,* 19(3) 473-82.

Mattson SN, Crocker N, Nyguen TT (2011) Fetal alcohol spectrum disorders: neuropsychological and behavioral features. *Neuropsychology review.* 2, 84-101.

Max J Castillo CS, Lindberg SD, Arndt S (1999) The Neuropsychiatric Rating Scale. Reliability and Validity. *J. Amer Acad. Child Adolesc. Psychiatry,* (3) 297-304.

Mc Donnell AM, Dang CH (2013) Basic review of cytochrome 450 system. *J Adv. Pract. Oncol.* July/Aug. (4) 263-268.

Mc Hugh RK, Wijderson S, Greenfield SF (2014) Epidemiology of substance abuse in reproductive –age women. Obstetrics and Gynecology Clinics of North America. 41(2) 177-89.

MC Kowen L (2020) *We are the Luckiest. The surprising magic of sober life.* Amazon on line, USA.

Mead EA, Sakar DK (2014) Fetal Alcohol Spectrum Disorders and their transmission through genetic and epigenetic mechanisms. *Front Genet.* 5, 154.

Menninger K (1938) *Man against Himself,* Harvest Books. USA.

Miranda RC (2012) MicroRNAs and fetal brain development. Implications for ethanol teratology during 2nd trimester period of neurogenesis *Front Genet,* 3, 77.

Monnott M, Lovallo WR, Nixon SJ, Ross E (2002) Neurological basis of deficits in affective prosody comprehension among alcoholics and fetal-alcohol exposed adults. *J Neuropsychiatry, Clin Neurosci,* 14, 3, 321-328.

Mukarjee R. (2014) Fetal Alcohol Spectrum Disorders. Exploring Prevention and Management, Mukarjee R copyright, Maastricht, published PhD thesis.

Mukarjee RAS, Layton M, Yacoub E, Turk JT, 2011) Autism and autistic traits in people exposed to heavy prenatal alcohol: data from a clinical series and nested case control study. *Advances in Mental Health and Learning Disability* 5(1) 43-49.

Nasser M (1995) The rise and fall of anti-psychiatry. *Psychiatric Bulletin,* 19, 743-746.

Neuchterlein KH, Phipps-Yonas S, Driscoll R, Garmezy N (1992) Vulnerability factors in children at risk: anomalies in social behavior, Chapter 20, 445-479, *Risk and Protective factors in Development of Psychopathology*, Eds, Rolf J, Masten AS, Ciccetti D, Neuchterlein KH, Weintrub S, Cambridge University Press, Cambridge UK, New York, USA.

Nicita F, Verotti A et al. (2014) Seizures in Fetal Alcohol Spectrum Disorders Evaluation of clinical, electro-encephalopathy and neuroradiologic features in pediatric case series, Epielpsia, Jan. 55(6) 60-6.

Ngai YF, Salistyoningram DC, O'Neill R, Innis SM, Weinberg J, Devlin AM (2015) Prenatal alcohol exposure alters methyl metabolism and programs serotonin transporter and glucocorticoid receptor expression in the brain. *Am. J Physiol. Integr. Comp. Physiol., Sept.* 309 (5) 613-622.

Norton, A. (2018). Discourses of motherhood and stigma production: FASD public awareness-raising in British Columbia, 1979–2015. Retrieved from https://dspace.library.uvic.ca//handle/1828/9320.

Offer D, Sabshin M Eds. (1991) The Diversity of Normal Behavior. Further Contributions to Normality. Basic Books, USA.

O'Higgins A, Sebba J, Luke M (2015) What is the relationship between being in care and the educational outcomes of children? Rees Centre for Research in fostering and Education. University of Oxford, UK, ISBN: 978-0-9929071-8-1.

Olson HC (2015) Advancing recognition of Fetal Alcohol Spectrum Disorders; The proposed DSM 5 diagnosis of neurobehavioral disorder associated with prenatal alcohol exposure. *Curr. Dev. Disord. Rep.* 2(3) 187-198.

O'Malley KD (2003) Youth with Co morbid Disorders, Chapter 13 IN The New Community Psychiatry, eds Pumariega A, Winters, Jossey Boss Publishers, San Francisco, USA.

O'Malley KD, Rich S (2012) Clinical Implications of a link between Fetal Alcohol Spectrum Disorders (FASD) and Autism or Asperger's Disorder: A neurodevelopmental frame for helping and understanding and management Chapter 20, in *Recent Advances in Autism Spectrum Disorders,* Vol 1, (FIitzgerald M., ed.) www open. intech.

O'Malley KD (2014) *The Knotted Cord. Transgenerational Alcohol Related Neurodevelopmental Disorder*. Nova Science Publishers, New York.

O'Malley KD (2014) Developmental Psychiatric Disorders in children, adolescents and young adults with fetal alcohol spectrum disorders. A transgenerational approach to diagnosis and management. Chapter 19, 241-261, in Carpenter B, Blackburn C, Egerton J, FASD, Interdisciplinary Perspectives, Routledge Publishers, London, New York.

O'Malley KD (2016) The psychopharmacology of children and adolescents with NDPAE, previously FASD. Presentation available, Intellectual Disability conference, 'Pros and cons of using medication in children and adolescents with developmental disorders'. RSM, London, January 22nd.

O'Malley KD (2018) Travelin' Still Poetry collection, Dornan Printers, Belfast.

O'Malley KD, Owens A (2018) NDPAE in child as marker for early mortality in birth mother. Presentation, NDPAE Diagnosis and Management, Intellectual Disability Conference, RSM, London May 18th.

O'Malley KD (2020), Book chapter, The positive role of medication in FASD, or NDPAE in Prevention, recognition and management of Fetal Alcohol Spectrum Disorders. A Practical Guide. Mukarjee R, Alton N Eds. Springer Europe Publishers, IN PRESS.

O'Neill E (2011) Pre and postnatal growth deficiencies in FAS. *Embryo Project Encyclopedia,* 05-04, http/ermbryo-asu.edu/handle/10776/2099.

Patten A, Brocardo PS, Mohapel JG, Christie BR (2014) oxidative stress in fetal alcohol spectrum Disorders-Insights for the development of antioxidant-based therapies. *Systems Biology of Free Radicals and Antioxidants.* 645-667.

Peterson J, Kirchner HL, Xue W, Mines, Singer LT, Bearer CF (2008) Fatty acid esters in meconium are associated with poor neurodevelopmental outcomes to 2 years of age. *J Pediatr.* 152 (6) 788-92.

Pham-Huy LA, He H, Pham-Huy C (2008) Free Radicals, Antioxidants in Disease and Health. *Int. J. Biomed. Sci.,* Jun. 4 (2) 89-96.

Plant M (1987) Women, drinking and society. Tavistock Publications, London.

Plant M (2014) Woman's alcohol consumption in the UK. Chapter 4, 39-50, IN Carpenter B. Blackburn C, Egerton Eds. FASD, Interdisciplinary Perspectives, Routledge Publishers, London, New York.

Plant M (2018) Women and alcohol presentation, Royal Society Medicine, Intellectual Disability Conference on NDPAE. May 21st, London.

Rae HE, O'Malley KD (2017) Foetal Alcohol Spectrum Disorders and Neurodevelopmental Disorder Prenatal Alcohol Exposure. What Podiatrists need to know. Podiatry Now, Aug., 20(8) 14-16.

Ramanathan R, Wilkemeyer MF, Mittal B, Perides G, Charness ME (1996) Alcohol inhibits cell-cell adhesion mediated by human L1. *J. Cell Biol.* 133(2) 381-90.

Rasmussen C, Martens KK, Denys K, Badry D, Henneveld D, Wyper K, Grant T (2012) The effectiveness of a community-based intervention program for women at risk to a child with FASD. Comm. *Mental Health journal,* 48, 12-21.

Rennick J, Asker R (1983) Ethanol sensitive times for the human conceptus. *Early Hum. Dev.*, 8(2) 99-111.

Rich S (2016) The Silent epidemic. A child psychiatrist journey beyond death row. Understanding and treating NDPAE. Lulu Publishing/Amazon, USA.

Rogers C, Luby J (2011) Sensory Over-Responsivity: A Diagnosis Whose Time Has Come? Editorial; *Journal Amer. Acad. Child Adolesc. Psychiatry* Vol 50, no 12, Dec. 1205-1206.

Rowland M, Tozer TM (2011) Clinical pharmacokinetics and pharmacodynamics. *Concepts and Applications*. 4th Ed. Baltimore, Lippinicott Williams and Williams.

Royal Society Medicine (2015) The pros and cons of using medication with children and adolescents with developmental disorders. Intellectual Disability Section Conference, January 22nd, London Power point presentations available.

Royal Society Medicine (2019) Conference, Parental Mental Illness and its impacts. London, Dec 13th, Presentations available.

Russell, R. (2018). Addressing Fetal Alcohol Spectrum Disorder: Problem intractability and the search for solutions. Retrieved from https://eprints.utas.edu.au/23918/.

Rutter M (1992) Psychosocial resilience and protective mechanisms. Chapter 9, 181-214, *Risk and Protective factors in Development of Psychopathology*. Eds., Rolf J, Masten AS, Cicchetti D, Neuchterlein KH, Weintrub S, Cambridge University Press. Cambridge UK, New York USA.

Rutter M (1998) Some research considerations on intergenerational continuation and discontinuation: comments on the Special section. *Developmental Psychology,* 34, (6), 335-364.

Rutter M, Kumsta R, Schlotz W, Sonuga Burke E (2011) Longitudinal studies using a "natural experiment" design.: The case of adoptees from Romanian Institutions. *J Amer Acad Child Adoesc. Psychiatry,* Vol 51, No 8, 762-768.

Ryan S, Chionnaith MN (2006) On the Spectrum: Similarities and Differences between students with Fetal Alcohol Spectrum Disorders and Autism Spectrum Disorders in Ireland, *Journal Special Needs Education,* 9, 43-52.

Sameroff AJ, Seifer R (1992) Early contributors to developmental risk. Chapter 3, 52-66, *Risk and Protective factors in the Development of Psychopathology*. Eds. Rolf J, Masten AS, Cicchetti D, Neuchterlein KH, Weintrub S, Cambridge University Press, Cambridge UK, New York USA.

Sampson PD, Streissguth AP, Bookstein FL, Barr HM (2000) On Categorizations in analysis of alcohol teratogenesis. *Environmental Health Perspectives,* doi.org/10.1289/ehp.00108s3421.

Shankar R, Ashby S (2019) Sudden unexpected death in Epilepsy (SUDEP) in people with intellectual disability and/or Autism. Willful blindness? Intellectual Disability Conference on Autism, November 11th, RSM, London.

Shalev A, Merranko J, Goldstein T, Miklowitz DJ, Axelson D, Goldstein BI, Brent D, Monk K, Hickey MB, Hafeman DM, Sakolsky D, Diler R, Birmaher B, (2019) A Longitudinal Study of Family Functioning of Parents Diagnosed with Bipolar Disorder. *J Am acad. Child Adolesc. Psychiatry,* Vol 58, No 1-0, 961-970.

SIGN (2019) *Scottish Intercollegiate Guidelines Network.* Edinburgh. Scotland. www.signs.ac.uk/sign-156-children-and-young people-prenatally exposed to alcohol.

Stalcup B (editor) (2000) Ethics. Greenhaven Press. San Diego, USA.

Stein A. Prof. (2019) Paper presentation, The Influence of perinatal depression on child development. understanding mechanisms. Conference, Parental Mental Illness and its impacts. RSM, London, Dec 13th.

Stoller JM, Holmes, LB (1999) Under recognition of prenatal effects of infants of known alcohol abusing women, *Journal of Pediatrics,* 135(4) 430-436.

Stafford Clark D (1969) Psychiatry for students. George Unwin and Unwin Publishers, UK.

Stratton K, Howe C, Battaglia F (eds.) *Fetal Alcohol Syndrome: Diagnosis, Epidemiology, Prevention and Treatment*. Washington DC, National Academy Press,

Streissguth AP, Landesman-Dwyer S, Martin J, Smith D (1980) Teratogenic effects of alcohol in humans and laboratory animals, 18 July, Science, Vol. 209, 353-361.

Streissguth AP, Barr HM, Sampson PD (1990) Moderate prenatal alcohol exposure: effects on child IQ and learning problems. *Alcoholism: Clin. and Exp Res.* Vol 14, Issue 5, 662-669.

Streissguth AP, O'Malley KD (2000) Neuropsychiatric sequelae and long term consequences of fetal alcohol spectrum disorders. *Seminars in Clinical Neuropsychiatry.* 5, 177-190.

Stern DN (1983) *The interpersonal world of the infant: A view from Psychoanalysis and developmental psychology.* New York, Basic Books.

Tomkins DM, Sellers EM (2001) Addiction and the brain: the role of neurotransmitters in the cause and treatment of drug dependence. *CMAJ,* Mar 20th, 164(6), 817-821.

Triet S, Beaulieu C (2018) Imaging Brain structure in Fetal Alcohol Spectrum Disorders. In *Ethical and Legal Perspectives in Fetal Alcohol Spectrum Disorders.* doi.10.1007/978-3-319-71755-5.6.

Volkow N. Koob G (2015) Brain disease model of addiction: why is it so controversial? *Lancet,* August, Vo 2, 677-678, www.lancet.com/psychiatry.

Walkup J (2019) AACAP, Positive Parenting Practices. Lecture on line training. Washington DC, USA.

Wells JL, Sawaya AL, Wibaek R et al. (2019) The Double Burden of malnutrition. Aetiological pathways and consequences for health. *Lancet,* Vol.395, Jan. 4th, 75-88.

Wessel J, Endrikat J, Buscher U. (2002) Frequency of denial of pregnancy results and epidemiological significance of a 1-year prospective study in Berlin. *Acta Obstet. Gynae. Scand.*, 81 (11) 10212-7.

Weyrauch D, Schwartz M, Hart B, Klug MG, Burd L (2017) Comorbid mental disorders in fetal alcohol spectrum disorders: a systematic review *Journal of Developmental and Behavioral Pediatrics,* May, 38 (4) 283-291.

Wilhelm CJ, Guizzetti M (2015) Fetal Alcohol Spectrum Disorders: An overview from the glial perspective. *Front Integr. Neurosci.,* 9, 65.

Wilson EO (2000), Biological imperative Cause People to Act Ethically, in *Ethics,* ed. Stalcup B, 29-36.

Windham GC, Von Behren J, Fenster L, Schaefer C, Swan SH (1997) Moderate alcohol consumption and risk of spontaneous abortion. *Epidemiology,* Vol. 8, No 5, 509-514.

Winnicott D (1984) *Through Paediatrics to Psychoanalysis.* Collected Papers. Hogarth Press, London.

Working Moms Canadian TV series started 2017, Wolft Rabbit Entertainment, Reitman C and Steinberg P, originators.

Young C, Shantar R et al. (2016a) Does intellectual disability in epilepsy (SUDEP) increase risk seizure. *European Journal of Epilepsy.* Vol 25, 112-116.

Young S, Absoud M, Blackburn C, Branney P, Colley B, Farrag E, Fleisher S, Gregory G, Gudjonnson GH, Kim K, O'Malley KD, Plant M, Rodriquez A, Ozer s, Takon I, Woodhouse E, Mukarjee R (2016) Guidelines for identification and treatment of individuals with ADHD and associated Fetal Alcohol Spectrum Disorders., based on Expert Consensus. *BMJ Psychiatry,* 16, no 324. doi 10.1086/s12888-016-1027-y.

Zero to Three (2005) *Diagnostic Classification of Mental health and Developmental Disorders of Infancy and Early Childhood* (revised edition), Washington DC, Zero to Three Publications.

Zieff CD, Schwartz –Bloom RD, Williams M (2016) *Understanding Fetal Alcohol Spectrum Disorders.* A Comprehensive Guide for Pre-K8 Educators. Chapter 3, Effects of prenatal exposure on brain development and postnatal function.

Key References for Epilogue in the Knotted Cord. An Update on Transgenerational Alcohol. 2020.

Barros NG, Ribot LM, Boronot S, Mangado L, Furnado V, Mendionoz J, Vacquez E, Montnez AS, Martin N, Jacos C, de Capo Casanelles M (2016). Psychiatric disorders in a sample of Russian adopted children with Fetal Alcohol Spectrum Disorder. Paper presentation, International European FASD conference, Royal Holloway Hospital, London.

Bateson G, Jackson DD, Haley J, Weakland JH (1963) A Note on the Double Bind-1962, *Family Process,* Vol.2, 154-161.

Biddle Z, O'Callaghan FV, Finlay-Jones AC, Reid NE (2020). Caregivers of children with FASD: psychosocial factors for self-compassion as a potential intervention target. *Mindfulness,* 11, 2189-2198.

Blair RJR (2003) Neurobiological basis of psychopathology. *Editorial, Brit. J. Psychiatry,* 182, 5-7.

Bolhuis K (2019) Editorial. Conduct Disorder as a neurodevelopmental condition: white brain mattermicrostrucrture and the importance of gender, callosal triats and development. *Journal Amer. Acad. Child and Adolesc. Pyschiatry,* Vol 58, no 12, 1154-1155.

Figley C (1995) Coping with Secondary Traumatic Stress disorder in those whom treat the traumatized. Publishers Brunner/Mazel, New York.

Gelo J, O'Malley KD (2003) Family stress in parenting a child or adolescent with FASD. *Iceberg,* Vol. 13, No 1, 1-4.

O'Malley PP (1999) Can psycopaths be treated? *Editorial. The Irish Medical Journal,* Vol. 39, no 4, 124-126.

O'Malley KD (2012) Reactive Attachment Disorder. PTSD and FASD. Do they commonly exist in inter-counrty adopted children? Invited Plenary, Inter –Country Adoption Conference, Cork, January 19th.

Raine A, Leney T, Biherle S, La Casse L, Calletti P (2001) Reduced prefrontal gray matter volume and reduced autonomic function in Antisocial Personality Disorder. Arch. Gen. Psychiatry, 57, 119-127.

Siever LJ, Davis KL (1991) A psychobiological perspective on the Personality Disorder. *Am. J Psychiatry,* 148, 1647-1658.

References (Appendix)

A.D.D. *Warehouse,* (2011-2012) current web site. USA.

Byrne, S, (2013). *"The Irish drink problem is hidden in plain sight, and it's escalating."* Evening Herald, Comment, Monday February 25th, Ireland.

Densmore, R (2011). *FASD Relationships. What I have learned about Fetal Alcohol Spectrum Disorder,* Published by Freisens Corporation, Altona, MB, Canada.

H.S.E. (2013). *Study on Costs to Society of Problem Alcohol Use in Ireland.*

Kulp, J (2004). *Our Fascinating Journey.* 2nd Edition, Better Endings. New Beginnings. Publisher, Brooklyn Park, MN, USA.

Malbin D. (2012). Fetal Alcohol/Neurobehavioral Conditions. Understanding and application of a brain –based approach. *A collection of information for parents & professionals.* 3rd Edition, FASCETS Inc. Portland, USA.

O'Malley KD (Editor) (2008). *ADHD and Fetal Alcohol Spectrum Disorders*, 2nd Edition. Nova Science Publishers, New York, USA.

O'Malley, KD (2010). *Fetal Alcohol Spectrum Disorders,* 175. *Encyclopaedia of Psychopharmacology,* Publishers Springer-Verlag, Berlin Heidelberg.

O'Malley KD (2011). Chapter 24, 'Fetal Alcohol Spectrum Disorders' in *The Sage Handbook of Developmental Disorders*. London, California, New Delhi, Singapore.

Orakwue, N, Curran, L, Savage, M, O'Malley, KD (2012). *Fetal Alcohol Spectrum Disorders. Pre-Training Evaluation: What the Irish Social Workers are Saying.* The Irish Social Worker, 17-21.

Statton KR, Rowe, CJ, Battaglia, FC (1996). *Fetal alcohol syndrome: diagnosis, epidemiology, prevention and treatment in medicine.* National Academy Press, Washington DC. USA.

Streissguth AP (1997). Fetal Alcohol Syndrome. *A Guide for Families and Communities.* Paul. H. Brookes Publishing, Baltimore, London, Toronto, Sydney.

Tanner Halverson, P (1997). *Strategies for parents and caregivers of children with FAS or FAE,* www. nofas.org/main/strategy.htm, USA.

ABOUT THE AUTHOR

Dr. Kieran D. O'Malley, M.B., B.CH., B.A.O., D.A.B.P.N.

Child and Adolescent Psychiatrist

Slievemore Clinic, Stillorgan, Co. Dublin, Ireland

Email: kierandomalley@gmail.com

Kieran Darragh O'Malley was born in Belfast, N. Ireland, & attended Clongowes Wood College School in Naas. Co. Kildare. He went to Medical School at University College Dublin, Ireland and qualified in 1972, with honours in Paediatrics and Psychiatry.

Post-Graduate Training: He completed formal registrar training in Community Medicine at South East Thames Regional Health Authority, Croydon, Bromley Area Health District and Guys Hospital Health District, London, UK. (1975-1977).

Also he completed formal postgraduate residency training in Family Medicine at The Royal Alexandra Hospital, Edmonton, Alberta, Canada (1978), and has practiced as a Family Physician in both Canada & Ireland. He was a member of the Canadian College of Family Physicians (1977-1983) He delivered & managed over 250 pregnancies, and was the GP member of the Royal Alexandra Hospital Perinatal Committee (1978-83).

His Adult Psychiatry training was done at Mc Gill University, Montreal, Quebec & University of Alberta, Edmonton in Canada. His Child Psychiatry & Fellowship Training was done at Cornell Medical School, New York, USA & Alberta Children's Hospital, University of Calgary, Alberta (Completed in 1987). He did MSc in Clinical & Theoretical Psychoanalytic Psychotherapy through University of East London and Centre for Psychotherapy, Belfast (2008-2009).

Awards: 1971 Ciba/Geigy Fellowship Award, McGill University, 1986 Best Psychiatric Resident Paper, 1996 Monnex/Alberta Medical Association Scholarship, 2001 Catcher in the Rye Award, AACAP, Work Group on Community Systems of Care, 2002

& 2004 One of America's Top Psychiatrists, Consumers' Research Council of America, 2011 Starfish International FASD Award.

Academic: He is a Board Certified Psychiatrist & Board Eligible Child Psychiatrist. Was a Visiting Scholar in the Department of Psychiatrists & Behavioral Sciences, University of Washington, Seattle, based in the Fetal Alcohol & Drug Unit from 1997-2000 & subsequently was appointed Acting Assistant Professor from 2000-2004, later a Lecturer in the Department of Psychiatry & Behavioral Sciences at the University of Washington (2004-2006). He has presented invited lectures, seminars & workshops on FAS/FASD in Canada, USA, Ireland, UK, Finland, France, Italy, Belgium, Holland and Australia. These include the Mater Hospital, Belfast & Trinity College, Dublin (April 2005), Alaska Psychiatrists mtg. Girdwood, Alaska (April 2006), All Ireland Psychiatrists Mtg. Belfast (Nov. 2006), 2nd International FASD conf. (Vancouver 2008), European Commission, Strasbourg (Sept. 2008), 3rd Int. FASD conf. Victoria (Mar.2009), European Commission, Brussels (Sept. 2009, Sept.2010), Dublin, Lucena CAMHS (Dec. 2009, Mar.2010), Rolduc Holland, 1st European FASD mtg. (Nov. 2010) Belfast Nasenni Teachers Conf. (Nov. 2010), 4th Vancouver Int. FASD Conf. (Mar 2011), UK FASD Trust mtg. Oxford (Oct 2011), Toronto CADDRA, ADHD mtg. & Joint AACAP/CACAP mtgs. (Oct 2011), Strasbourg 2nd FASD European mtg. (Dec 2011), Cork, 2012, Kamloops BC (Oct.2012), FASD Level II, Mayo, 5th Vancouver Int. FASD conf. (Feb 2013). Co – organizer (with Dr. Ama Addo Consultant Child and Adolescent Psychiatrist, Glasgow), and speaker on "The pros and cons of using medication with children and adolescents with developmental disorders." Intellectual Disability section, RSM, London, January 2016; Co-organizer Conference (with Carolyn Blackburn PhD), and speaker on "Neurodevelopmental Disorder Prenatal Alcohol Exposure, (NDPAE)." Intellectual Disability section, RSM, May 2018, London; Co-organizer Conference with Dr. Ama Addo, Consultant Child and Adolescent Psychiatrist, on "Management of Complex Behavioral Phenotypes: An update." Intellectual Disability Section, May 2019. London.

Clinical: He was a Child & Adolescent Psychiatric Consultant for the Belfast Trust, working at The Young Peoples Centre & the Royal Victoria Hospital and ran a Developmental Disability & co-morbid Psychiatric Disorders Clinic (2006-2009). Now Charlemont Clinic Dublin specializing in Psychiatric Developmental Disability & Locum Child & Adolescent Psychiatric Consultant at Our Lady's Children's Hospital Crumlin (2010-2013). Belfast Developmental Disability Clinic dealing with FASD 2007-12. (Irish Medical Council no: 08167, College of Psychiatrists of Ireland CPD no.11476).

70-75 Publications, 11 book chapters, has co-authored a book with Frances Kapp PhD called "Watch for the Rainbows." True stories for Educators & other caregivers of children with Fetal Alcohol Spectrum Disorders (Published in 2001) and edited a book "ADHD &

FASD" for Nova Science Publishers, New York, published 2007, 2nd printing 2008. Book Chapters, 'FASD. Diagnostic dilemmas and challenges for a modern transgenerational management approach.' Novick Brown N, & Streissguth AP in Bentham On –Line Publishing, USA & 'FASD', Chapter 24, Sage Handbook of Developmental Disorders(2011) 'Clinical implications of ASD/FASD link' Intertech on line (2013).

Research: Experience includes Principal Investigator in a USA/Canada Multi-Centre Trial of liquid Risperidone for children with Disruptive Disorder (1997-1998), as well as Psychiatric Consultant on the 25 year follow-up of the Seattle Longitudinal Prospective Longitudinal Study of Alcohol in pregnancy (Seattle 500), with Professor Ann Streissguth as PI. Has formally submitted to NIMH a research study proposal to scientifically evaluate the safety & efficiency of Dextroamphetamine, Methylphenidate & placebo in 6-12 year old children with FASD. Consultant on MSC, FASD Training pilot project, Dr. Nnekka Arakwue, RCSI, Dublin, & PhD, Sharon Elias, University of Limerick, using Parenting Stress Index, WISC & Vineland Adaptive Behavioral Scales in FASD.

He was on the Advisory Committee of The National Indian Justice Centre, Santa Clara, CA, which was assessing Native American Youth with FASD, involved with The Criminal Justice System (2002-2006), funded by The Centers for Disease Control (CDC). Also, he was involved with the American Academy of Child & Adolescent Psychiatry (AACAP) Work Group on Community Systems of Care (1997-2006), in the developmental & research evaluation of new standardized Mental Health Assessment instruments for service intensity needs. The CAS11 (for children & adolescents) & the ESC11 (for infants, toddlers & children under 5).

Teaching: Experience included Psychiatric Consultant in the National FAS Training for Indian Health Service, based at University of Washington (1997-2005), Didactic course with Ann Streissguth PhD for Psychiatric Residents 1V on Dual Diagnosis (developmental disability & psychiatric disorder)(2001-2005), as well as Adjunct Faculty, Canadian Studies Centre, at the Jackson School of International Studies, University of Washington, teaching a 3 credit course on Comparative Health Care Practices in Canada & the USA. (2000-2005). Clinical teacher/lecturer in Belfast & Dublin.

Dr. O'Malley is a *reviewer* for the *Can. Child & Adolescent Psychiatry Review, Psychiatric Services, Archives of General Psychiatry, J. Pediatrics, Alcoholism: Clinical & Exp. Research & Neuropsychology.*

Medico-Legal experience includes at least 80 Reports &/or Court Appearances as an Expert Witness in Child/Adolescent/Family Psychiatry. These have been in Edmonton & Calgary, Canada. More recently he has been an Expert Witness in both Canada & the USA for complex cases with FASD. Expert Witness legal work Belfast, Dungarvan, Dublin linked to Dev. Psychiatric interest in FASD.

He is a member of the American Academy of Child & Adolescent Psychiatry, Canadian Academy of Child & Adolescent Psychiatry, Royal College of Psychiatrists. NI Section (2006-2010), Society for the Study of Behavioral Phenotypes, Board member, Royal Society of Medicine, Fellow.

Professional Affiliations:

Distinguished Life Member American Academy of Child and Adolescent Psychiatry (since 2017).

Fellow Royal Society Medicine (since 2010).

President Intellectual Disability Section Royal Society Medicine (RSM), 2017-2018.

Council Member Intellectual Disability Section RSM (since 2014).

Member College of Psychiatrists of Ireland (since 2011).

Member Learning Disability Faculty College of Psychiatrists of Ireland.

Member Canadian Academy of Child and Adolescent Psychiatry for over 20 years from 1994.

Member Society Study of Behavioral Phenotypes (SSBP) for 20 years from 1997.

Presentations:

(2012), Royal College of Psychiatrists, Learning Disability Section, Invited Talk with Prof. Jeremy Turk on "Genetic and Acquired Developmental Disorders." Manchester, Sept.

(2013), *All Ireland Psychiatrist's Meeting*, Invited Talk on "Implications of a link between FASD & ASD/Asperger's Disorder." Malahide, Dublin, Nov.

(2016), Invited Talk. *7Th National Biennial Conference on adolescents and adults with FASD* entitled "From medication to participatory research to stop overmedication-sleep-wake behavior assessments of medicated adolescents with FASD-a round table discussion." Vancouver. BC. Canada, April 6th.

(2016), *International European FASD Conference*, Royal Holloway Hospital paper on "Clinical phenotypes of Russian adopted children and adolescents with NDPAE living in Ireland." London, September 12th to 14th.

(2016), Royal College of Psychiatrists, Learning Disability Section, Invited talk with Dr. Raja Mukarjee on "Diagnosis and Management of FASD or NDPAE." Cardiff, Sept.

(2018), British Medical Association Invited talk on "Mental Health and Learning Disabilities, GP training, Clinical and Legal Issues Neurodevelopmental Disorders." Feb 20th.

(2018), *Conference call planning meeting* (Kay Kelly organizer) with Lummi Tribe, Washington State on "FASD/NDPAE school intervention initiative."

(2019), British Medical Association, Invited talk "GP training. Fragile X Syndrome. Implications for management for GP and family," Aug 21st.

(2020), *College of Psychiatrists of Ireland, Annual Meeting. Workshop*: "The Healing Power of Poetry." Kilkenny, March 26th. POSTPONED.

International and National Academic Presentations on FASDs or NDPAE 2014-2019: In Tallin Estonia, San Antonio TX, San Diego CA, Oakland CA, (USA), Vancouver, BC. London, Manchester, Liverpool, Cardiff, Belfast, Ballycastle (UK), Dublin, Malahide, Limerick, Cork, Mullingar, Tuam, Kilkenny (Ireland).

Other Life Interests include a passion for theatre, poetry & rugby, playing rugby for 30 years: Malone Colts, Dublin Pirates, Montréal Irish, London Irish, Edmonton Leprechauns, Cornell Med. Calgary Irish.

Directed 60 plays over 25-30 years in Canada, USA:

Travesties, Medea, Play, Faith Healer, The Chairs, The Subject was Roses, Relache, Sive, The Plough and the Stars, and including 8 years Staged Readings of Joyce's Ulysses, Seattle, & 3 recent shows for Wild Geese Returned in Dublin. Previous Artistic Director; WalterdaleTheatre, Edmonton, Liffey Players and Visual Tribe, Calgary, Wild Geese Players Seattle (Also their Founder).

Poetry Books:

A Sun's Eye, 2012, and, Thinking of, 2014, Travelin' Still 2018, Air 2019, Earth, 2021 in press.

He married Siobhan in 2008 and they have 7 adult children and 3 grandchildren between them.

INDEX

B

C

E

H

I

K

L

M

N

O

P

Q

R

S

T

U

V

W

Y